COPING
WITH
TRAUMA

Hope Through Understanding

Second Edition

COPING
WITH
TRAUMA

Hope Through Understanding

Second Edition

JON G. ALLEN, PH.D.

Helen Malsin Palley Chair in Mental Health Research and
Professor of Psychiatry, Menninger Department of Psychiatry and
Behavioral Sciences at the Baylor College of Medicine
Senior Staff Psychologist, The Menninger Clinic,
Houston, Texas

Washington, DC
London, England

Copyright © 2005 American Psychiatric Publishing, Inc.
ALL RIGHTS RESERVED

Manufactured in the United States of America on acid-free paper
17 16 15 14 13   5 4
First Edition

Typeset in Adobe's Berkeley and HelveticaNeue

American Psychiatric Publishing, Inc.
1000 Wilson Boulevard
Arlington, VA 22209-3901
www.appi.org

Library of Congress Cataloging-in-Publication Data
Allen, Jon G.
    Coping with trauma : hope through understanding / Jon G. Allen.—2nd ed.
        p. cm.
    Includes bibliographical references and index.
    ISBN 1-58562-169-2 (pbk.)
        1. Post-traumatic stress disorder. 2. Psychic trauma. I. Title.

RC552.P67A45 2005
616.85'21–dc22

                                                                    2004055334

British Library Cataloguing in Publication Data
A CIP record is available from the British Library.

To Susan,
with whom I have shared
the treasure of attachment

CONTENTS

Part I
FOUNDATIONS

Part II
EFFECTS OF TRAUMA

Part III
TRAUMA-RELATED PSYCHIATRIC
DISORDERS

Part IV
HEALING

ABOUT THE AUTHOR

Jon G. Allen, Ph.D., holds the positions of Helen Malsin Palley Chair in Mental Health Research and Professor of Psychiatry in the Menninger Department of Psychiatry and Behavioral Sciences at the Baylor College of Medicine, and Senior Staff Psychologist in The Menninger Clinic, Houston, Texas. Dr. Allen received his B.A. degree in psychology at the University of Connecticut and his Ph.D. degree in clinical psychology at the University of Rochester. He completed postdoctoral training in clinical psychology at The Menninger Clinic. He conducts psychotherapy, diagnostic psychological testing, consultations, psychoeducational programs, and research, specializing in trauma-related disorders and depression. He has taught and supervised students at the University of Rochester, Northern Illinois University, the University of Kansas, Kansas State University, and Washburn University of Topeka. He is past editor of the *Bulletin of the Menninger Clinic* and a member of the editorial boards of the *Journal of Trauma & Dissociation* and *Psychiatry* and serves as a reviewer for several professional journals and book publishers. He is the author of *Traumatic Relationships and Serious Mental Disorders,* coauthor of *Borderline Personality Disorder: Tailoring the Therapy to the Patient* and *Restoring Hope and Trust: An Illustrated Guide to Mastering Trauma,* and coeditor of *Diagnosis and Treatment of Dissociative Disorders* and *Contemporary Treatment of Psychosis: Healing Relationships in the "Decade of the Brain."* He has authored and coauthored numerous professional articles and book chapters on trauma-related problems, depression, psychotherapy, hospital treatment, the therapeutic alliance, psychological testing, neuropsychology, and emotion. He is also a jazz pianist and composer.

FOREWORD

During the past twenty years the study of trauma and its treatment has grown dramatically. Empirical research has been undertaken, new therapeutic modalities have emerged, and groundbreaking theoretical works and their applications have been published. Clinicians from all theoretical persuasions are utilizing these advances for the benefit of thousands of patients all over the world. Given the worldwide need to confront the short- and long-range effects of the multifarious forms of abuse and to comfort the victims of catastrophic events of natural disaster, genocide, and war, millions more can also benefit from this scientific progress. One crucial and cost-effective tool for the relief of the sequelae of trauma, asserts Dr. Jon Allen in this second edition of *Coping With Trauma: Hope Through Understanding,* is the empowering and powerful method of patient education.

A gifted clinical psychologist, distinguished researcher and educator, and student of comparative philosophy, Dr. Allen is uniquely qualified to explore—and explain—the many aspects of trauma to a wide audience. Basing his book on classes he has taught to patients and insights he has derived from carefully listening to their feedback in those groups and in individual therapy hours, he traverses the landscape of trauma with breadth and depth. Clear, incisive, and revealing, his chapters on each major domain of trauma are essential reading for patients, their family members, and clinicians. In this second edition of his popular text, he has thoroughly updated and expanded information on aspects of the aftermath of trauma—and the wealth of emotional, interpersonal, brain-based, psychopharmacologic, and psychotherapeutic dimensions of recovery.

Dr. Allen's understanding of the causes and effects of trauma, the detritus of the comorbid and ancillary difficulties that lie in its wake, and the potential for healing based on current approaches and new ones on the horizon make this volume a veritable treasure trove of state-of-the-art information and clinical wisdom. Although the subject of trauma is a somber one for even the most enthusiastic and knowledge-hungry reader, Dr. Allen has sagaciously attenuated any potential for devolvement into the gloomy by including case studies of patients who have weathered the maelstroms of trauma's consequences. He uses examples of patients who have begun to pull together a new and better life for themselves, in part derived from understanding themselves and their illness more thoroughly by the educative method. These lessons are also leavened with the author's extensive knowledge of and appreciation for what philosophy and ethics can offer the individual who desires to make positive and long-lasting change. He laces his text with the "wisdom of the ages" as much as with the data derived from scientific protocols to help uplift the patient and inspire a state of hopefulness on the journey to a better life.

In the 25 years that I have known Dr. Allen, it is clear he brings both passion and compassion to every aspect of his work. In this volume, he extends his reach from the narrower clinical and academic realms to the wider world of patients and their family members. This serious work of heart and mind teaches and helps build skills for overcoming serious trauma and guides the individual toward more intimate relationships and improved self-care. These skills can heal the wounds of many sufferers. They offer patients and their loved ones a better future. This brilliant and compelling book leaves me feeling hopeful about the possibility for growth and generativity for those who have sustained trauma—and inspired by what contemporary psychiatry also offers to help them flourish.

Kathryn J. Zerbe, M.D.
Professor of Psychiatry and Obstetrics & Gynecology, Vice Chair for Psychotherapy, and Director of Outpatient Services, Department of Psychiatry, and Director of Behavioral Medicine, Center for Women's Health, Oregon Health Sciences University, Portland, Oregon

PREFACE

In the decade since the publication of the first edition of this book, clinicians and researchers devoted to helping traumatized persons have generated a wealth of new knowledge. In addition, the field continues to be transformed periodically by changing manifestations of trauma—for example, by the attacks of September 11, 2001, and the ensuing national preoccupation with terrorism, itself an ongoing trauma. These developments notwithstanding, I naively set out with the modest goal of updating the first edition, incorporating the latest scientific and clinical information in the process. But I quickly realized that I needed to rethink and rewrite the book, even though I've retained some parts in near-original form.

Although war and terrorism now preoccupy us nationally and internationally, my initial focus on attachment remains, because the quality of early attachments contributes substantially to the individual's capacity to cope with trauma of any sort later in life. Moreover, recent developments in attachment theory have greatly enriched my understanding of trauma, reshaping the whole book, not just the chapter on attachment. In addition, extensive contemporary research on emotion—which is becoming a science unto itself—prompted me to recast the chapters on emotion and emotion regulation. I've reorganized the material on the neurobiological understanding of trauma into the chapter on illness. A new chapter on depression was added because it's a pervasive trauma-related problem that poses a number of catch-22s for recovery. I've consolidated material on various forms of self-destructiveness—substance abuse, eating disorders, and deliberate self-harm—which I construe as coping strategies that backfire. In this context, I've also addressed suicidal states and self-defeating aspects of personality disorders. Finally, I've concluded with a new chapter on maintaining hope—by all accounts the most crucial challenge for traumatized persons.

Acknowledgments

While my primary debt is to all the patients I've had the privilege to teach, I remain indebted to my early mentors with expertise in trauma: Alice Brand-Bartlett, Bonnie Buchele, and Bill Smith. And both editions of this book have benefited substantially from my collaboration on all clinical matters with David Console, who directed the Trauma Recovery Program at The Menninger Clinic in Topeka. I'm especially grateful to several colleagues who have joined me enthusiastically in conducting trauma education groups at the clinic in recent years, including AnnMarie Glodich, Maria Holden, Janis Huntoon, Kay Kelly, Lisa Lewis, Ella Squyres, and Alice Rogan. I've benefited greatly from AnnMarie Glodich's creatively extending this educational program to the adolescent age group and into the public school system. I've also profited from the opportunity to work with Kay Kelly for nearly a decade in co-leading groups in partial hospital and outpatient services as well as from her extending the educational intervention to workshops for family members of traumatized persons. I'm also grateful to Lisa Lewis and Kay Kelly for developing a condensed version of the educational course for patients in the Professionals in Crisis program at The Menninger Clinic, from which Lisa, Kay, and I developed a concise psychoeducational book for trauma survivors, *Restoring Hope and Trust: An Illustrated Guide to Mastering Trauma*, published by the Sidran Foundation. All these extensions of the initially specialized trauma education program have been enthusiastically received, attesting to the widespread need to understand the nature of trauma, its impact, and its treatment.

The second edition of this book is the fruit of a midlife intellectual growth spurt stemming from my good fortune to have the opportunity to work with Peter Fonagy, who regularly sojourned from London to Topeka and more recently to Houston to direct research in the Child and Family Program of The Menninger Clinic. Peter Fonagy's pioneering work is reshaping the field of attachment theory and research, and, profiting greatly from his uncommon intellectual generosity, I've been able to incorporate these contemporary developments into my teaching and writing. Peter Fonagy also brought to our shores an international consortium of exceptionally talented colleagues, including George Gergely, Jonathan Hill, and Mary Target, from whom I've also learned a great deal. I'm also grateful to Efrain Bleiberg for masterminding this research evolution at Menninger and for his continuing role in our collective intellectual development. This book has also been enriched by my collaboration with Efrain Bleiberg, Toby Haslam-Hopwood, and April Stein in educating patients about a variety of attachment-related topics beyond trauma. Finally, I owe a special debt to my friend and colleague Helen Stein, with whom I collaborated on a daily basis in research, teaching, writing, and clinical practice during the Child and Family Program's tenure in Topeka.

I've had the benefit of significant professional help along the way to writing this book, most importantly from Richard Munich, Medical Director and Chief of Staff of The Menninger Clinic, who was instrumental both personally and professionally in creating a position that enabled me to make the move from Topeka to Houston to continue this work. Similarly, I'm grateful to Stuart Yudofsky, Chairman of the Menninger Department of Psychiatry and Behavioral Sciences at the Baylor College of Medicine, for his thoroughgoing support throughout this transition. I am also grateful for the support of the Helen Malsin Palley Chair in Mental Health Research, which has afforded me the opportunity to do this work. And I thank Susan Allen, Peter Fonagy, Edith Funk, Jerome Groopman, Toby Haslam-Hopwood, Leonard Horwitz, Richard Munich, Alice Rogan, and Stuart Yudofsky for reviewing various parts of this manuscript and thereby helping me to refine it.

Lastly, I am deeply grateful to Robert E. Hales, M.D., Editor-in-Chief for Books, American Psychiatric Publishing, Inc., for his strong encouragement to do a second edition of this book; I'd not have done so otherwise. And I'm appreciative for Editorial Director John McDuffie's expert guidance in preparing the final manuscript as well as for the good fortune to have Pam Harley's and Ann Eng's talented editorial direction in these editions.

INTRODUCTION

Trauma will not go away. In the past few decades public attention has shifted from one source of trauma to another, for example, from war to domestic violence and maltreatment of children. Now terrorism grips the national psyche, while combat and abuse of women and children continue unabated. Now more than ever, we must understand psychological trauma for the sake of prevention as well as healing. Fortunately, professional knowledge about trauma and its treatment has burgeoned since the American Psychiatric Association formalized the diagnosis of posttraumatic stress disorder (PTSD) in 1980. Yet professionals must make this knowledge available to those who most need it: trauma sufferers and those who care for them.

For more than a decade, I've been conducting educational groups for traumatized patients at The Menninger Clinic. If you were to sit in on one or two of these group meetings, you'd draw the obvious conclusion: he's teaching them about trauma. Yet, if you were to observe a group over a few months' time, you'd see it differently: *they're teaching him* about trauma. Both are true. We pool our expertise, and we've continued to refine our understanding over the past decade. The time is right to make this evolving knowledge available beyond the clinic.

This book differs from educational groups in being a monologue rather than a dialogue, although it has plenty of dialogue behind it. Endeavoring to preserve the teaching spirit, I refer to the reader as "you," with the trauma sufferer in mind throughout. But I learned from the first edition that the book also appealed to an unintended audience: therapists and other health professionals. While continuing to address the traumatized person directly, this edition is intended for a wider audience—anyone seeking a comprehensive yet readable account of current professional knowledge that meshes with patients' experience. Given the pervasiveness of trauma, to varying degrees the "you" fits us all.

It is my fondest hope that, like the first edition, this book will be of help to traumatized persons. Yet I would not call it a "self-help" book. Perhaps a "self-education" book would be more apt. As you can tell from the weight of this book, it's not a quick read. And it's not light reading either. In conducting educational groups, I've found that trauma sufferers aren't content with simple explanations and pat answers. Aspiring to teach all I know, I have created something akin to a college course. This is the textbook—albeit one addressed to the reader's personal concerns.

Although this book isn't light reading, you needn't have taken any psychology courses to understand it. You'll grasp it on the basis of your personal experience. I've included the necessary background in psychology and psychiatry in the book. But we must go beyond psychology and psychiatry to understand trauma fully. We need help from biology, because trauma is a physical illness. And we need help from philosophy, because trauma confronts us with existential concerns that far exceed the reach of science and medicine.

A GUIDE TO READING THIS BOOK

I've organized this book explicitly, making liberal use of headings and sub-headings throughout. So you can easily pick and choose, finding topics of most interest. Yet the book is designed to be read front to back, because later chapters build on information and concepts introduced in earlier chapters. I've included ample references to the professional literature as well as to a number of scholarly books written for a general audience. To keep the number within a manageable limit, the references to the scientific literature are illustrative rather than exhaustive. To spare readers from searching through the nonetheless long list, I've included a short list of suggested readings at the end of the book, following the references. There's also a glossary of technical terms used throughout the book in the event that you lose track of the meaning from one part of the book to another (or you've failed to heed my plea to read it from start to finish).

The plan is simple, starting with understanding trauma and its diverse sources. Attachment theory also lays the foundation, because emotional bonds play a paramount role in coping with trauma. One idea from attachment theory provides the conceptual glue for the whole book, from the first chapter on trauma through the last chapter on hope: healing entails making sense of trauma in the context of secure attachment relationships.

The book covers the effects of trauma from two perspectives. From the psychological perspective, I discuss the impact of trauma on emotion, memory, the self, and relationships, as well as incorporating research from neuroscience to make the case that trauma is a physical illness. From the psychiatric perspective, I discuss various trauma-related disorders and symptoms: depression, PTSD, and dissociative disorders, along with a range of self-destructive behaviors to which trauma can make a contribution. Finally, I discuss various facets of healing, starting with ways of regulating emotions, then reviewing current treatment approaches, and concluding with the foundation of all healing, hope.

This book is intended to be intellectually challenging, drawing on current knowledge in psychology, psychiatry, neuroscience, and philosophy to stimulate new ways of thinking. Yet, if you're in the throes of coping with trauma, you may also find the book emotionally challenging. Reminders of trauma commonly evoke traumatic memories and painful emotions. Some readers have told me they must take the book in small doses. Others are taken aback by how closely the book fits their personal experience—disconcertingly, they see themselves in the pages, just as they see their experience on the blackboard in educational groups. I make no claim to clairvoyance; through countless discussions in educational groups, trauma sufferers have contributed to the book as they have to the educational groups. But the fact that the material hits home carries an advantage: trauma is alienating, and it can be reassuring to find that your experience is wholly human, shared by many others.

Part I

FOUNDATIONS

Chapter 1

TRAUMA

Why read about trauma? Avoidance is such a common reaction that it's a defining feature of posttraumatic stress disorder. If you've been traumatized, you're likely to steer clear of anything that reminds you of the traumatic events. Thinking about traumatic experience stirs up painful emotions. Avoidance is utterly natural, but it can keep you stuck. Blotting the traumatic experience out of your mind can prevent you from coming to terms with it. To cope with trauma and to get past it, you need to think about it. If you've been traumatized, congratulate yourself for reading this. You're not avoiding; you're coping.

Many individuals who struggle with trauma are extremely frustrated with themselves. They're highly self-critical, adding insult to their injuries. They fail to take account of the serious impact of their traumatic experience, and they don't make sufficient allowance for the limitations of their all-too-human nature. Many feel that they are "crazy." On the contrary, here's my thesis: *persons who have been traumatized are responding in ways that are natural and understandable, given their previous experience.*

The main purpose of this book is to foster self-understanding. Greater self-understanding should help you feel less crazy. But I have an even more ambitious agenda. I want to encourage self-*acceptance*. Ideally, by better understanding and appreciating the impact of trauma and your efforts to cope with it, you may develop greater compassion for yourself.

Trauma Happens

We often use the word, *traumatic,* loosely to refer to stressful events—losing a job or getting a divorce. *Webster's New Twentieth Century Dictionary*[1] defines trauma more narrowly as a violently produced wound and as an emotional shock with a lasting effect. Think of the types of injuries that are treated in specialized emergency departments called trauma centers. The counterpart that we will consider is a violently inflicted *psychological* wound with lasting effects. And, as we'll see, the lasting effects are physiological as well as psychological.

It's helpful to distinguish *exposure* to potentially traumatic events, such as being in a car wreck, from the resulting trauma, namely, the *lasting adverse effects,* such as being too fearful to drive. A young man referred to our trauma education group protested that he didn't belong there. He reported that he'd been dealing cocaine and had witnessed numerous stabbings and shootings, as well as having numerous brushes with death. But he was partly right about not belonging in the group: he found the violence exciting and denied that he'd been traumatized. Thus he'd been exposed to many *potentially* traumatic events—I certainly would have been traumatized by them!—but he did not suffer trauma. One concern of this book is why the same kinds of events traumatize some persons and not others.

As our young cocaine dealer's viewpoint attests, the same *objective* events—witnessing violence—may have different *subjective* effects. For purposes of diagnosing posttraumatic stress disorder (PTSD), traumatic events are defined specifically as including both objective and subjective aspects.[2] Objectively, the person was exposed to events involving death, serious injury, or a threat to the physical integrity of self or others. Subjectively, the person responded with feelings of fear, helplessness, or horror. The cocaine dealer was exposed to objectively threatening events without the subjectively terrifying experience.

What are the lasting adverse effects we call trauma? The *intrusion of the past into the present* is one of the main problems confronting persons who have developed psychological symptoms and psychiatric disorders as a consequence of traumatic experience. Those who've been traumatized may be plagued by distressing memories, flashbacks, and nightmares; they may continue to struggle with the powerful emotions they experienced at the time of the trauma; and they may continue using the same self-protective means that they initially learned so as to shield themselves from the traumatic experience. This combination of intrusive and avoidant symptoms is the essence of PTSD (see Chapter 9, "Posttraumatic Stress Disorder"). And trauma also contributes to other psychiatric disorders, for example, depression and substance use disorders. But trauma isn't confined to psychiatric disorders.

Traumatic experiences can result in cynicism, bitterness, distrust, alienation, hatred, vengefulness, demoralization, loss of faith, and loss of hope. All these are ways we can be traumatized by terrifying events that ought not to happen.

Coping with trauma entails separating the past from the present and gaining control over both the painful emotions and the self-protective defenses erected against them. Many traumatized persons are urged, "Move on," "Put the past behind you," or worse, "Get over it!" Easier said than done. The problem is *how* to move on, which is the subject of this book.

Trauma happens. Traumatic events are ubiquitous. Just turn on the news. A typical day's fare may include floods, tornadoes, earthquakes, fires, car crashes, plane crashes, train wrecks, rapes, kidnappings, assaults, murders, school shootings, terrorist attacks, and war-related mayhem. In a half-hour's news you see a tiny fraction of the day's traumatic events. And that's just the fraction that's *reported*. The day's news excludes all the traumatizing events that take place in private, behind closed doors, and that are kept secret. The scope of these more hidden sources of trauma—childhood maltreatment and domestic violence—has now come out into the open.

Trauma comes in many forms. There are also vast differences among individuals who undergo trauma. "Coping with trauma" is an ambitious subject for a single book. But considering all forms of trauma together is justified, because there are similarities in patterns of response that cut across different types of trauma and different individuals. Nevertheless, the challenges of coping with trauma and the risk of psychiatric disorder vary substantially from person to person, depending on the nature of the trauma.

Types of Trauma

To provide a foundation for the rest of this book, I'm about to stake out the territory of traumatic events, and I'm going to highlight the domain of attachment trauma, that is, trauma in attachment relationships. I know from conducting educational groups that thinking about different types of trauma—as you're about to do—may evoke disturbing memories. You should feel free to skim or skip whatever you wish; the last thing you need is excess immersion in trauma. Small doses, interspersed with calming or pleasurable activities, might be best. Yet there's something to be said for thinking clearly about different aspects of traumatic events. Just giving pain a name can relieve and transform it.[3] The goal is to render traumatic experience thinkable and speakable; for that, you need words and concepts to help you sort it out and make whatever sense can be made of it. No one reading this book needs to be convinced of the significance of trauma, so I'll keep this survey brief.

Single-Blow Versus Repeated Trauma

On the basis of her extensive studies of traumatic experience in children, psychiatrist Lenore Terr[4] distinguished *single-blow* traumas from *repeated* traumas. Single shocking events may produce enduring traumatic reactions in some individuals. Natural disasters are an example. These include earthquakes, tornadoes, avalanches, fires, floods, hurricanes, and volcanic eruptions. The severity of symptoms that people report after disasters varies widely from one study to the next. Depending on the scope of the destruction and the degree of threat to life and limb, anywhere from a small minority to a large majority of persons exposed to such disasters may be traumatized, suffering lasting effects.[5]

Closely related to natural disasters are technological disasters, such as dam breaks, building collapses, plane crashes, chemical spills, and nuclear reactor failures. But there's an important difference between natural and technological disasters: the community pulls together around natural disasters; people help and support each other. Technological disasters, on the other hand, tend to be more socially divisive, because much attention is diverted to finding fault and fixing blame.[5]

Criminal violence also involves single-blow trauma. Examples are burglary, robbery, aggravated assault, rape, and homicide. Violent crimes not only have a direct impact on victims but also have an indirect—and frequently traumatic—effect on those who witness them and on those whose loved ones are injured or killed. Unfortunately, a substantial majority of victimized persons have been exposed to more than one crime,[6] and the traumatic effects can be cumulative.

The loss of a loved one is certainly traumatic, in the broad sense of the term. A great deal of overlap is shared between grief and posttraumatic symptoms; both potentially involve painful intrusive feelings, such as pangs of grief, and denial of the loss or other efforts to avoid these feelings.[7] Although all losses may be traumatic in the general sense, loss and trauma can be combined when the loss is sudden or unexpected and particularly horrifying, such as witnessing the violent death of a loved one.[8] Such traumatic losses may be experienced with a combination of intense fear or horror and painful grief.

As traumatic as single-blow events may be, the traumatic experiences that result in the most serious psychiatric disorders are prolonged and repeated, sometimes extending over many years. For example, combat entails multiple traumatic events over many months. Being a prisoner of war, a political prisoner, or a concentration camp inmate all involve continual trauma over months and years. Sexual, physical, and emotional abuse in the family may span the whole of childhood development. Even worse, a history of childhood maltreatment may be followed by years of battering in adulthood, making for a lifetime of trauma.

Extent of Interpersonal Involvement

As the previous examples illustrate, there's a range of interpersonal involvement in trauma. Although it makes no sense to rank one type of trauma as worse than another—trauma is trauma—the extent of interpersonal involvement often plays an important role in the nature and extent of the effects.

I array the extent of interpersonal involvement along a spectrum as follows:

impersonal trauma→ interpersonal trauma→ attachment trauma

Impersonal trauma happens by accident, for example, as a result of acts of nature such as earthquakes and tornadoes. Interpersonal trauma, such as trauma resulting from an assault, is deliberately inflicted by other persons. Trauma that results from deliberate acts by others, at worst with malevolent intent, is often hardest to bear. Some events, such as car crashes caused by drunk drivers, result in trauma that falls between impersonal and interpersonal trauma. Such "accidents" can be construed as crimes because they result from negligence, and persons whose loved ones are killed by drunk drivers are as vulnerable to posttraumatic symptoms as the loved ones of homicide victims.[9]

The combination of repeated traumatic events and intense interpersonal involvement occurs in attachment trauma, a term psychiatrist Kenneth Adam and his colleagues[10] coined in conjunction with research on traumatized adolescents. *Attachment trauma* occurs in relationships in which there is a close emotional bond and a significant degree of dependency. Trauma resulting from child abuse is a glaring example. The impact of such trauma can be especially far-reaching, because it can affect the capacity for trusting relationships. I devote much of this book to the impact of attachment trauma, because attachment trauma can set the stage for vulnerability to other forms of trauma, and attachment relationships play a paramount role in healing from trauma.

Varieties of Interpersonal Trauma

The range of events resulting in interpersonal trauma varies as widely as the range of violence and recklessness. As traumatic as accidents and natural disasters may be, trauma stemming from deliberate or negligent actions by other persons can be especially hard to bear.

War

Much trauma occurs on a massive scale in wars, and much of our understanding of traumatic reactions has come from persons who have survived prolonged combat experience—but not unscathed. The diagnosis of PTSD was formalized in the aftermath of the Vietnam War.[11] War-related trauma is potentially severe, repeated, and prolonged. Intrinsic to combat is risk of death and injury. Many soldiers in Vietnam were involved in hundreds of firefights. For many, there was little respite; guerrilla warfare meant continually being on guard for unpredictable attacks. But the traumatic experiences in war are not only repeated, they are multiple. While your own life is at stake, you are liable to witness violence, death, and mayhem on a large scale. You may suffer repeated losses. You live with many privations, far from home.

For the vast majority of us who have been spared from combat experience, the horrors of war are virtually incomprehensible. The trauma of war comes not only from being a passive victim of violence, but from being an active participant. Such war trauma is compounded not only by the danger of being injured or killed, but by the acts of injuring, maiming, and killing. Particularly devastating is the maiming and killing of civilians, including women and children. Participating in war and becoming a "killer" do violence to one's identity.[12] And the legacy of active involvement in such horrific events can be a lifetime of guilt.

War is not the only culturally sanctioned source of trauma. We are in the midst of a worldwide epidemic of human rights abuses. Politically inspired violence includes kidnappings, disappearances, indiscriminate maiming and killing, political imprisonment, brutal interrogation, and torture.[13] Many victims who survive are forced into exile, which piles trauma on top of trauma. While we are opening our eyes to the trauma that results from domestic violence and child abuse, we remain relatively blind to the effects of pandemic human rights violations.

Terrorism

September 11, 2001, suddenly brought international terrorism to United States soil on a massive scale, although it was preceded by the horrific homegrown terrorism of the bombing of the Alfred P. Murrah Federal Building in Oklahoma City in 1995. The goal of terrorism is to inflict psychological trauma, albeit for political ends. The exploitation of terror for political purposes is hardly new: historian Charles Townshend[14] dates the origin of the modern political concept of terrorism to 1793, when the French government employed terrorism to buttress the revolution. Although recent events lead us to associate terrorism with attacks on governments, Townsend points out that state-sponsored terror has dwarfed the terrorist attacks of rebels throughout the modern era.

The line between war and terrorism is blurry, because deliberately terrorizing the enemy on a large scale is a common strategy in war. Strategic bombing in World War II, including the bombing of Hiroshima and Nagasaki, is a glaring example in the twentieth century; the "shock and awe" strategy in the second Iraq war is a twenty-first-century example. Yet terrorism is most clearly marked by the selection of random targets and the indiscriminate maiming and killing of noncombatants—innocent civilians. Townshend thus construed terrorism as an assault on reasonableness. The inherent unpredictability and senselessness of terrorism makes it particularly terrifying and traumatizing. Senselessness reaches its extreme in random assaults such as the 2002 sniper attacks in the Washington, D.C., area, which did not appear to have a political agenda but seemingly resulted from malice for its own sake.

We're now terrorized on a grand scale by weapons of mass destruction, a phenomenon Townshend puts under the rubric of Superterror. As the Cold War and the last half-century's threat of nuclear war attests, this phenomenon is not new. Freud[15] saw it coming; in 1929, long before the Cold War but at the dawning of the Holocaust, he wrote, in his masterwork *Civilization and Its Discontents*:

> Men have gained control over the forces of nature to such an extent that with their help they would have no difficulty in exterminating one another to the last man. They know this, and hence comes a large part of their current unrest, their unhappiness and their mood of anxiety. (p. 112)

We're not novices at creating terror on a large scale, but we continue to get better at it, and we're paying the price: the traumatic legacy of heightened fear and anxiety.

As we witness on a daily basis, terrorism begets counterterrorism, and psychological trauma is compounded by trauma to society. Terrorism often succeeds in threatening liberal democracy by promoting repressive measures that undermine hard-won liberty and spawn intolerance. We face dangers from without and dangers from within. On a personal and societal level, we risk being traumatized to the extent that terrorism succeeds in leading us to live in fear and erodes our freedom. As we'll see in discussing PTSD, the bane of the traumatized person is avoidance. Contemporary British philosopher A.C. Grayling[16] counseled that investing too much energy in safety risks limiting opportunity and growth; he advocated living more freely, albeit somewhat more dangerously. Thus September 11th's traumatic legacy includes not just fear but also eroded freedom.

Criminal Violence

As the daily news attests, being a victim of violence is not a rare event. Not only do many persons experience physical or aggravated assault but many also suffer the loss of family members and friends as a result of criminal and vehicular homicide. Rape victims probably constitute the largest group of people with PTSD in this country.[17] One survey found that nearly a quarter of the women respondents gave a history of having been raped and that, of women with PTSD, nearly half had a history of rape.[6] Especially alarming was the finding that a substantial majority of women with a history of incest have been subjected to rape, a far greater proportion than among those without an incest history.[18] As alarming as these statistics are, they undoubtedly underestimate the prevalence of rape, because rape is notoriously underreported. In a similar vein, sexual harassment is not typically included in the domain of trauma,[19] but it should be. Sexual harassment is potentially associated with a wide range of psychological, health, and job-related problems.[20] In addition, the process of filing complaints and the ensuing legal proceedings are notoriously stressful.[21]

Attachment Trauma

As I construe it, there are two senses to the concept of attachment trauma. First, as stated earlier, the term refers to trauma that occurs in attachment relationships—not just in childhood but also in adulthood. Second, as will become clearer in the next chapter, this form of trauma is especially important for us to understand, because it can hamper our capacity to form secure attachment relationships, and this capacity must be restored.

Child Abuse

More than two decades ago, Karl Menninger[22] wrote the following passage:

> A great deal remains unknown about ideal parenting, although there have been millions of experiments and prescriptions. Some parents learn their task, some never do, and often by the time some find wisdom, their children are no longer children. We know that there are some terrifyingly wrong parental behaviors. Children are beaten, burned, slapped, whipped, thrown about, kicked, and raped daily. Children have been objects of discipline and

punishment and senseless cruelty for centuries, since civilization began. Is there any form of physical abuse that they have not been subjected to?

Worse yet, children are abandoned and neglected and mistaught, lied to, and misinformed. The more we investigate the details of family life in recent centuries of "civilization"—and even in previous centuries and other cultures—the more we find that child abuse, which is thought of as a modern evil, has been prevalent for eons and eons in older European cultures. Child abuse is a long-standing stain on the record of the human race. Children are weak and small, parents are strong and big; parents can get their way by sheer force, proving (to the child) that "might makes right."

No one actually knows or can even imagine how much children are made to suffer by parents who—at least at times—are heartless, sadistic, brutal, or filled with vengeance nursed since their own childhood days! (p. 329)

The scope of childhood maltreatment is staggering, and its forms are various. Building on the work of British psychologist Antonia Bifulco and her colleagues,[23] I find it helpful to distinguish among three forms of abuse (physical, sexual, and emotional) and two forms of neglect (physical and psychosocial) as summarized in Table 1–1.

TABLE 1–1. Experiences leading to attachment trauma

Abuse	Neglect
Physical	Physical
Sexual	Psychosocial
Emotional	Emotional unavailability
Antipathy (rejection)	Cognitive neglect
Psychological abuse (cruelty)	Interpersonal neglect

Physical Abuse

Family violence takes many forms and has profound consequences. Children are direct targets, and they are also deeply affected by witnessing violence between adults and violence directed toward their siblings.

Physical abuse of children is not new but was brought into glaring light in the 1960s with the identification of the *battered child syndrome*,[24] with children under 3 years of age being at greatest risk. The extent of injuries is variable but includes permanent damage and, at worst, death. Attentive to the psychological trauma associated with physical abuse, Bifulco and her colleagues[23] emphasized the extent of *threatfulness* involved, which includes the degree of violence, extent of physical injury, frequency of the incidents, and the relationship to the perpetrator—as well as the perpetrator's state of mind. Particularly frightening is physical abuse by a caregiver who is dangerously out of control, in a wild rage.

Extensive research shows physical abuse to be a widespread problem, although the prevalence is difficult to pinpoint, given the wide range of actions included and variation from one sample studied to another.[25] Research on the potentially traumatic impact of physical abuse shows a wide range of psychiatric and behavioral problems extending from childhood to adulthood. These problems include not just a higher likelihood of aggression and violence but also increased risk of substance abuse and depression, along with self-injurious and suicidal behavior.[26,27]

Witnessing violence, even if you are not directly involved in it, also can be extremely traumatic. Seeing anyone being beaten is extremely stressful. The greater your attachment to the victim of violence, the more extreme the stress is likely to be. Commonly, in situations of family violence, siblings observe each other being terrorized and injured. Especially terrifying is violence directed against a primary attachment figure, such as a father's violence toward a mother. In such cases, the distress of witnessing violence is compounded by the threat of losing a primary source of security. Tragically, many children in this country witness the homicide of a parent, with profoundly traumatic results.[28]

Sexual Abuse

Little wonder that sexual abuse has garnered so much attention: it's not rare, and we continue to become increasingly aware of its scope. More than two decades ago, psychiatrist Judith Herman[29] summarized research suggesting that between one-fifth and one-third of women had had some sexual encounter in childhood with an adult male. As with physical abuse, sexual abuse covers a wide range of actions ranging from fondling to sexual intercourse and may occur in a variety of relationships, ranging from strangers to neighbors, teachers, clergy, siblings, stepparents, and biological parents. Accordingly, estimates of prevalence are highly variable, although extensive subsequent research has confirmed Herman's concerns regarding the widespread occurrence of sexual abuse.[30] As with physical abuse, in gauging the traumatic impact of sexual abuse, the extent of threatfulness must be taken into account.[23] Key factors include age inappropriateness, the stressful and threatening nature of the activities, degree of coercion, abuse of power and trust, and the nature of the relationship with the perpetrator. Psychologist Jennifer Freyd[31] aptly construed trauma resulting from sexual abuse in an attachment relationship as *betrayal trauma*, highlighting the abuse of trust.

As Herman[29] reported, the vast majority of victims of sexual abuse are female, and the vast majority of offenders are male. Yet sexual abuse of boys is not uncommon[32] and is often extremely traumatic. Like girls, boys are most often sexually abused by men. The scope of sexual abuse of boys by priests is now blatantly evident, and Freyd's concept of betrayal trauma applies here as well. The trauma includes not just damage to relationships with persons in authority but also the undermining of faith and confidence in religious institutions.

We are witnessing a skyrocketing increase in reports of sexual abuse of children. Is this a new epidemic? Is sexual abuse now occurring more frequently, or are we just becoming more aware of it? A group of researchers scoured the literature to compare data from the survey by Kinsey and associates[33] in the 1940s with comparable data from more recent surveys.[34] These authors concluded that the prevalence of sexual abuse has *not* increased in the past four decades, a finding supported by another more recent review.[30] Rather, we're more aware of sexual abuse because it's now more often reported.

Among the various forms of traumatic experience, sexual abuse is now in the spotlight, and we must be careful about making generalizations. Sexual abuse, like other sexual behavior, takes an infinite variety of forms. And sexual abuse does not occur in a vacuum; it's often coupled with other forms of stress and traumatic experience—much of which occur in the family.[35] Because of the variety of forms and contexts of sexual abuse, its effects are extremely variable. There's no question, however, that sexual abuse poses a major public health problem, with trauma evident in the form of diverse symptoms and psychiatric disorders, including PTSD, depression, behavior problems, and sexual disturbance.[36,37] Because sexual abuse is typically intertwined with extensive family disturbance, however, it's often difficult to disentangle the impact of sexual abuse from the other adversities in which it is embedded.[38,39]

There's no question that sexual abuse significantly increases the *risk* of having psychological problems and psychiatric symptoms. But adverse effects are not inevitable. Reviews of research suggest that about one-third of sexually abused children have no symptoms, and a large proportion of those who do show disturbance recover from it—although a minority get worse.[40] In addition, less than one-fifth of adults who were sexually abused as children show serious psychological disturbance.[41] Of course, more psychological trauma is associated with more severe abuse—occurring over a longer duration; involving force, penetration, helplessness, or fear of injury or death; perpetrated by an attachment figure; and coupled with a lack of support or followed by negative consequences arising from disclosure.[40] To reiterate, at worst, sexual abuse involves betrayal trauma and attachment trauma, and it's evident that sexual abuse by biological fathers is especially traumatic for this reason.[36]

Emotional Abuse

Emotional or verbal abuse can be distinguished from physical and sexual abuse. Many patients insist that it was worse to be beaten with words than with belts. Just imagine the effects of your parent screaming, "I wish you had never been born!" or "I wish you were dead!" And imagine hearing it hundreds of times over many years. Like other forms of abuse, such emotional abuse encompasses a wide range of actions. Bifulco and her colleagues[23] usefully distinguished between antipathy and psychological abuse, although there's a gray area between them. *Antipathy* entails rejection, often shown in the form of criticism and disapproval but also reflected in coldness and ignoring the child, sometimes in the context of favoritism toward another child.

Psychological abuse goes beyond antipathy, involving cruelty toward the child. Sadly, such abuse takes many forms. Examples from Bifulco and colleagues' investigations[42] include humiliating and degrading the child, terrorizing the child (e.g., playing on fears), depriving the child of basic needs (e.g., for sleep or food) or valued objects (e.g., precious mementos or a pet), inflicting extreme distress or discomfort (e.g., force feeding), emotional blackmail (e.g., threats of harm to a sibling or parent if abuse is revealed), and corruption (e.g., forcing the child to take drugs, steal, or engage in prostitution).

Although much interpersonal trauma stems from the eruption of passions—violent rages, greed, or lust—psychological abuse illustrates that the severest forms of trauma can be inflicted deliberately. Calculated cruelty can be far more terrifying than impulsive violence. Psychiatrist Jean Goodwin[43] identified the extreme end of the spectrum of psychological abuse as *sadistic abuse,* and psychoanalyst Eric Fromm[44] held that the sadist terrorizes for the purpose of gaining absolute control over the victim. As psychologist Theodore Millon[45] documented, there are different types of sadists: explosive, tyrannical, enforcing, and spineless; plainly, children can be traumatized by sadistic parents of all sorts. Not surprisingly, psychological abuse puts the victim at risk for a wide range of problems and symptoms, including shame, low self-esteem, depression, suicidal behavior, anxiety, and dissociation.[46] Yet, to reiterate a point that pertains to all forms of maltreatment, psychological abuse is typically associated with other forms of abuse and neglect, such that its effects are difficult to disentangle from the rest.

Neglect

Over the course of the past several decades, various forms of child abuse have garnered well-deserved attention. Ironically, the attention to abuse in the trauma literature has arisen in tandem with the neglect of neglect.[47] Neglected children represent the largest segment of child protective services cases,[37] and the adverse impact of neglect may equal or even exceed that of abuse.[48] In general, abuse entails acts of commission, and neglect entails acts of omission. *Physical neglect* includes both failure to provide for basic needs (e.g., food, clothing, shelter, health care) and lack of supervision that puts the child in harm's way.[49] We have contrasted physical neglect with *psychosocial neglect,*[50] which includes *emotional neglect* (unresponsiveness to the child's emotional states), *cognitive neglect* (failure to support the child's cognitive and educational development), and *social neglect* (lack of attention to the child's social and interpersonal development).

Many patients in treatment for trauma-related problems give a history of emotional neglect and suffer from a sense of emotional deprivation. The concept of *psychological unavailability*[48] aptly describes their experience with caregivers. The psychologically unavailable parent is unresponsive to the child's signals, especially the child's pleas for warmth and comfort. Although physically neglected children are often emotionally neglected as well, psychological unavailability often takes place in the context of adequate physical care. Plainly, psychological unavailability results in attachment trauma, and it's not surprising that such emotional neglect leads to problems in attachment relationships as well as problems in relationships with peers. Indeed, psychological unavailability may be the most subtle yet most severe form of maltreatment.[51]

Domestic Violence

Surveying a vast literature on trauma, psychologist Deborah Rose[52] concluded that the home, which we idealize as a refuge, is the most dangerous place to be. The concept of attachment trauma pertains to adult relationships as well as to parent-child relationships, and the statistics are equally alarming, for example, indicating that from one-fifth to one-third of women are liable to be assaulted by an intimate male partner.[53] In her classic work, *The Battered Woman,* psychologist Lenore Walker[54] identified a three-phase cycle of violence: 1) the gradual escalation of tension around minor incidents, 2) the acute battering incident, and 3) the kind and contrite behavior in the aftermath of the battering incident. The loving kindness and contrition cements the attachment relationship. To reiterate a now well-worn point, estimates of the prevalence of battering vary widely from one study to another, but there's no question that marital violence is a major problem worldwide.[55] And, although women are reportedly as disposed as men to physical aggression in intimate relationships, male aggression is far more intense and damaging. Moreover, whereas men typically behave aggressively to dominate and control women, women typically resort to aggression for defense and retaliation.[56]

Sadly, as Walker's work attests, not just physical abuse but all other forms of abuse to which children may be exposed and that can result in attachment trauma—sexual abuse, antipathy, psychological abuse, and emotional neglect—are characteristic of traumatic attachments in adulthood. And attachment trauma of all forms in adult relationships also is associated with psychiatric symptoms and disorders. Marital rape is far more common than rape by a stranger, and it is equally violent. Moreover, marital rape is especially likely to extend over a period of hours and to be repeated.[57] Antipathy and psychological abuse is also part and parcel of battering relationships, and verbally abused women are nearly as likely as physically battered women to develop PTSD.[56] At worst, a battered woman may be captive to sadistic abuse and subjected to coercive control, which may take the form of threats of violence to herself and to others—children, parents, and friends.[58] Isolation from other potential sources of support further cements the traumatic attachment, as the battered woman becomes increasingly dependent on periods of loving-kindness that provide a brief safe haven and respite from assault. Thus finding other sources of support is a crucial pathway out.

Stress Pileup

This brief survey reveals the wide range of events that can be traumatic and provides a glimpse of the kinds of trauma wrought by exposure to these events. Although trauma is trauma, we have seen that many factors contribute to the severity of the impact. The effects are liable to be most pervasive when the trauma is interpersonal, repeated, unpredictable, multifaceted, inflicted with sadistic or malevolent intent, undergone in childhood, and perpetrated in an attachment relationship.

To capture the vulnerability created by exposure to traumatic events, I have borrowed the concept of *stress pileup* from the family systems literature.[59] This concept fits hand in glove with one of the best-documented research findings in the field of trauma: the *dose-response* relationship.[60] Think of alcohol: the more you drink, the more intoxicated you become. So it is with stress: the higher the "dose" of trauma, the more potentially damaging its effects. The greater the stressor, the higher the likelihood of developing PTSD. The closer you are to the site of the volcano's eruption or the closer you are to the sniper, the more you are affected. A group of researchers clearly demonstrated the dose-response relationship in a well-controlled study of PTSD in Vietnam veterans.[61] They controlled for the veterans' genetic makeup and early experience by studying identical twins who were exposed to different levels of combat. They found that, all else being equal, the more combat exposure, the higher the risk of posttraumatic stress symptoms.

As it is in combat trauma, stress pileup is evident in attachment trauma. There's an extensive literature on physical and sexual abuse and a growing literature on psychological abuse and neglect—although these adversities rarely occur in isolation. Indeed, it's difficult to gauge the impact of any single form of childhood maltreatment because the various forms are so intertwined. For example, Bifulco and colleagues[46] found that psychological abuse typically occurs in conjunction with many other adversities, and we might think of psychological abuse not in isolation but rather as compounding the effects of other forms of abuse. The same compounding of multiple forms of abuse and neglect is inherent in adulthood battering relationships as well. Thus we must think of the dose-response effect not just in terms of the repetition of traumatic events but also in terms of the compounding of multiple forms of maltreatment. Especially in relation to attachment trauma in childhood, I emphasize the combination of abuse and neglect, believing that *the core of trauma is feeling afraid and alone.*[25] That is, a frightening experience is most difficult to bear when it is not followed by a comforting attachment experience that restores the feeling of safety and helps the child make sense of the experience. Sadly, the absence of such restorative experience is precisely what is traumatic about traumatic attachments.

Furthermore, we know that exposure to earlier traumatic experiences puts the individual at risk for exposure to later traumatic experiences, for example, when a history of childhood abuse is followed by a battering relationship in adulthood.[62] And it's not just attachment trauma that contributes to stress pileup: with a history of attachment trauma, any additional stressor—such as a car crash—can be the last straw in the process of stress pileup.

Moreover, it's not uncommon for a kind of stress pileup to unfold during the course of a "last straw" event:

> A woman with a long history of psychological problems who was doing well in psychiatric treatment for her anxiety disorder was working in the vicinity of the Oklahoma City bomb blast. Coping reasonably well with the immediate shock and horror of the event, she went to a nearby hospital to visit an injured child. Fleeing that hospital in the midst of a bomb scare, she was accosted by a security guard with a gun and interrogated. She continued to manage well until she went to get her car from the underground garage a couple of days after the bombing, at which point she saw the fatally injured occupants being hauled out in body bags. That last straw was her undoing; she was shaking uncontrollably and needed immediate psychiatric help. But she had developed a good support system, and she had a close friend to whom she was able to reach out, giving reason for optimism that she could weather this latest trauma.

Given the phenomenon of stress pileup, much of coping with trauma entails avoiding exposure to *additional* trauma.[63] As terrorist attacks most glaringly attest, much trauma is a result of fate and cannot be avoided. Hence the best one can do is to learn to decrease avoidable stress and to cope more effectively with unavoidable stress.

Derailed Development

As you've already glimpsed, throughout this book I'll be emphasizing the value of understanding trauma from a developmental perspective. A few examples will illustrate how stress pileup may unfold over long stretches of a lifetime:

Picture a happy-go-lucky girl on the threshold of adolescence. She doesn't have it easy. Her parents work long hours to support her and her brothers and sisters. Her mother is kind and loving, but she's not home much. Her father spends long periods working out of state. The youngster spends most of her free time playing with a couple of girlfriends. She dreams of getting married and having children of her own. She plays house. Perhaps *she* can have a family that spends a lot of time together.

One afternoon she's playing in her room while her parents and their friends are having a holiday celebration outside. It's noisy, and they're drinking. Her uncle comes into the room. He's always been nice to her; at first she's puzzled but not frightened. But then he picks her up roughly and carries her to her bed. He undresses her and starts molesting her. His sour breath smells of beer and peanuts. He puts his hand over her mouth and tells her to be quiet. She can't breathe, and she panics. She hardly knows what's happening. She's completely overpowered. She can't fight. She can't move, and she can't think.

He leaves. She's alone and frightened. She struggles out of bed, goes into the bathroom, and cleans herself up. The party's still going on. She's in shock; she feels dazed, and her thoughts and feelings are a jumble. She's afraid to tell anyone. She wouldn't know what to say. She feels ashamed. She might get in trouble. Who would believe it? Was it her fault?

So much for her dreams. Now she has nightmares. So much for playing house. Given what she did, no one would want to marry her. She's angry, and she becomes more bitter and rebellious. By mid-adolescence, she's learned well that alcohol calms her fears, temporarily. She's depressed. She discovers that marijuana allows her to escape, but she can't concentrate on her schoolwork. Her life goes downhill. Her parents can't understand why she can't stay away from drugs. She never tells a soul.

She meets a lot of men. Initially, she's attracted to them. Before long, she becomes sullen or hostile. Sometimes she's belligerent. Men can't figure her out. She drives them away as soon as she starts to get close; she's afraid of attachments. Eventually, she finds a man with whom she feels fairly safe and secure. After a couple of years of breaking up and getting back together, they become engaged and move in together. It's a far cry from what she'd imagined as a child. Her fiancé is good to her. But soon after they begin living together, they both think she's going crazy. She's tried to stay off marijuana, but she can't. When they start having sex, she sometimes flies into a rage, screaming at him—"Get away from me!" The trauma stemming from her uncle's assault has undermined her primary attachment relationship.

She's admitted to a psychiatric hospital, believing she's losing her mind. She's always known that she's got more than a drug problem. She goes to see a psychotherapist. She realizes that she needs to talk about being raped. For more than a decade, she's kept it to herself, but she's never forgotten it. It's not easy, but slowly she musters her courage and tells her therapist what happened. She begins to feel relieved. Just telling someone seems to help. She needed to get it out. Over the course of several therapy sessions, she begins to piece it all together. She sees how her fiancé's actions trigger memories of the rape. She can't stand the smell of beer or peanuts on his breath. He's a big man. When he's on top of her and she's excited, she becomes short of breath. She panics. She learns that she has PTSD. She understands more fully why she's been using marijuana and alcohol. She can see how her attitude toward life changed and how her life took a turn for the worse after the rape.

She wants her fiancé to understand. But she's afraid to talk with him, and she asks her social worker to help her. She's learned to talk openly with her therapist about her experience, and, despite her apprehension, she does a good job of explaining to her fiancé what has happened. The social worker helps her fiancé see that she's having flashbacks just like people who have been in combat. This is the first time she and her fiancé have talked about their sexual relationship without arguing.

In the hospital, she talks to her therapist, social worker, nurses, and other patients. She's not the only patient in the group who has experienced trauma. She makes some friends. She finds women she can confide in and women who confide in her. She finds strengths in herself that others rely on. She discovers that she enjoys writing poetry and that others like it. She's finding creative expression for her feelings that touches other patients. She begins to realize that she's no longer withdrawn, bitter, and isolated. On the contrary, she's enjoying being with people. She's establishing—or reestablishing—her capacity for secure attachments.

One day she comes to therapy pleased and somewhat bewildered. She says she's starting to feel like a different person. Her therapist has a different view. He sees that she's gotten back on course. She's not a different person; instead, she's recapturing some of her youthful character. The rape had derailed her development in young adolescence, and she's just now getting back on course in adulthood. She has many good qualities to rekindle.

Let's push the traumatic juncture up a few years:

Consider the 18-year-old who goes to Vietnam. He's graduated from high school. A star wrestler, he's tough. He's had a couple of girlfriends. He, too, contemplates marriage and a family. He's had summer jobs and has considered some career options that would require technical school or college. But, facing the prospect of being drafted into the Army, he joins the Marines.

He goes to war. He sees death and mayhem. He's tough and physically fit, but he's terrified. To defend himself, he must kill without thinking. At first, when he kills, he becomes disoriented and violently ill, which he manages to conceal from his fellow soldiers. His best buddy is killed. More buddies are killed. He becomes enraged. He starts to fight back recklessly, with little regard for his own life. The more he kills, the more powerful he feels. He's become a killer. But he can't entirely suppress his horror at it all—in quiet moments he painfully remembers the life seeping out of an enemy soldier he shot at close quarters, the assaults on civilians, and the mutilation of the bodies of enemy soldiers.

Wounded, he comes home. His physical injuries are evident to all, and they eventually heal. No one can see his psychological injuries, and there's no opportunity for them to heal. His parents are proud that he's now a man, but they urge him to forget about the war, or at least not to talk about it. Anyway, he feels that anyone who hasn't been there could not possibly understand. Who would *want* to understand? He's like a fish out of water—tense, jumpy, and irritable. He drinks. He can't stand noise and crowds. He doesn't feel like doing much of anything constructive. His friends from high school have all gone their own ways. He can't get close to anyone. His temper flares, he's still strong and tough, and he gets into bar fights repeatedly—flying into a blind rage, he sometimes comes dangerously close to maiming or killing anyone who is foolish enough to wind up at odds with him. Women find him remote. He's not all there. He often blanks out, as if he's off somewhere else, and misses half the conversation. When women urge him to open up, he breaks off the relationship. Who would want to know what he's been through—and the depth of the violence that still haunts him? What's become of his development? What are his prospects for healing attachment relationships?

Or we can push the trauma back to the beginning:

Consider the child whose development has faltered from the start. Since he was a baby, his mother generally ignored him. He never quite knew from one moment to the next who would feed or dress him—perhaps his mother, his sister, or his grandfather. Sometimes no one did. His mother may have been in bed, depressed. She may have been sitting by the window, staring into space. When his father was there, he was yelling at his mother, yelling at him, or hitting him.

The child never had any sense of security or stability. His family provided little foundation for development. He has no reason to think that relationships can be gratifying. There was scant encouragement, no recognition for learning or accomplishment. He learned just to grab whatever he could get. His development is not derailed; it never got on track. The track led straight to prison. His attachment relationships were not just disrupted; they hardly developed.

Some individuals overcome severe childhood trauma and do remarkably well in early adulthood, only to find that the prior trauma comes back unexpectedly to haunt them later in adulthood when the pileup of stress takes its toll:

> A woman managed to break away from her troubled family. She made it through childhood and adolescence by dint of determination, strong defenses, and high intelligence. Doing well in school and earning praise from teachers sustained her. She became a highly successful professional. She married a loving partner. Now she's liked, respected, and admired.
>
> But by the time she's 40 years old, the stressors have piled up. She's had a miscarriage, she's lost a friend to cancer, and she's had to move away from a home she loved. Recently, she's had to fend off her boss's sexual advances. The last straw is a car accident. She's not seriously hurt, but she's badly shaken. Inexplicably, her anxiety level skyrockets. She can't sleep. Long-buried childhood memories start to haunt her. She can't quite make sense of them, and she tries not to think about them. She's worn out from constant anxiety and lack of sleep.
>
> She becomes increasingly depressed. She loses her temper, and she bursts into tears. Her husband withdraws, spending more time out with his friends. She starts to wonder if he's having an affair. She's had a hard time concentrating at work, and she doesn't have the energy to keep up the fast pace. She's used up a lot of sick leave. She's been passed up for a promotion, and she's afraid she'll lose her job. In desperation, she takes an overdose of sleeping pills. She enters a psychiatric hospital where she begins to think and talk about her severely traumatic childhood. She can't go back to work, and she's not sure her marriage can be rescued. Her derailed development may take years to get back on track.

The Eye of the Beholder

To emphasize a point made earlier in this chapter, there are two components to traumatic experience: objective and subjective. Objectively, traumatic events pose a threat of death or serious injury to oneself or others. These threats are usually, but not always, external. Discovering that you have a serious disease also can be traumatic. When we talk about trauma, we usually focus on the objective events—the tornado, combat, rape, or beatings. But keep in mind that *the subjective experience of the objective events constitutes the trauma.*

Much psychological trauma entails direct bodily harm, and the diagnostic criteria for PTSD emphasize a threat to physical integrity of oneself or others.[2] Yet these criteria are too narrow: as the traumatic impact of psychological abuse attests, threats and injuries to *psychological* well-being—in the absence of physical danger—can be highly traumatic. And all too often, the physical and psychological threats go together. Regardless, there's a psychological wound. The objective event is subjectively interpreted. One person may appraise a situation as being far worse than it appears to another person.

The more you believe you're endangered, the more traumatized you'll be. Objectivity and subjectivity do not always match. Research with burn patients showed that the extent of emotional distress, not the severity of the burn, determined the posttraumatic symptoms.[64] You can be traumatized by someone with a fake gun. Psychologically, the bottom line of trauma is overwhelming emotion and a feeling of utter helplessness. Bodily injury may or may not be evident, but psychological trauma is coupled with physiological upheaval that plays a leading role in the long-range effects (see Chapter 7, "Illness").

Allowing for subjectivity, there's room for interpretation, and you can mislead yourself. You could exaggerate the seriousness of a situation and suffer unnecessarily. But I think many persons suffer unnecessarily from *minimizing* the seriousness of what they have undergone. Often I've heard, "What happened to me isn't really that bad, because something much worse happened to someone else I know." No matter how bad it was, it could always have been worse.

For example, some individuals clearly remember having been terrorized by their father's rages. They've been harangued and beaten. They've feared for their life. But they don't remember being sexually abused. They assume that sexual abuse must have occurred also, but they can't remember it. Sexual abuse becomes the smoking gun they need to account for their trauma-related symptoms. Sexual abuse may have occurred and been blocked from memory. But maybe not; being terrorized and beaten is enough.

Many individuals who have been abused, mistreated, or severely neglected throughout childhood have no yardstick for what's normal. Many were socially isolated. They had no reasonable standard by which to judge their experience. They may have lived in a world of family violence, having minimal contact with nonviolent families. They may have assumed that most other children were also subjected to such violent and chaotic experiences. They think that there's no reason for their symptoms, even when they've undergone what to others is obviously years of terrifying experiences. They discount the significance of clearly remembered traumatic experience. Having no explanation for their problems, they feel "crazy." For such persons, an important part of coping with a history of childhood abuse is learning what's reasonable, normal, and tolerable in relationships—and insisting on it henceforth.

Not All Symptoms Come From Trauma

Just as it may be harmful to minimize a clearly remembered traumatic experience, it can be harmful to assume without evidence that a traumatic experience is the cause of various problems and psychiatric symptoms. Some of the popular books on incest, for example, can be misleading if the reader infers, "I also have these problems, so I must have been sexually abused, even if I can't remember it." Even worse: "If I can't remember it, that just *proves* that I was abused." There's no escape.

You'll see in this book that a wide range of symptoms may be associated with traumatic experience—anxiety, depression, and substance abuse, for example. But if you're anxious, depressed, or struggling with substance abuse, does that mean that you have been abused? Of course not; these psychiatric symptoms are simply among the most common in the general population. Medical conditions, heredity, early losses, developmental factors, psychological conflicts, and interpersonal stresses contribute to such problems as anxiety, depression, and substance abuse. Several of these factors are commonly combined in the etiology (causation) of psychiatric disorders. Traumatic experience may or may not be a factor. Keep this basic principle in mind: *the cause cannot be inferred from the symptom.*

Not All Exposure to Potentially Traumatic Events Leads to Disorders

No one comes through potentially traumatic events unscathed. By definition, these events are overwhelming and psychologically injurious. But for many forms of exposure to extreme stress, recovery without ill effects is the rule. PTSD—or any other psychiatric symptom or disorder—is by no means inevitable. Exposure to stress places individuals *at risk* for psychiatric symptoms and disorders. There's a wide spectrum of risk. For some forms of trauma, such as that resulting from natural disasters, the risk is low. For trauma resulting from traumatizing experiences that are severe, prolonged, and high-dose, such as sadistic abuse, the risk is high. For children who witness the murder of a parent, the risk may approach 100%.[65] The level of risk depends not only on the severity of the trauma but also on the vulnerability and resilience of the exposed individual.

Before proceeding, you should know about *medical student's disease.* When medical students read about various symptoms in medical textbooks, they are likely to worry that they have a host of grave diseases. Be forewarned—this book describes just about everything that could possibly go wrong after you've experienced trauma. Much of my clinical experience has been with persons who have undergone the more extreme forms of trauma, so I'm accustomed to seeing the whole gamut of disturbances.

You'll notice that I keep insisting that various forms of difficulty are *natural* reactions to traumatic experience. To say that reactions are natural and understandable is not to say that they are *inevitable*. Don't feel compelled to find all these problems in yourself. I've included what *may* happen, so that if it *has* happened, you'll be able to learn something about it.

Chapter 2

ATTACHMENT

Imagine yourself going out for a walk in your neighborhood. About a mile from your home, two men in a pickup truck drive by, shouting obscenities. A few minutes later, they come back, pull up in front of you, get out, and come at you brandishing knives. You feel endangered, alone, and without protection. You scream for help but no one responds. Satisfied with having terrorized you, the assailants take off. You run for home unscathed physically but badly shaken emotionally. You come in the house trembling and tearful.

Now imagine two possible scenarios. Scenario 1: you're able to put your feelings into words, you have a good capacity to ask for support, and you have a close relationship that provides comforting. When you arrive home, your spouse hears you come in, immediately responds to your distress, and asks you to sit on the couch and tell her what happened. As you do so, you're held and assured that you're safe. Your children also come to your side and do their best to comfort you. You gradually calm down. Scenario 2: you're socially isolated. You come in to your empty house and are left to cope all on your own. You cannot think of anyone you can call or go to see. You can't think straight and can't figure out what to do to calm down. You take a drink—or several.

These two scenarios illustrate how indispensable attachment theory is for understanding trauma. The mother-infant bond is the prototype of attachment, but our need for attachment relationships is lifelong. We learn to feel safe and secure in the world—or fail to do so—in an attachment relationship. Trauma of any sort profoundly threatens our sense of safety and security. Recovery requires that we restore our sense of security, often with the help of an attachment relationship. Of course, we learn ways of comforting and calming ourselves without having to rely on others, but our ability to regulate our emotional states, too, is learned—or not—in the context of an attachment relationship.

To fully understand the impact of trauma of any kind at any age, we must adopt a developmental perspective, considering how trauma can affect the course of your life—and how coping can entail a course change for the better. Here are some reasons why attachment is so important to understanding trauma and how to cope with it: First, much trauma occurs in the context of attachment relationships. Second, trauma can disrupt your capacity to make use of attachment relationships. Third, attachment trauma earlier in life renders you more vulnerable to later trauma. Finally, as the two scenarios described earlier illustrate, secure attachment relationships play a major role in healing. Thus your ability to cope with trauma has strong foundations in your history of attachment relationships.[66]

The Foundation of Development

Psychiatrist John Bowlby developed attachment theory in the 1950s in the course of investigating the mental health implications of children's reactions to the traumatic experience of separation from their parents. He concluded that mental health depends on the child's experiencing a consistent relationship with a nurturing caregiver.[67] Attachment theory continues to inspire a major line of research in child development.[68]

Bowlby rooted his theory of the mother-infant bond firmly in biology, drawing from evolutionary theory and ethology. Attachment develops from *proximity*—the tendency of the youngster to stay close to the mother and vice versa. Bowlby believed that attachment behavior evolved because being close to the mother provided some assurance of safety. In evolutionary terms, proximity to the mother protects offspring from predators. When separated from their mother, offspring let out a distress cry that brings her to the rescue, reinstating proximity. As offspring develop, they learn to run back to their mother when they are separated from her.

The process works both ways: the infant is biologically prepared to form an attachment to the caregiver, and the caregiver is biologically prepared to form a bond with the infant. Offspring maintain proximity; mothers protect. The endangered child separated from the mother is distressed; the mother blocked from protecting her endangered child is distressed. Thus attachment is a reciprocal relationship; infant attachment behavior is intertwined with maternal bonding and caregiving. And, just like their children, caregivers need attachment relationships that provide a safe haven and a secure base to support their caregiving.[69]

Attachment is ancient. Neuroscientist Paul MacLean[70] asserted that the family as a biological institution goes back 180 million years, originating with the earliest mammals while they waited in the wings for 115 million years to take over from the dinosaurs. Bowlby[67] extended this heritage beyond mammals to include some ground-nesting birds. Attachment needs are as firmly rooted in our biology as our needs for food and water.

Attachment behavior and emotional bonding develop in conjunction with nursing and the relatively prolonged dependence of mammalian offspring on mothers. Although we humans are recently evolved mammals, we are at the top of the heap in the amount of parental care we require. The long period of parental care we require profoundly shapes our minds and brains, and it provides the foundation for all subsequent development. Ideally, parenting is the essential buffer against trauma. Yet parenting can fail to buffer trauma, and, at worst, it can be a source of trauma.

The Functions of Attachment

As Bowlby made plain, without the protection afforded by attachment, our species would not have evolved, nor would any of us survive as individuals. Early in life, we need to stay close to stay safe. But attachment provides far more than physical protection, particularly in us humans, where attachment is the crucible for the development of the mind. Core functions of attachment relate directly to trauma: attachment relationships provide a safe haven and a secure base, and they also foster our ability to regulate our physiological arousal.

A Safe Haven

Most obvious in what I've said so far about attachment is the *safe haven* that a secure attachment relationship provides. Along with physical protection, attachment provides a *feeling of security*. We need to be physically safe and to feel emotionally secure. Trauma undermines both; healing attachment relationships restore both. When we're distressed, injured, endangered, or in pain, we seek a safe harbor. Learning to do so was crucial to our physical survival, and being able to do so throughout life is crucial to our emotional well-being.

A Secure Base

The safe haven of an attachment relationship also provides a *secure base* for exploration of the world and thus for autonomy.[71] The toddler confidently explores the playground, occasionally glancing back to make sure his father's keeping an eye on him. As we grow older, we venture farther away from our secure base and for longer periods of time. But we continue to need a secure base in attachment throughout our lifetime. The concept of attachment as providing a safe haven and secure base has much in common with psychoanalyst Erik Erikson's[72] idea of *basic trust*. As I see it, Bowlby placed basic trust in its wider developmental context.

Bowlby[71] maintained that "no concept within the attachment framework is more central to developmental psychiatry than that of the secure base" (pp. 163–164). Without a secure base, we would not feel confident to explore and learn about the world. The secure base is a launching pad for independence. Ideally, life is a series of excursions from a secure base. Having the secure base, the youngster feels free to explore, always with a sense that security and safety are close at hand. Secure attachment not only promotes confident and playful exploration in good times but also fosters the ability to explore possible solutions to problems—including seeking help—in bad times.[73] Impinging on the sense of security, attachment trauma undermines exploration, initiative, and autonomy. Thus traumatized youngsters may be unable to avail themselves of the rich environment needed to foster healthy development, especially the social environment.

Regulating Physiological Arousal

Stress and trauma can wreak havoc with physiology. As I'll discuss in Chapter 7 ("Illness"), trauma evokes the fight-or-flight response, which entails a high level of physiological arousal associated with sympathetic nervous system activation. Every major organ system is involved in this response. Recall that the safe haven of secure attachment promotes a feeling of security. This feeling parallels the dampening of arousal on the physiological level. Soothing is an inextricable part of the caregiver-infant bond, and it occurs in conjunction with the emotional attunement between the two individuals. The distressed infant seeks out the mother for comfort; when in contact, the infant is quieted. Separation from the mother is a primary cause of distress and physiological arousal; reunion both calms emotions and restores physiological equilibrium. Attachments also can provide needed stimulation, alleviating boredom or depression. Thus attachment serves to maintain a balance, keeping arousal within an optimal range.

Attachment promotes a *psychobiological synchrony* between organisms as behavioral and physiological systems become attuned to each other.[74] Synchrony is evident, for example, in sleep-wake cycles and feeding cycles, when mothers' and infants' schedules and rhythms become mutually adapted. Emotional attunement and physiological synchrony operate in tandem. Ideally, caregivers and infants are on the same wavelength.

Early attachment is embedded in maternal caregiving that regulates the infant's physiological development.[75] The infant is born with stable biological systems, but these systems are fine-tuned by caregiving, and they become disruptively perturbed without it. The mother's touch—holding, rocking, warming, and providing a wealth of sensory stimulation—affects physiological, endocrine, and neurochemical functioning. Thus attachment relationships play a key role in the healthy development of the nervous system.[76] On the other hand, psychiatrist Martin Teicher and colleagues[77] proposed that early trauma in attachment relationships puts the brain into an alternate developmental pathway; albeit well adapted to a stress-filled world, this adaptation comes with the cost of high stress sensitivity (see Chapter 7).

Optimally, the external regulation of physiological functioning by sensitive caregiving gradually becomes internalized, such that the developing child becomes increasingly able to self-regulate. With adequate emotional attunement from the caregiver, the youngster has the repeated experience of his or her arousal being soothed and then develops the capacity for self-soothing.

Just as trauma disrupts the secure base and basic trust, it also disrupts physiological regulation. Often a kind of double whammy results here: the traumatic experience generates hyperarousal (fear, panic, pain), and the individual is abandoned or neglected after being injured and aroused. Arousal beyond normal bounds is coupled with a lack of soothing or comforting. Most problematic is what my colleagues British psychologists Peter Fonagy and Mary Target aptly characterized as a *dual liability*.[78] First, the obvious point, attachment trauma evokes extreme distress. Second, the more subtle point, attachment trauma undermines the *development* of the capacity to regulate that distress. Fortunately, secure attachment relationships later in life provide the foundation for developing better capacities for emotion regulation (see Chapter 12, "Emotion Regulation").

Mentalizing

Knowing that secure attachment provides a safe haven and secure base as well as the interpersonal foundation for regulating physiological arousal, we have ample grounds for emphasizing the role of attachment in healing from trauma. Yet there's an even more important reason, and it is being explored by Peter Fonagy and his colleagues.[79,80] Their findings are revolutionizing our understanding of the functions of attachment and its relation to trauma. Here's the core insight: the secure base of attachment not only facilitates exploration of the outer world but also promotes exploration of the *inner world*—the world of the mind; that is, one's own mind and the mind of others. Bowlby[71] laid the groundwork for this insight in proposing that, akin to the mother who provides a secure base for her child, the psychotherapist's role

> is to provide the patient with a secure base from which he can explore the various unhappy and painful aspects of his life, past and present, many of which he finds it difficult or perhaps impossible to think about and reconsider without a trusted companion to provide support, encouragement, sympathy, and, on occasion, guidance. (p. 138)

In this passage, Bowlby described the essence of healing from trauma: exploring painful feelings with a trusted companion.

Building on Bowlby's thinking, Peter Fonagy and his colleagues are exploring scientifically how the secure base of attachment provides the developmental foundation for learning about the mind—indeed, *for coming to have a mind* and a self in infancy. Following Fonagy,[81] I've adopted the term, *mentalizing*, which neatly pinpoints the process of fathoming mental states, such as emotions, in oneself and others.[82,83] When you think about what you're feeling, or you wonder what someone else might be thinking, you're mentalizing. When you're empathizing, you're mentalizing.

Of all the technical terms I'm employing in this book, mentalizing is the one I'm most eager for you to incorporate into your own thinking, because it goes to the heart of healing: making sense of trauma in secure attachment relationships.[25] More broadly, mentalizing renders behavior intelligible; it's the basis of self-awareness and sensitivity to others. And I'm hoping that this book, by helping you understand the psychology of trauma and drawing your attention to the related mental states and their meaning, will promote your ability to mentalize in the trenches, when you're struggling with trauma-related feelings—what I'll call mentalizing emotionally.

A Primer on Mentalizing

You can get plenty of mileage out of the concept of mentalizing by considering just one major facet: *thinking about feelings*. As I'll explain in Chapter 3 ("Emotion"), if you have a solid grasp of a person's emotional state—or your own—you know a great deal. As you've already gathered, in much of this book I encourage thinking about feelings. Yet there are some complexities that we must address to make full use of the concept of mentalizing; hence, the following primer is provided.

- Simply put, mentalizing entails awareness of mental states and processes in oneself and other persons. But we have a wide *variety of mental states and processes:* emotions are foremost, but we're also aware of needs, desires, motives, intentions, goals, hopes, thoughts, beliefs, attitudes, fantasies, dreams—the list is nearly endless.

- The *time frame* of mentalizing can vary. You can mentalize about specific mental states in the *present* (e.g., what you're feeling at the moment), the *past* (e.g., figuring out after the fact what you felt when you did something), or even the *future* (e.g., anticipating how you might feel if you actually do something you're considering). Your ability to mentalize about the past—understanding your mental states in hindsight—helps enormously in enhancing your ability to mentalize in the present. In this book, I capitalize on that fact with the aim of increasing your self-understanding.

- The *scope* of mentalizing can vary with your breadth of perspective. You can focus narrowly on a person's feeling at a given moment (e.g., she looks irritated). And you can be aware of the broader context of that mental state (e.g., she thinks I lied to her), even to the extent of taking into account a broad swath of the person's history (e.g., she's extremely sensitive to any sign of betrayal because of her father's recurrent untrustworthy behavior). Thus, expanding the scope of mentalizing may take into account a broader time frame as well as the wider network of interactions and relationships that influence an individual's mental states. The same applies to your own mental states. Self-understanding often requires you to broaden the scope of mentalizing, considering the wider context beyond the present moment. Understanding how past trauma influences current feelings is a prime example.

- This broad-scope view illustrates a key point about mentalizing: we render the actions of other persons and our own actions intelligible by putting them into a *narrative* context. We ceaselessly create stories involving thoughts and feelings. Think of a time when you had to justify your actions to someone. Think about how you explain your emotional reactions to someone else's behavior. Better yet, think about how squabbling children behave when a parent confronts them. Each one comes up with a different story. We begin learning to mentalize early in life by creating stories to account for actions. For better or for worse, you continually tell yourself stories about yourself in your own mind, and these stories influence who you are. Self-critical stories, for example, can undermine your self-confidence. Ideally, mentalizing, like storytelling more generally, is *creative*: mentalizing, we come up with fresh perspectives that integrate past knowledge with present information and observations.

- Furthermore, the act of mentalizing involves a broad range of *mental processes*. For example, you can *perceive* a mental state; you can *pay attention to, recognize, think about, remember, interpret, make sense of,* or attempt to *explain* mental states. You also can *mirror* mental states, feeling something akin to what another person feels when you empathize. And you can *respond* to others' mental states without being aware of doing so. For example, you might respond to nonverbal cues that signal you should keep your distance from another person. You might not be aware of these cues or even your backing off, perhaps having only the most vague sense of discomfort.
- As I've just implied, we can mentalize more or less consciously, explicitly and implicitly. Mentalizing *explicitly* is a conscious process in which we think deliberately about the reasons for actions—often when we are puzzled: Why would she have said that? How could I have done that? We mentalize explicitly when we put our feelings into words, whether we are trying to make sense of ourselves or need to express what we are feeling to others. Most often, however, we don't have time to mentalize explicitly when we're interacting with others. We're mentalizing *implicitly*, that is, spontaneously and intuitively, without thinking about it. When your friend tells you about a major disappointment, you automatically adopt an expression combining sadness and caring, leaning forward to make emotional contact. Thus the natural empathy we have for one another is based on our ability to mentalize implicitly. We also mentalize implicitly when we hold a conversation, keeping the other person's perspective in mind and taking turns naturally.
- Importantly, we mentalize more or less *effectively*. Mentalizing is a *skill*. As Peter Fonagy and his colleagues are learning, attachment relationships play a crucial role in acquiring skill in mentalizing. To mentalize accurately we need an open-minded attitude of interest and curiosity, whether we're mentalizing another person or ourselves. Additionally, effective mentalizing also requires *knowledge*. Knowledge about other individuals and their contexts plays a major role in our ability to mentalize effectively. For example, when you know a person well, you're in a better position to broaden the scope of your mentalizing—able to create a richer narrative understanding and more accurate stories about mental states. The same applies to yourself: self-knowledge is crucial to accurately apprehending your own mental states. And we're all capable of self-deception, of mentalizing inaccurately.
- Most challenging, we mentalize *emotionally* and *interactively*. In much of this book, we are concerned with mentalizing emotionally—remaining self-aware in the midst of strong emotions. Oftentimes, interactions in close relationships evoke strong emotions and thus tax our ability to mentalize effectively. Consider the challenge of mentalizing interactively:

each person has their own mind *and* the other person's mind in mind, even in the midst of strong emotions. Mind boggling.

- Finally, we often *need others' help to mentalize* most effectively. No doubt, we're able to some degree to sort out confusion about our own and others' feelings and actions by thinking about them. Yet I'm increasingly impressed by the limitations of our ability to make sense of experience on our own. Effective mentalizing typically requires dialogue with others; you'll often make best sense of what you're feeling by talking to a trusted friend who can help you take a more objective view. You might start out just feeling vaguely "upset" and, over the course of the conversation, come to recognize that you're feeling hurt, ashamed, and resentful. Fundamentally, as we've already glimpsed, mentalizing is an interactive process.

What could be more important than having the psychological *freedom* to mentalize? This freedom is crucial to developing self-knowledge as well as to understanding other persons. A secure base in attachment promotes this freedom, and trauma can impinge on it. Most problematic, trauma in early attachment relationships can compromise the *development* of skills in mentalizing, thus interfering with learning self-awareness and sensitivity to others. Fortunately, secure attachment in later relationships can get this development back on course.

Development of Mentalizing

Ordinarily, we learn to mentalize like we learn language, naturally and effortlessly. We take our mentalizing capacity for granted, but, like language, it's a remarkable evolutionary achievement. And, as in language, skill in mentalizing is the culmination of a long period of development that occurs in the context of relationships. My colleague Hungarian psychologist George Gergely has studied how mentalizing develops in infancy, focusing on the development of emotional awareness in attachment relationships. Gergely and Watson[84,85] proposed that, initially, we learn what we feel through a process of *social feedback*, and attachment relationships are a primary source. The emotional response of the mother to the infant's distress provides such feedback: the infant sees his emotional state reflected in his mother's face and hears it reflected in her voice; as a result, he develops more keen awareness of what he feels inside. We all rely on such social feedback throughout life to enhance our awareness of our feelings. When you're distressed, being mentalized—having a sense that a caring person has your mind in mind—is affirming, reassuring, and calming. It helps you to know just what to make of what you're thinking and feeling.

It's hardly surprising that we learn to mentalize best in secure attachment

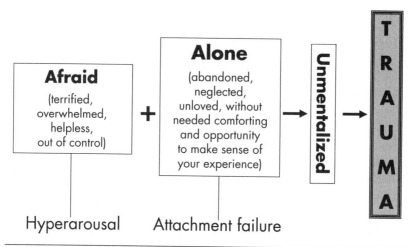

FIGURE 2–1. Facets of attachment trauma.

relationships.[86,87] Secure attachment in childhood also promotes healthy relationships with peers that in turn promote mentalizing in a wider sphere of relationships.[88] Thus mentalizing provides the foundation for both self-awareness and healthy relationships. But, just as secure attachments promote mentalizing, traumatic attachments may undermine it: the child who feels hated shies away from awareness of the parent's mind and blocks awareness of his own painful emotional states.[78] Moreover, to mentalize, we need to be in a state of optimal arousal—alert but relatively calm—and the hyperarousal associated with traumatic states thus blocks mentalizing.[82] Thus, as depicted in Figure 2–1, the combination of feeling extremely frightened and *alone*—without any opportunity to make sense of the experience in a safe relationship—interferes with mentalizing. The failure of mentalizing, in turn, plays an important role in making the experience traumatic: going through frightening events alone makes it especially hard to come to terms with the experience.

But all is not lost. We also know that, given other opportunities, traumatized persons can learn to mentalize more skillfully. And Fonagy's research[89] has shown that the development of mentalizing in the face of trauma promotes *resilience*, that is, the capacity to cope with adversity. That's why I place so much emphasis on mentalizing in this book.

Patterns of Attachment

If you've been traumatized, you know what it's like to be without a safe haven and secure base. A number of attachment patterns fall far short of the biological ideal of safe proximity. We've learned a lot from research on these different patterns. Bowlby's collaborator, Mary Ainsworth, developed an ingenious method to study attachment patterns in infants.[90] Because she wanted to observe attachment behavior in action, Ainsworth created the *Strange Situation* to study infants' and mothers' reactions to separation and reunion. The basic scenario is this: the infant and mother are brought into an unfamiliar but comfortable room filled with toys. A stranger enters, and the mother subsequently departs, leaving the infant in the room with the stranger. Then the mother comes back into the room, pausing to allow the infant a chance to respond to her return. After a while, the stranger leaves the room. Then the mother leaves the infant all alone in the room, subsequently to return a second time.

Ainsworth's Strange Situation has provided a goldmine of information about different patterns of attachment. Thousands of Strange Situations have been studied throughout the world.[91] We now appreciate how optimal caregiving promotes secure attachment and how less-than-optimal caregiving contributes to insecure attachment. Four basic patterns of attachment are summarized in Table 2–1. Two patterns of insecure attachment are less than ideal but nevertheless fall within the normal range: *avoidant* and *resistant* attachment are contrasting adaptive strategies for dealing with stressful or problematic mother-infant relationships. At worst, neglect, maltreatment, and abuse may lead to *disorganized* attachment, in which the infant has no workable strategy for relating to the attachment figure. I'll review these different patterns of infant attachment, because they throw attachment into bold relief, and we can easily appreciate their adulthood counterparts.

In discussing the origins of attachment patterns, I'll emphasize the caregiver's contribution, with the mother-infant relationship as the prototype. Plainly, the infant's temperament also makes some contribution to attachment;[92] for example, distress-prone infants' irritability makes them more difficult to soothe and more likely to develop insecure attachments. Of course, multiple factors also influence the parent's capacity to provide optimal caregiving, including the parent's own trauma history, personality characteristics, psychiatric disorders, current life challenges and stressors, and—not least—supportive attachment relationships.[93] Yet, whatever influences may bear on the infant's and caregiver's behavior, *the infant-caregiver interaction* is the final common pathway for attachment.

Secure Attachment

Secure attachment is the antidote to trauma. Secure attachment characterizes the majority of infants studied in the Strange Situation. Securely attached infants are highly sensitive to their mother's presence and keenly

TABLE 2–1. Attachment patterns

Pattern	Characteristics
Secure	Confidence in availability and emotional responsiveness of caregiver; basic trust
Avoidant	Anticipation of rejection and avoidance of contact with attachment figure when distressed
Resistant	Frustration in seeking comfort when distressed; "kick-and-cling" pattern
Disorganized	Lack of stable strategy for relating to attachment figure; fright without solution

aware of her leaving the room. Depending on their temperament, securely attached infants may be more or less distressed when left alone with the stranger. They may protest or try to follow their mother. Regardless of their level of distress, they rely on their relationship with their mother for comfort. They rapidly seek proximity when she returns; they may make eye contact or approach and greet her. They're easily reassured. They alternate smoothly between exploring and seeking contact with their mother. When threatened or distressed, securely attached infants seek proximity and find comfort; when security is reestablished, they return quickly and confidently to playing and exploring their environment.

The mother's key contribution to secure attachment consists of her accessibility and sensitive responsiveness to her infant's attachment needs.[90] Securely attached infants are likely to have mothers who are able to see things from their baby's point of view and are attuned to their baby's needs. They can accurately perceive the infant's signals and respond promptly to them. They respond to the infant on the basis of the infant's needs rather than by imposing their own needs on the infant. They're responsive to both positive and negative feelings. In short, they're accessible and dependable. But don't get the idea that secure attachment requires perfect mothering. This ideal may be sustained only for 20 minutes of being observed in a research laboratory! Mothering doesn't need to be perfect; it just needs to be good enough.[94]

Like the securely attached infant, the securely attached adult reaches out for contact and comfort in times of distress, confident that the attachment figure will be accessible and emotionally responsive. Secure in your attachment relationship, you anticipate that your attachment figure will have your mind in mind. The relationship will be calming and restoring, emotionally and physiologically. You'll be able to make sense of your distress. You'll mentalize and be mentalized.

Avoidant Attachment

In the Strange Situation, the avoidant infant explores and plays without evident concern for the mother's whereabouts and does not appear to be distressed by her absence. When the mother returns, the infant appears to be indifferent, turns away, or may want to be put down if picked up. Yet the avoidant infant's seeming nonchalance is misleading; heightened physiological arousal persists after the reunion, suggesting that the avoidance is defensive.[95]

Studies of mother-infant interactions suggest that avoidance is a strategy to cope with rejection of the infant's bids for contact and comfort; responding to rebuff, avoidant infants have learned to detach and suppress their attachment needs.[96] Similarly, the avoidant adult is dismissive of attachment,[97] adopting a self-sufficient stance—at the extreme, with a sense of not needing anyone to provide comfort. This avoidant or dismissing stance works reasonably well, in childhood or in adulthood, as long as the distress remains within bounds. It's hardly an effective strategy for coping with traumatic stress.

Resistant Attachment

In the Strange Situation, resistant infants are preoccupied with attachment to the exclusion of interest in exploration and play.[90] They're more focused on their mother than the toys in the playroom. In direct contrast to avoidant infants, they're alert to danger and overtly sensitive to separation, and they become highly distressed when their mother leaves. Yet they are not easily comforted by her return. Their attachment behavior is intermingled with ambivalence and anger. They may seek proximity but angrily resist comforting. Whereas avoidant infants turn down the dial on their attachment needs, resistant infants turn it up—but their heightened needs only fuel conflict in their interactions with the caregiver.

Resistant attachment arises in response to inconsistent caregiving.[97] Mothers of resistant infants may be insensitive to the infant's needs, they may regard the infant as a nuisance and respond belatedly, they may be withdrawn, and they may provide insufficient stimulation. The infant's inclination to maximize attachment behavior can thus be seen as an adaptive effort to attract the attention of the unresponsive or inconsistent caregiver. Yet the infant's ambivalence interferes with soothing whenever the mother is more forthcoming.

Preoccupied attachment is the adult counterpart to resistant attachment in infancy.[97] Adults in preoccupied attachment relationships are highly ambivalent; feeling anxious and in need, yet feeling vulnerable to abandonment and resentful of the attachment figure's failings. Hence their attachments are marked by a combination of dependency and hostility, and, fraught with conflict and discord, their attachment relationships tend to be stormy. In our educational groups, my colleague, psychologist Helen Stein, called this the *kick-and-cling* pattern of attachment, a term that traumatized patients readily appreciate.

Disorganized Attachment

You can begin to see how problematic attachments lead to interpersonal difficulties. Rejection and inconsistent responsiveness can lead to isolation and ambivalence. What happens when attachments are downright traumatic?

Over many years, researchers who studied mothers and their infants in the Strange Situation consistently observed many unclassifiable cases—ones in which the attachment pattern is not clearly secure, avoidant, or resistant. Researchers then developed a meaningful understanding of these unusual patterns of attachment behavior, which now fall under the rubric of *disorganized* attachment.[98]

In the Strange Situation, the behavior of disorganized infants lacks clear goals and is contradictory. The infant may alternate among proximity seeking, avoidance, and resistance. For example, on reunion, the infant may approach the mother as if to make full physical contact and then suddenly turn away. Or the infant's seeking of proximity may be interrupted by a sudden outburst of aggression. These contradictions may be expressed even more dramatically when the infant simultaneously approaches and avoids the mother, inhibiting attachment behavior as it occurs. For example, the infant may approach the mother by backing toward her with his head averted. Or the infant may nestle in the mother's lap but look away with his head down while maintaining a dazed expression. The disorganized pattern also entails a more severe version of the avoidant pattern. The infant may become frightened or distressed but make no effort to seek out the mother. Or the infant may even be *frightened of the mother.* Then the infant may show periods of freezing, as if psychologically paralyzed. Or the infant may be profoundly apathetic.

The disorganized pattern is often associated with more severe forms of maltreatment, including physical, sexual, or emotional abuse, or extreme neglect in some cases.[99] But attachment disorganization is not always a sign of maltreatment. Mothers of disorganized infants are either *frightening to* the infant or *frightened of* the infant.[100] The mother's frightened or frightening behavior may include invading the infant's space, looming over the infant, being afraid or timid in relation to the infant, playing frightening games with the infant, or being extremely sensitive to rejection by the infant. The mother's behavior may result from her own traumatic experience, whether it be a traumatic loss in her own background or her own history of maltreatment. Thus, reminding her of her past, the infant's attachment needs may evoke a post-traumatic state in the mother, which is, in turn, alarming to the infant.[25]

A frightened or frightening mother puts the infant in a situation of intolerable conflict: *the safe haven is alarming.* This contradiction is the core experience in many traumatic relationships. The disorganized infant is in a dilemma, and there's no way to adapt successfully. Put between a rock and a hard place, the infant's resulting behavior appears chaotic, contradictory, and disorganized. Similarly, the adult with a history of traumatic attachment relationships may have no workable strategy for maintaining attachment relationships and may be confined to a fearful pattern of being highly anxious and yet isolated from attachments.[101]

Developmental Changes in Attachment

From the research I've just reviewed, you might infer that attachment patterns are stamped in for life as a result of the mother-infant interaction. Not so. Even in infancy, the pattern of attachment depends on the quality of the particular relationship: if the quality of the mother-infant interaction differs from the father-infant interaction, the infant will show different attachment patterns with each parent, potentially being secure with one and insecure with the other.[93] Taking mother-infant attachment as the prototype is not entirely off the mark, however, because research findings suggest that maternal attachment exerts greater developmental impact.[102,103]

As with any other major area of development, attachment undergoes monumental changes over the course of childhood and into adulthood. At first, attachment in infancy is largely tied to infant-caregiver interactions. Gradually, however, the developing capacity to hold relationships in mind, for example, to derive comfort from the memory of an interaction with an attachment figure, enables the child and adult to sustain attachment relationships during increasingly long physical separations. Second, the potential range of attachment figures expands dramatically over the course of a lifetime. Of course, the infant's range of attachments is contingent on the composition of the household and the caregiving arrangements. Generally, attachments cover an ever-widening sphere, developing with nonparental caregivers, siblings, and peers. Given the variations in contemporary family composition and caregiving, it's fortunate that attachment behavior is so flexible.

The finding that the infant's pattern of attachment depends on the behavior of the caregiver is extremely important. Keep in mind that the infant is *biologically disposed to form a secure attachment.* My clinical work has led me to appreciate the profound resilience of the attachment system. I've had countless opportunities to admire individuals' persistence in working their way toward more secure attachments. This relentless search begins early in life. Even in the presence of pervasive family violence or abusive experience, the infant and youngster will find and make use of islands of security. And youngsters will often form relatively secure attachments outside the family, for example, with peers, teachers, coaches, grandparents, neighbors, or clergy.[104] It's rare for a person to arrive at adulthood without *some* capacity to form a positive, close, and secure attachment.[101]

And we do not just form attachments with individuals; we also develop a sense of belonging to institutions and groups. For some people, affiliation with groups provides a primary source of attachment and security.[105] Affiliation begins developing in relation to the family unit and then extends to other groups. Like attachments with individuals, affiliation with groups can alleviate distress and sustain self-esteem. From this perspective, it's little wonder that groups are so helpful in the treatment of individuals who have been traumatized (see Chapter 13, "Treatment Approaches").

Also, we should not minimize the significance of attachments to animals.[106] Particularly in the context of trauma, pets such as cats, dogs, and rabbits may be emotional lifesavers for children and adults. They're our mammalian kin,[70] and they have attachment capacities akin to ours. So it's little wonder that we can form affectionate bonds with them. Besides, they're furry, providing a much-needed comforting touch. It's not surprising that traumatized persons may find refuge in strong bonds with pets,[101,107] and these bonds are to be encouraged, as long as they do not substitute for attachments with other persons.

In thinking about the diversity of attachments that can form over the lifetime, we should not overlook the importance of attachments to familiar places and inanimate objects. This phenomenon of bonding to places has been called *site attachment*.[108] Children coping with trauma invariably seek a safe place in the environment, such as their room, their closet, their bed, or a spot in the woods. Just as children rely on familiar inanimate objects (stuffed animals, a security blanket), so, too, do adults. It's important to be able to go to a tangible place of safety. But it's also possible to seek shelter in your imagination. Traumatized individuals often find it helpful to visualize an imagined or actual safe place. Relaxation and hypnosis can be used to enhance such visualization, which can be enormously powerful. Picturing oneself in a safe place can be a key component of self-soothing.

In sum, we have extensive evidence for both stability and change in attachment patterns over the course of development.[109] Naturally, the more stable the quality of the attachment relationship, the more stable the attachment pattern. A secure attachment pattern can be disrupted by family stress that adversely affects the quality of caregiving. Conversely, the opportunity to form a close relationship with a sensitively responsive attachment figure offers the possibility of change from insecure to secure attachment.[110] We consider attachment to be somewhat fluid: an individual may show different patterns of attachment with different attachment figures at a given point of time, as well as different patterns of attachment with the same attachment figure at different points in time, depending on the nature of the interaction at the time.[101,111] We are counting on the possibility of change when we view secure attachment relationships as crucial to healing from trauma. And we know from our research that the majority of traumatized persons do not give up on finding some level of security in attachment relationships.[101]

Rerailed Development

We humans are a highly adaptable species, but we have limits. We can develop and thrive in a wide range of environments—but not *all* environments. Psychologist Sandra Scarr[112] spelled out what she considered to be the necessary conditions to promote human development: protective parenting adults, a surrounding group of family members and peers, and ample opportunities for social learning that promote normal development. Scarr emphasized that, under optimal conditions, children actively choose and construct their own environments. Children evoke responses in their caregivers, and they seek out situations that fit their needs, abilities, and interests. Yet those who suffer severe childhood trauma may not have as much choice. They may be deprived of growth-promoting opportunities, and they may not be able to escape developmentally destructive influences. But sooner or later, many persons *are* able to leave traumatic environments. They *can* find environments conducive to putting their development back on course. Even if you've undergone prolonged trauma, you can potentially choose and construct a healthier environment for yourself. The new environment will foster new learning: the world is dangerous; people are dangerous—but not *that* dangerous. The world can be relatively safe, and many people can be trusted.

Just as there are vicious circles, there are benign circles. Learning to calm yourself enables you to see the world as a safer place; seeing the world as safer, you can relax even more. Learning to trust one person enables you to trust others; your capacity to trust blossoms. Learning to stand up for yourself and to prevent others from exploiting you allows you to feel better about yourself; as your self-esteem improves, you stand up for yourself even more. Every step in the right direction can lead to further steps; the challenge is to bring development back on course.

Part II

EFFECTS
OF TRAUMA

```
+-------------------------------------------------------+
|   •      C h a p t e r    3       •                    |
|-------------------------------------------------------|
|                                                       |
|               EMOTION                                 |
|                                                       |
+-------------------------------------------------------+
```

EMOTION

A 10-year-old boy reaches for a glass to get a drink of juice. His hands are wet, and the glass slips, falling to the floor and smashing. His father flies into the kitchen, his face contorted with rage. The boy cowers in terror. His father screams at him to clean it up; the boy's hands shake so badly that he cuts himself in the process. In disgust, his father takes over, hands his son a knife, and tells him to go outside to cut a switch. The boy is trembling with fear, and he's also furious at his father. Holding the knife, he fleetingly imagines stabbing his father, but he quickly pushes the thought aside and goes outside as commanded. He tries to find a branch with only a few sharp spikes on it. He brings the switch to his father, who's standing out on the porch. His father makes him pull down his shorts and begins whipping him. The boy tries not to cry or yell, but he can't help it. He sees the two neighbor girls watching through the bushes. He turns his face away in shame. His father sends him to his room. After a while, the boy calms down some, but he doesn't feel okay. He's been through scenes like this many times before, and he feels despair, certain that things will never change. The boy doesn't have much choice about how he feels. Fear, anger, shame, and deep sadness are all natural reactions to this kind of intensely emotional episode.

If we were to follow this boy's trajectory into adulthood, we'd not be surprised to learn that he struggles with intense emotions. He responds intensely to men in positions of authority, for example, being unreasonably afraid of his boss's criticism and sometimes infuriated by it. Following in his father's footsteps, he occasionally lashes out at his son in anger and then feels guilty and ashamed. Such intense reactions—especially to any reminders of the traumatic events—are the emotional legacy of trauma. And the opposite occurs too: many traumatized persons complain that their emotions are blunted; for example, they cannot feel angry or loving. Thus they may struggle with a combination of too much and too little emotion: panic, terror, rage, and despair, alternating with feeling numb, empty, or emotionally dead.

Understandably, if you often feel overwhelmed, you may want to rid yourself of your emotions. I think of this approach as stoicism: striving to show strength in the face of misfortune by remaining unemotional. This stoic strategy can be fostered early in life, when children are rebuked or punished for showing emotion—even as they're being emotionally provoked. If you've developed this strategy, you have a venerable precedent, going back two millennia to ancient Greek philosophy. Arising in about 300 B.C.E., Stoic philosophy held sway for a number of centuries, and it continues to permeate our attitudes toward emotion. Epictetus, a philosopher in the Roman Empire, represented the Stoic perspective well.[113] The basic principles are familiar: we must distinguish what is in our control from what is not. External events—traumatizing events included—are not within our control. Desiring to control external events sets us up for anxiety, frustration, and misery. For the sake of our mental tranquility, we must let go of our desire to control events. Within our control, Epictetus believed, are our *interpretations* of external events—how we think and feel about them. In sum, our emotions stem from our desires and judgments; although we are not in control of external events, we are in control of our desires and judgments. By developing the proper desires and making the proper judgments, we can control our emotions and maintain peace of mind.

If you feel overwhelmed by your emotions, you might find Stoicism appealing. But consider this Stoic aspiration:[114] "Remember ... when you embrace your child, your husband, your wife, you are embracing a mortal. Thus, if one of them should die, you could bear it with tranquility" (p. 7). Self-control is taken to the extreme. In the wisest passage on emotion I've come across, contemporary philosopher A.C. Grayling[16] put Stoicism in perspective:

> Although this teaching was designed to help people bear vicissitudes bravely, and in its inspiration is one of the tenderest and most thoughtful of philosophies, it misses a very important point. This is that if one is frugal with one's emotions—limiting love in order to avoid its pains, stifling appetites and desires in order to escape the price of their fulfilment—one lives a stunted, muffled, bland life only. It is practically tantamount to a partial death in order to minimise the electric character of existence—its pleasures, its ecstasies, its richness and colour matched by its agonies, its wretchedness, its disasters and grief. To take life in armfuls, to embrace and accept it, to leap into it with

energy and relish, is of course to invite trouble of all the familiar kinds. But the cost of avoiding trouble is a terrible one: it is the cost of having trodden the planet for humanity's brief allotment of less than a thousand months, without really having lived (pp. 167–168).

Of course, no one will take issue with the idea that we must exert some emotional control. We'd best refrain from acting in harmful ways in intense emotional states—lashing out in a rage. Such blatant failures of emotional control are the cause of much trauma. Yet we must not predicate our general attitudes toward emotion on such extremes.

I'm taking a 180-degree turn from Stoicism: *healing from trauma requires cultivating emotion, not squelching it.* Trauma tends to narrow the range of emotions—you may be stuck in fear or resentment, unable to experience positive emotions. Healing from trauma entails feeling and expressing more, not feeling and expressing less. Cultivate emotions. Think of emotions like a flower garden, with all kinds of plants—maybe weeds, thorns, and cacti sprout up among glorious blossoms. Or think of a modern painting—a Kandinsky—with many vibrant colors and hues, black and bright red alongside beautiful pastels. A symphony will also do. It's the variations and subtleties I'm emphasizing, without putting on rose-colored glasses and glossing over the darker and more intense emotions that are anything but pretty.

Cultivating emotions—mentalizing emotionally—is the best path to avoiding emotional excesses. Persons who suffer with trauma often find themselves blindsided by sudden eruptions of emotion: they go from zero to 100 m.p.h. in a split second. Yet I believe that they're blindsided because they've been *suppressing* their feelings, which gradually intensify until they can no longer be suppressed; then they're expressed in disruptive ways. Cultivating greater awareness of your feelings is preventive: you cannot influence what you do not know.

For the sake of cultivation, we must understand emotion well, and we're fortunate that psychologists, neurobiologists, and philosophers have put so much effort into this endeavor. Because emotion is central to trauma, I begin this chapter with a primer on emotion. Postponing discussion of enjoyable emotions to Chapter 12 ("Emotion Regulation"), here I'll consider several emotions that play a major role in trauma: fear, anger, shame, guilt, disgust, and sadness. I conclude the chapter with further thoughts about how greater emotional awareness—mentalizing emotionally—can help prevent untoward eruptions.

A Primer

If you're troubled by your emotions, it's worth your while to become knowledgeable about them and to appreciate their complexity and diversity as well as their adaptive value. And there's a practical point here: becoming more attuned to your emotions will help you regulate them more effectively.[115] But you should be forewarned that I've packed a great deal of information into this primer on emotion. You may find it slow going, but I believe that understanding your emotions thoroughly is worth the effort. And I'm campaigning for a positive view of emotion that you might find somewhat alien, so I'm pulling out all the stops.

Emotions Are Adaptive

More than a century ago, Darwin[116] recognized the survival value of emotions, which psychologists now take for granted. Fear and anger exemplify the self-protective value of emotions: when threatened, we automatically become energized to react quickly and vigorously, running or counter-attacking, depending on the circumstances. Cold logic won't do.

As I've already hinted, however, our emotions promote far more than mere survival. Contemporary philosopher Martha Nussbaum[117] proposed that emotions are evaluative judgments regarding the status of our goals and projects; they're not just concerned with our survival but with all aspects of our *flourishing* in the world (see Chapter 14, "Hope"). We judge the world emotionally, and our emotional judgments are at once informative and motivating. We're inclined to prize logic and reason, but, without the guidance of our emotions, our actions are liable to be unreasonable. Neuroscientist Antonio Damasio[118] has shown how our gut feelings continually guide our actions. When brain damage severs our access to gut feelings, we lose the ability to act in a way that suits our best interests—even in a situation as mundane as gambling, which requires prudence guided by emotion. Alcohol does the same, neutralizing fear, rendering us insensitive to risks, potentially allowing us to put ourselves in harm's way, for example, by driving drunk with misguided confidence.

Geared toward our flourishing, emotions set our priorities. But they do far more: emotions organize our actions. When someone blocks you from reaching a goal, for example, you're likely to become angry. The anger shows on your face, your blood pressure rises, your muscles tense, and you're prepared for a confrontation to alleviate the interference. If you have a history of trauma, you may be horrified by the sudden eruption of anger. But step back for a moment and think of this process from another angle: this complex emotional response is nothing short of amazing. In an instant—far more quickly than you can think about it—your emotion mobilizes you to take appropriate action. Thinking of emotions as organizing may be jarring if you're feeling disorganized by your strong reactions. You might think of it this way: emotions abruptly interrupt your ongoing activity, reordering your priorities and reorganizing your functioning accordingly.[119] By design, emotions are disruptively reorganizing.

To claim that emotions evolved as adaptive solutions to basic problems of survival that confront our species is not to claim that they are perfectly adaptive. Rather, emotions have the *potential* to be adaptive,[120] a potential that we must actively cultivate. Evolution never leads to perfection,[121] and the vast majority of species that ever lived has become extinct.[122] Our evolved abilities, including emotional abilities, don't always work properly—and then we need to work on them.

Emotions Are Organizing

We can best appreciate the organizing quality of emotions by considering them to be complex *packages* of responses.[123] These packages are so sophisticated that we can only glimpse their complexity. *Emotion* is the umbrella term, and the major components of emotions are physiological reactions, expressions, actions, thoughts, and feelings.

To illustrate, let's stick with anger. Anger mobilizes us to respond vigorously to threat or interference, and vigorous action must be supported by elaborate *physiological* activation—all of which must occur in a split second. The brain orchestrates a pattern of activation in the sympathetic branch of the autonomic (involuntary) nervous system.[124] This activation includes, for example, increases in heart rate and blood pressure that provide fuel for the large muscles, the heart, and the brain itself, while also reducing blood flow to gastrointestinal organs—directing energy to where it is most needed at the moment. Physiological activation in a wide range of organ systems is accompanied by automatic changes in emotional *expression*, most obviously in the face and the voice. This social-communicative function of emotion, too, is adaptive: we automatically signal our emotional states to others to guide their behavior. They may instantly get the message: back off!

Many emotions also trigger purposeful *actions*, or at least an inclination to act. When we are angry, we feel like striking out and may do so. These physiological reactions, communicative expressions, and emotional actions can occur quickly, before we have a chance to think. But emotions invariably trigger *thoughts*. When we are angry, for example, we may think about the unfairness or blameworthiness of someone's actions: "How could he have done that?!" And the direction of causation goes both ways: emotions trigger thoughts, and thoughts trigger emotion. Hence emotions are triggered by internal events—thoughts and memories—as well as external events.

Emotions Are Informative

We often equate feelings and emotions, but it's helpful to make a distinction: *feelings* are one component of emotions, namely, our conscious experience of our emotional states. As Damasio[125] put it more technically, our feelings are composite mental images of the changes wrought by emotion in our body and brain. That is, we have conscious access to our emotional states because we feel them: we feel the physiological arousal and our behavioral responses and tendencies, including sensory feedback from our facial expressions. Our feelings provide evaluative information about our goals and projects: they can serve as a signal (I'm being thwarted) and a guide to action (I must stand up for myself).

Separating feeling and emotion helps us think about the (not uncommon) occurrence of being out of touch with our emotions. Feelings are but one aspect of an emotional state, and we can have emotions without feeling them. You can be angry without being aware of it. Someone might notice irritation in your face or tone of voice when you're not feeling angry. If the anger is brought to your attention, you might begin to feel it. If you're afraid of your anger, you may not be able to feel it without someone else's drawing your attention to it. Regardless, you'll be angry *before* you feel it: the emotional state must coalesce before you can form a mental image of it.

Emotions Are Processes

I've said emotions are amazing—and potentially blindsiding—because they unfold so fast. Yet their quickness obscures their complexity: we shouldn't lose sight of the fact that emotions, however brief, are complex *processes* that unfold over time. For basic emotions like fear and anger, the whole cascade of reactions I've described can unfold in a second or two.[126] Sometimes the burst of emotion also subsides quickly. You feel afraid in an instant when a car suddenly pulls in front of you, and you feel relieved after you've averted the crash and realize that it was a near miss. You feel a flash of anger when someone shoves you, then you calm down when you realize it was just an accident. Of course, when the provocative event continues, so will the emotions. And you can prolong your emotional states with your imagination, thinking in ways that fan the flames of worry or resentment. You might stew in anger about the driver's being so reckless or about the carelessness of the person who bumped into you.

Recognizing that there are gray areas, we can distinguish emotion from moods and temperament, which are more enduring.[127] As just described, emotions are generally brief, lasting seconds or minutes. *Moods*—feeling irritable or blue—may last for hours or even days. Depressed mood can become so severe and prolonged as to be diagnosed as a *mood disorder* (see Chapter 8, "Depression"). Fortunately, we can be in cheerful moods as well as irritable, anxious, and depressed moods. Moods lend a coloring to all our experience, even if we're not aware of them continuously. We may not always feel them, although others may be affected by them. We might think of emotions as brighter colors and moods as pastels. Moods set the stage for heightened readiness to respond with emotions: in an irritable mood, you're more prone to erupt in anger.

We often use the word "temperamental" to refer to moodiness. But *temperament* has a more technical meaning, referring to biologically based personality characteristics. While we all share a common human nature, each of us has an individual nature, which is partly based on genetic makeup. There are many different facets of temperament, not all of which relate directly to emotion. Some children are more active, more impulsive, or more sociable than others.[128] Yet many temperaments are emotional. We can be temperamentally prone to anxiety,[129] aggression,[130] depression,[131] or cheerfulness.[132] Given the biological contribution to temperament, some temperamental traits are evident early in infancy. Many temperamental differences seen in humans are also clearly evident in primates and other mammals.[128] Like moods, which they also influence, temperaments render you more likely to respond with the associated emotions.

Emotions Are Directive

Given the potential subtlety of our experience, we have a rich language for emotion, distinguishing exuberance from excitement and pique from irritation. But we don't always have such refined ideas about what we feel. Quite often, when I observe a patient in the midst of an emotional state, I inquire what she is feeling, and she accurately responds that she doesn't know—even though she's clearly feeling something. Sometimes our emotions are not well defined,[133] and we can rightly say that we're just feeling "emotional," or perhaps "upset" or "distressed." Something's wrong, and we don't know what. Then we try to refine the feelings so as to have a better understanding of what's going on. The effort is worthwhile: we need to decipher our feelings so we can take direction from them.

Most broadly, our emotions evolved to steer us toward whatever might benefit us and away from whatever might harm us. Thus emotions direct and motivate approach and avoidance behavior. Accordingly, many emotion researchers make a global distinction between positive and negative emotion. This distinction works as long as we don't confuse positive with good and negative with bad—all emotions are useful. Rather, think of positive and negative like magnetic poles, attracting and repelling.

This global positive-negative distinction has proven very useful.[134] We differ from one another in our general tendencies toward positive emotionality and negative emotionality, the general inclination to seek reward or avoid harm. Being partly temperamental, these individual differences can be observed early in infancy—in behavior, autonomic arousal, and corresponding patterns of brain functioning. As measured by electroencephalographic (EEG) readings of frontal lobe activity, for example, negative emotion is reflected in relatively high activation of the right cerebral hemisphere, whereas positive emotion is reflected in higher activation of the left hemisphere.

I'll distinguish among different forms of positive emotion in Chapter 12, "Emotion Regulation"; here I want to consider positive emotionality in general. To reiterate, positive emotions are adaptive in motivating us to approach whatever may be beneficial to us. We curiously explore art exhibitions and new cities. We eagerly anticipate a good meal. Positive emotions energize this approach behavior and also provide a feeling of reward. Some persons are blessed, by temperament and experience, with the personality disposition of positive emotionality; they're characteristically cheerful, optimistic, and outgoing—highly engaged with the world around them and with other people. As we'll see in Chapter 8, "Depression," the opposite occurs as well: depressed mood can be understood as a low level of positive emotionality—nothing holds any interest or promises excitement—and pleasure is hard to come by.

Whereas positive emotions facilitate approach behavior, negative emotions prompt avoidance and withdrawal from whatever may be harmful to us. Positive emotions promote engagement, and negative emotions promote disengagement. Notably, anger doesn't fit well into this scheme, because it's a negative emotion that may promote aggressive approach or engagement (attack) as well as avoidance. Anxiety, fear, and disgust are prototypical of negative emotionality. Like positive emotionality, negative emotionality is a personality characteristic, which entails proneness to anxiety and distress. Persons characterized by negative emotionality are directed by caution: they tend to be relatively inhibited and avoidant, highly sensitive to threat and the prospect of criticism or punishment, and inclined to focus inward, more disposed to ruminating than taking action.

This broad distinction between positive and negative emotions has proven enormously fruitful in illuminating the biology of emotion, personality differences, and early development. But we face two main problems with this view. First, we need to think about emotion in a more refined way: positive and negative emotions have vastly different forms, and we should not just lump them all together. Second, as I've already stated, the term negative emotions is prejudicial: although they're painful and may cause serious problems, negative emotions are not inherently bad. At this crux the Stoics, long antedating Darwin, took a wrong turn: they did not consider that negative emotions are (potentially) adaptive. And we differ from one another in our feelings about feelings. Some persons feel pleasure in sadness (e.g., nostalgia) or gratification in anger (e.g., a sense of power). Granted, many challenges of survival, and the emotions that support them, are hardly enjoyable.

But we need fear, anger, and disgust for self-protection. We must cultivate them, not plow them under.

Emotions Are Universal

Emotion researchers have taken a big step beyond the global distinction between positive and negative emotions by exploring the possibility of universal agreement on a small set of *basic emotions*. These basic emotions evolved to cope with fundamental adaptive challenges that go beyond mere approach and avoidance.

One particularly fruitful strategy to discovering basic emotions has been examining the extent of cross-cultural agreement on categorizing emotions from pictures of facial expressions.[126] Based on this research, we have a short list: fear, anger, sadness, disgust, surprise, and happiness. Researchers are actively exploring the extent of correspondence among different components of these emotional packages, investigating how well the discrete facial expressions correspond to specific patterns of physiological arousal as well as to conscious feelings of emotion.[123,135] Paralleling research on facial expression, psychologists are also studying the extent to which various emotions can be distinguished in the voice, a similarly rich and subtle vehicle for communicating emotion.[136] In recognition of their themes and variations, some of the basic emotions are best construed as *families,* each encompassing a wide range. Anger varies from irritation to rage, and fear has many shades from apprehension to terror.[126]

Paralleling research on facial and vocal expressions, neuroscientists are distinguishing among basic emotions by linking different forms of emotional behavior to specific patterns of brain activity and corresponding neurotransmitters and hormones.[137] Like research on expressive behavior, brain research demonstrates that many of our fundamental emotional responses have been hardwired over the course of evolution. As Darwin made plain more than a century ago, we share much of this basic emotional circuitry with our mammalian kin, along with our attachment proclivities, as dog and cat lovers will readily attest.

To understand the emotional impact of trauma, we must fully appreciate the hardwired, automatic quality of the basic emotions, particularly fear and anger. But crucially important for coping with trauma is understanding how basic emotions couple hardwiring with learning and regulatory controls. With hardwiring and no controls, we'd be completely at the mercy of our emotions, and they'd lose their adaptive potential.

Emotion researcher Robert Levenson[119] neatly distinguished between *core emotion programs* and the *control mechanisms* that surround them. Imagine yourself trying to finish a difficult task under time pressure and being interrupted by a coworker who needs your help. Your core emotion program responds to the interruption of your activity, and you feel a flash of irritation. Then your control mechanisms kick in as you quickly realize your coworker has a legitimate need and it'll only take you a few minutes to help him.

The core programs of each basic emotion match prototypical situations to adaptive responses—danger to fear, thwarting to anger, loss to sadness. As the example of a flash of irritation illustrates, perceptions of prototypical situations launch core emotion programs rapidly and automatically. Then control mechanisms immediately come into play as we bring our history of learning to bear on the situation. We learn to exert control in two ways. First, we can change the *input*—the provocation—to the core programs by reappraising situations. For example, after a second thought, we realize the situation is easily manageable. Alternatively, we can inhibit the *output,* that is, intervening in the transition from action tendencies (feeling like hitting) to actions (hitting). As our intuition attests, inhibiting the output requires great effort, which is evident in a high level of physiological arousal (e.g., in elevated blood pressure) and muscle tension (e.g., in clenched fists and jaws).

One additional point about emotional learning: evolution designed us to respond to survival-related triggers with basic emotions—for example, to respond to falling with fear. Yet we continually learn new triggers—we're likely to fall on ice. We're designed, however, to learn more readily than to unlearn. Traumatized persons will best appreciate Ekman's[126] point that we're designed to get emotional triggers in, not out.

Emotions Are Social

The short list of basic emotions hardly begins to capture the richness of our emotional experience. I'll use the term, *social emotions,* quite loosely to encompass a somewhat broader range of emotions. And I'll be discussing two of these, shame and guilt, in greater detail shortly. For the moment, I want to emphasize that most of the adaptive challenges we face are interpersonal. First and foremost, our emotions guide us in relating to each other: forming and maintaining attachments, developing alliances, competing for resources, and so forth. Without emotional guidance, we'd be utterly lost in relating to others, as the condition of autism sadly attests.[138]

We can think of the basic emotions as being more biologically hardwired and the social emotions as being more culturally shaped. But I don't want to push this distinction too far. As the Stoics rightly saw, we respond emotionally to things we can't control, and other persons—being inherently unpredictable and uncontrollable—are prominent in this emotional field. Moreover, all the basic emotions are social emotions in the sense that their communicative expressions are recognized universally, and these expressions evolved because they serve a social function. In addition, the expression of basic emotions is powerfully shaped by cultural factors: we can learn to inhibit our display of fear, anger, or sadness—to a degree. And, as discussed in the previous chapter on attachment, emotional learning takes place in the context of social relationships[139] and attachment relationships in particular.[79] Conversely, the social emotions are no less biological; we'd hardly be able to experience them without a brain and a body. But they're not tied so narrowly to specific brain circuitry, autonomic nervous system activity, or actions.

The prototypical social emotions—embarrassment, shame, guilt, and pride—begin developing in the second year of life, as we become sensitive to others' reactions to our behavior. Hence these emotions are also regarded as the *self-conscious emotions*.[139] Sympathy and empathy are not specific emotions but rather reflect emotional responsiveness to a wide range of emotions in others. Yet sympathy and empathy are worth noting in the sphere of social emotion, because they are highly adaptive in promoting helpful behavior.[140]

Social psychologist Jonathan Haidt[141] usefully expanded the realm of social emotions to include *moral emotions,* namely, those connected with the welfare of other persons or society as a whole. He enumerated several categories that overlap basic and social emotions: other-condemning emotions include anger, disgust, and contempt; self-condemning emotions include shame, embarrassment, and guilt; other-suffering emotions include compassion and distress at another's distress; and other-praising emotions include gratitude, awe, and elevation (being deeply moved by exemplary acts of others). Haidt also includes *schadenfreude,* that is, feelings of pleasure in response to others' misfortunes; schadenfreude peaks when you feel they're getting their comeuppance. And, while we're in the social-moral realm, we might also add the troublingly ubiquitous emotions of jealousy and envy.[142] Not uncommonly, for example, traumatized persons feel envious of others who do not have to struggle with such painful and difficult problems—and they feel ashamed of their envy.

Emotions Are Intelligent

The emotions I've enumerated just begin to reflect the rich texture of our evaluative relation to the world and to each other. I've highlighted the adaptive nature of emotions but wish to go one step further: emotions are not just adaptive, they're potentially intelligent.

Continuing a long philosophical tradition, we're accustomed to contrasting reason and passion, viewing emotions as irrational. This occasional truth—more than occasional if you've been traumatized—should not unduly influence our thinking about emotion. Contemporary philosophy and psychological science are converging on a different view: emotion synthe-sizes reason and passion. Rather than pitting reason against emotion, we should think of their syntheses: reasonable passion and passionate reason. We're accustomed to wanting to think clearly; as one of our educational group members commented, it's also desirable to *feel clearly*.

Philosopher Robert Solomon[143] views emotion as ordering experience and putting our priorities right, equating emotion with rationality. Martha Nussbaum, in her magisterial book *Upheavals of Thought: The Intelligence of Emotions*,[117] construes emotions as intelligent responses to the perception of value; emotions are a way of seeing and a way of knowing. But they are pow-erful and profound ways of knowing, knowing beyond words. She likened the upheaval of grief at the news of her mother's death to a nail being driven into her stomach, concluding that emotional knowing can be downright vi-olent. We know most deeply when we know emotionally.

The sheer speed of intense emotional reactions misleads us. Emotions can seem to take you by brute force: you may not know what hit you; you feel blindsided. But emotions are not blind: they are complex interpreta-tions—amazingly fast interpretations. Thus the Stoics were right to construe our emotional responses as based on our interpretations of situations. But they were misleading in implying that we can rid ourselves of negative emo-tions by changing our interpretations. It's not that we ordinarily deliberate on an interpretation then have an emotion (although we sometimes do): our emotions *are* interpretations. They're often faster than conscious thought. Of course, we oftentimes alter our emotions by reinterpreting the situation—after the fact.

In modern psychological theory of emotion, these interpretations are called *appraisals*. Appraising a situation as dangerous, we feel fear. Recogniz-ing it as a near miss, we reappraise the situation as posing no danger and we calm down. The rapidity of appraisals is astounding. You can begin to ap-praise situations unconsciously, in a fraction of a second, much faster than you can think. By the time you're aware of the near miss in the car, you've already hit the brakes and turned the steering wheel; then you realize you're alarmed and shaken up. A crucial point: our appraisals are not separate from the emotion or prior to emotion; they are components of the emotional package.[133]

Our emotional reactions are launched with an initial appraisal, but the ap-praisal process is ongoing. Decades ago, stress researcher Richard Lazarus[144] distinguished *primary appraisals* of the situation (I'm in danger) from *second-ary appraisals* related to our ability to cope with the situation (I can avoid this fight if I walk away). Secondary appraisals play a major role in the course of emotion: your response to a dangerous situation will vary, depending on whether you feel helpless and overpowered or confident that you can get yourself to safety. But you don't just have a single primary appraisal followed by another secondary appraisal. Your complex emotional reactions involve a continual cascade of appraisals—a dozen or more can unfold in parallel in a split second.[133] And this cascade includes appraisals of your own emotional responses, emotional reactions to your emotions: you can feel endangered or empowered by your building anger. Your shifting appraisals lead to rapid shifts in your emotions: you can be angered by someone's rudeness then realize that you're likely to be hit and become afraid. All the while, with changing appraisals, the emotional packages change: your physiology, facial and vocal expressions, actions, and feelings are shifting, quickly adapting and readapting to the evolving challenges of the whole emotional episode.

We can best capture the full intelligence of emotions by appreciating their narrative structure.[117] Think of each emotional reaction as containing a story. The plot may be simple (suddenly dodging flying debris) or enormously complex (suddenly learning about a spouse's affair). Oftentimes the story can be signaled in a quick burst of feeling, but articulating the story will take a lot longer. The story may be obscure. You may not know why you feel irritated, anxious, or depressed. Then you must work to construct a story—and there's no guarantee of validity. You're not always keen on the truth, for example, when you feel envy or schadenfreude, all too human as these emotions may be.[142]

Moreover, each emotion has a history. The intelligence of our emotions—the sophistication of their stories—derives from our evolutionary history as well as our individual history. We all share a common story—we become angry when our goals are thwarted. But each of us becomes attuned to certain cues that reflect our individual twist on that story. In Ekman's[126] terms, emotions contain themes and variations. You may be sensitized to thwarting by men or by women or by persons in authority. An emotional reaction can bring out this story—and its history—in a split second. Then you enact the next scene in the evolving story. Of course, sometimes the old story doesn't fit the current situation, and you need to reappraise the situation deliberately so as to move the plot in a more realistic direction.

I'm making the case that we do best when we cultivate rather than suppress our emotions, embracing and befriending them rather than avoiding and squelching them. This is not to say we will enjoy them—quite the contrary. But we can profit from their wisdom. We can profit most, however, when we attend to them. We can mentalize emotionally, that is, feel and think about our feelings at the same time.[79] Mentalizing emotionally is one facet of the continual reappraisal process that occurs during emotional episodes, as we take our own emotional state into account. Moreover, given that most of our emotional episodes are interpersonal, mentalizing others' emotional states—empathizing—is also crucial to our continual reappraisals. No doubt, mentalizing emotionally is a big challenge in the context of trauma, where emotional responses are quick and intense.

Fear and Anxiety

> Imagine a girl whose mother is alcoholic. Whenever her mother drinks, she loses her temper and goes on a rampage. The girl is in her bedroom playing, aware that her mother is in the kitchen drinking. She knows that the tide has turned when she hears her mother yelling. She runs to the closet; it's hot, stuffy, and dark. Her mother is looking for her and screaming her name. The girl feels trapped, sweaty, and panicky. If she goes to her mother, she might get yelled at or beaten. But the longer she hides, the more her mother will be enraged. She's in a dilemma. She feels helpless, and her anxiety escalates as she tries to make up her mind what to do. But her mother storms into the room and yanks open the closet door. Then the danger's clear and imminent, and she feels fear.

We could draw out this emotional episode and distinguish a wide spectrum of emotions in the fear family: apprehension, anxiety, fear, panic, and terror. I'll focus on fear, anxiety, and panic, and then briefly discuss coping strategies.

Fear

Of all the emotions, fear is most central to trauma. Posttraumatic stress disorder (PTSD) is classified among the anxiety disorders, placing it in the fear family. Fear is a response to threat of being harmed, physically or psychologically. Basic triggers include something hurling toward you through space, sudden loss of support, and the threat of physical pain.[126]

Fear conditioning contributes substantially to reexperiencing trauma.[145] You may be familiar with classical conditioning from Pavlov's pioneering research.[146] Dogs learn to salivate at the sound of a bell, after being exposed to repeated pairings of the bell with the scent of food. The food is an *unconditioned stimulus* for salivation, automatically eliciting an involuntary response. Through learning, the bell becomes a *conditioned stimulus* for salivation. A charging bear—or a looming, angry parent—is an unconditioned stimulus for fear. Fear conditioning associates previously innocuous stimuli with frightening events: the smell of alcohol on a parent's breath could be associated with episodes of rage, and alcohol could then become a conditioned stimulus, triggering the fear response in the absence of direct physical threat.

As you probably know from painful experience, conditioned fear responses are amazingly fast, faster than thought processes. These fear responses can misfire when triggered by isolated stimuli in situations that are not actu-

ally dangerous. For fear to serve its adaptive function, learning must go beyond associating one facet of a situation with another—the smell of alcohol on
the breath with the danger of being hit. We must learn to distinguish safe situations (e.g., being out with the family in a restaurant) from dangerous situations (e.g., being at the dinner table at home). This more complex learning is
called *contextual conditioning*. Unfortunately, trauma can undermine this more
discriminating pattern of responding, with the result that fear may fire off too
intensely at the wrong time—what's called *context-inappropriate responding*.[147]
There's nothing wrong with the response; it's just not occurring in the right situation. One isolated cue that serves as a reminder of trauma —the scent of alcohol or the sound of a loud voice—might set off the fear response. But the
cue is occurring without the full dangerous context. My colleague, social
worker Kay Kelly, colloquially dubbed context-inappropriate responding the
90/10 reaction: it's as if 90% of the emotion comes from the past trauma and
10% from the present trigger.[148] In the throes of a 90/10 reaction, you can regain control by mentalizing emotionally: you can consciously think through
your emotional reaction in light of the current context, for example, reassuring yourself that you're safe in the present. Admittedly, this is much easier said
than done.

Anxiety

Whereas fear is a response to clear-cut imminent danger, anxiety is a more
diffuse state of preparation for future danger. When we're anxious, our attention is directed toward any indications of threat in the environment.[149]
Thus anxiety tends to feed on itself: what threats we can't see, we can imagine.

We can understand anxiety by considering its opposites: predictability,
control, confidence, and familiarity—circumstances and situations unfolding as expected and desired. Want to pull yourself out of an anxiety state?
Find something you are good at. Do it. Get absorbed in it. Anxiety stops us
in our tracks. It's linked to novelty, the unexpected, and loss of control. Or
something that used to work that doesn't work anymore. Anxiety signals
danger: punishment, pain, and distress ahead. It signals us to put everything
on hold while we try to figure out what to do next.

The complex circuit in the brain that supports fear and anxiety has been
aptly named the *behavioral inhibition system*.[150] This circuit continually
checks to see that things are going according to plan; when they don't, the
behavioral inhibition system kicks in, bringing us to a screeching halt:
Freeze! Stop, look, and listen, and get ready for action. The circuit can check
progress many times in just a second; we can become anxious quickly when
things don't go according to plan.

Anxiety signals a state of arousal, and it functions to ensure readiness for coping. Anxiety is adaptive to the extent that the behavioral inhibition system disrupts ineffective behavior and prompts an immediate search for a better solution. When you're anxious, you're stirred up, prepared to cope, but you don't know just *how* to cope. Alert, you look for danger, yet feel helpless or out of control. Being anxious, you're likely to focus inward on your own discomfort.[151] Then you may become distracted, more preoccupied with controlling your anxiety than with the external problem that you need to confront.

Momentary anxiety is adaptive; chronic anxiety is not. Cues associated—however remotely—with past traumatic experience can trigger anxiety. You feel quickly and unconsciously that something is not working, that danger lurks nearby. At worst, you can wind up in a chronic state of anxious apprehension.[151] Nothing is ever quite right; you never feel completely safe.

As stated earlier, anxiety seems to feed on itself. That's because anxiety is linked to anticipation. You don't have to do everything to see how it will work; you can *think* it through, anticipating consequences. In the lingo of computers, you are able to run *simulations* in your head instead of having to rely on actions in the world.[152] Evolution has provided you with a mixed blessing. You can also drive yourself crazy with this marvelous capacity to simulate! You can fuel your anxiety by running all kinds of frightening simulations; this process is akin to sitting through a bunch of horror movies. Simulation can rapidly become self-defeating. You may feel more anxious and helpless rather than better prepared to cope. Ideally, you'd use your facility for simulation only for constructive purposes—planning ahead.

Panic

A *panic attack* is an extreme fear response. In the context of horrific traumatic experience, even the word "panic" fails to convey the intensity of the experience. *Terror* may be a better term than panic.[58] Unlike fear, panic often occurs without any conscious reason. If you suddenly encounter a bear in the woods and flee in terror, we would not say that you had a panic attack. If you behave in the same way in a shopping mall without any clear reason, then we call it a panic attack. In the context of trauma we might use the term, *terror attack*.

Stress and trauma are common in the backgrounds of persons who develop panic disorder,[153] as well as those who experience *nocturnal panic*, that is, panic attacks that intrude into sleep.[154] Persons who have been traumatized are likely to have panic attacks, because the terror that was appropriate to the traumatizing situation is set off suddenly, without warning, for reasons that may not be clear. The panic attack may be set off instantaneously and unconsciously by some environmental cue associated with past trauma.

A panic attack may also be set off by an *internal* physiological cue, such as a change in heart rate, "butterflies," or shortness of breath, if those physiological sensations were also part of the original traumatic experience. Just as we're reminded of trauma by external events, we're also reminded of trauma by internal sensations. Thus treatment of traumatized persons struggling with panic attacks may include interventions that desensitize them to these physiological sensations.[155] That is, you can purposely induce the sensations (e.g., increasing your heart rate by exercise or making yourself dizzy by spinning around in a chair) and learn not to fear them.

Anxious Temperament

Many patients beset by trauma wonder: Why me? They know that others—perhaps siblings—have gone through similar events without suffering such extreme fear. I'm convinced that, for many persons, temperament plays an important role in the impact of exposure to potentially traumatic events. As noted earlier, temperament is part of our biological predisposition to emotional disturbance, and, as part of the fear family, anxious temperament is most relevant to trauma.

Developmental psychologist Jerome Kagan[129] has extensively studied the differences between *inhibited* and *uninhibited* children. He observed that about 20% of children show an inhibited profile, whereas about 40% show an uninhibited profile. Recall that the behavioral inhibition circuit makes us stop, look, and listen. The hallmark of anxious temperament is an inhibition to the unfamiliar—whether the unfamiliar is people, situations, objects, or events. Inhibited children, on exposure to the unfamiliar, show avoidance, distress, or subdued emotion. For example, on the first day of preschool, the inhibited toddler is likely to sit alone in a corner cautiously, whereas the uninhibited toddler will immediately jump into play with other children. The inhibited toddler's behavioral inhibition system is easily turned on in novel, unfamiliar, or stressful situations. This proneness to arousal is partly a result of genetic factors.

Children who are inhibited in infancy will not necessarily remain inhibited for the rest of their life; they may learn to overcome their inhibited temperament. Yet temperament puts constraints on development: while initially inhibited infants may move out of the inhibited range into the middle ground, they won't move into the uninhibited range. But Kagan proposes that temperamentally inhibited children who are exposed to more stressful environments are likely to *remain* inhibited and anxious. He has also noted, however, that excessive maternal protection—intended to spare the inhibited child from frustration and anxiety—may backfire by hampering the child's development of coping mechanisms. But overprotection is not the primary problem for children who are mistreated. It's reasonable to suppose that individuals with an inhibited temperament, who are prone to distress, would be most sensitive and reactive to traumatic experience. Sadly, I think that such individuals, who may be more quiet and compliant, may be more likely to be intimidated and exploited than those who are temperamentally more feisty and obstreperous.

Temperament refers to partly inborn characteristics that are evident early in life. We all share in human nature, and we all have our individual natures—temperament. Stretching the meaning of the word, one could think of temperament as not only shaping responses to trauma but also being altered by traumatic experience. There's no doubt that prolonged stress can have a lasting effect on the nervous system. Thus, a child who is temperamentally calm and sociable may become characteristically more distressed and withdrawn as a consequence of repeated trauma.

Coping With Anxiety

Broadly speaking, there are two general approaches to mastering fear and anxiety. One involves efforts to calm yourself and to lower your general anxiety level by various techniques such as relaxation and exercise. The other involves deliberate exposure to the anxiety-provoking situation—in safe circumstances. I'll discuss these approaches more fully in the context of emotion regulation (Chapter 12, "Emotion Regulation") and treatment (Chapter 13, "Treatment Approaches"). Here I want to emphasize the strategy of cultivating rather than squelching emotion.

One of the major problems with fearfulness and anxiety is *anxiety sensitivity*, worry that anxiety will have grave consequences.[156] This *fear of fear* can create a snowballing of anxiety, for example, as fear of increasing heart rate can escalate into a panic attack. Healing from trauma involves learning that anxiety and fear, as emotional states, are not dangerous—no matter how unpleasant they may be. Exposure therapies—getting back on the horse that threw you—entail confronting fear in a safe context, and part of the desensitization process entails diminished fear of fear. When you're less frightened of your anxiety—as well as less frustrated with it, less ashamed of it, and less embarrassed by it—your anxiety diminishes.

I've heard countless traumatized patients, beset by fear and anxiety, refer to themselves as being a "wimp" or a "coward" when I think of them as strong and courageous. I think they are being unduly stoic and are misunderstanding courage. To be courageous is not to be fearless; that's recklessness. On the contrary, as Grayling[157] avers, "Courage can only be felt by those who are afraid.... The quaking public speaker, the trembling amateur actor, the nervous hospital patient submitting himself to needles and scalpels, all are manifesting courage" (p. 22). To be traumatized and afraid, and to carry on nonetheless, is courageous. Reaching out for help and seeking treatment is courageous.

Anger and Aggression

Anger is also one of the basic emotions that are supported by much hard-wired brain circuitry that we share with other mammals.[137] Fear and anger are closely intertwined as part of the fight-or-flight response; both promote survival as part of the defense reaction.[124] When escape is impossible, we must rely on attack for self-protection. Hence anger's action is aggression.

The common theme in the instigation of anger is thwarting—that is, any interference with our goals and projects.[126] A sense of injustice and unfairness are ubiquitous triggers. Thus frustration commonly triggers anger and aggression. More fundamentally, anger stems from anything that causes distress and displeasure, including physical pain, high temperature, and loud noise.[158] The arousal of anger produces an inclination to attack and hurt—if not the person responsible for the thwarting or distress, at least someone or something. We call attacking indirect targets, usually those in a subordinate or less powerful position, *displaced aggression*. For example, when stressed in a multitude of ways, men are more prone to abuse their children and batter their spouse.

Just as anger and aggression play a major role in traumatizing behavior, being subjected to anger and aggression inflicts trauma. As evident in battling couples and warring nations, anger and aggression beget anger and aggression. Ample evidence shows that child abuse promotes aggression in childhood and adulthood.[159] Physical abuse of children constitutes a double whammy, providing instigation to aggression as well as a model for how to behave when angry—aggressively.

Many persons who have been traumatized have severe conflicts about their angry feelings and about expressing their anger. Fear of anger is a common experience. For children and adults who are being abused or attacked, expressing anger and being aggressive can result in being hurt worse. Thus abused persons may attempt not only to inhibit their *expression* of anger, they may also try to avoid *feeling* anger. Furthermore, particularly if you have a history of abuse, and you've witnessed the destructiveness of anger, you're likely to feel guilty and ashamed when you experience and express anger. Then anger can do violence to your sense of self, creating shame—abhorrence in feeling identified with an abusive parent.

Having severe internal conflicts about an inevitable, natural response to provocation and frustration—often as a result of being punished for it—is itself a major problem. Hence healing from trauma entails promoting greater comfort with anger, which can help with the control of aggression. Yet we cannot advocate cultivating anger without distinguishing between its benign and destructive forms.

Benign Anger

The level of violence within homes and among groups worldwide makes it hard to think of anger as benign. And this is not a new problem: in the sixth century, Gregory the Great listed anger as one of the seven deadly sins (the others being pride, greed, lust, envy, gluttony, and sloth). Centuries before, anger was a primary target of the Stoic philosophers. Yet anger evolved for self-protection, and we still need it for that reason. Deadly sin notwithstanding, it helps to think of anger as a good thing. Psychologist Harriet Lerner[160] began her best-selling book, *The Dance of Anger,* declaring that anger sends a message: we're being hurt; our needs are not being met; something's not right. We must heed this emotional message.

To reiterate, anger is potentially adaptive. From infancy onward, anger provides fuel for overcoming obstacles.[161] Have you ever become irritated when you try to open a door that's stuck? Your irritation energizes you to yank it open with more force. So it is with interpersonal obstacles. Like anxiety and fear, anger is a source of arousal. It prepares us physiologically for actively coping, confronting, resolving controversy, and defending ourselves. Think of anger as power. Assertiveness, for example, is an effort to make your case and get your way. When you run into an obstacle, assertion can become infused with anger, which increases the vigor of your coping.

I remember talking about different forms of constructive anger years ago in a trauma education group and having a wise patient protest that I'd missed one: *outrage.* She was certainly right: given the scope of traumatizing maltreatment, oppression, violence, and large-scale mayhem in the world, we sorely need this empowering form of angry protest. In outrage, we have another form of what Nussbaum characterized as violent knowing: "This is *outrageous!*" Indignation and outrage can instigate change in personal relationships as well as in society more broadly. We're now confronting so many sources of trauma that we're hard pressed to prioritize targets of outrage.[162]

Destructive Anger

As is all too clear in our daily lives and in the world at large, anger and aggression can readily get out of hand, going beyond resolving controversy and ensuring self-protection to become destructive. Common examples of uncontrolled aggression are vengefulness, cruelty, and sadism. Persons who are treated cruelly are provoked into being hostile themselves, and they are likely to have significant conflicts about their own sadistic feelings—feelings that are virtually inevitable in light of their past experiences.

Psychiatrist Henri Parens,[163] an astute observer of anger in infancy and childhood, spelled out a useful continuum of anger. At the benign end of the continuum, he put *irritability* (beginning anger) and *anger* (a moderate level)—both of which he regarded as helpful and self-protective. I'd add outrage to this list. Then he went on to define three levels of destructive aggression: hostility, hate, and rage. When anger rises to the intensity of *rage,* it's liable to be unmanageable and disorganized, then likely to lead to destructive aggression, as in blind rage. Rageful aggression can become a malignant passion, sought out for the pleasure it provides.[44] Persons who have developed such destructive levels of anger may find it extremely gratifying to trash a room or to intimidate someone. They may reject such nondestructive substitutes as vigorous exercise because such substitutes are less gratifying to their passion.

Like anger, rage involves a burst of emotion. But the anger family also includes smoldering emotions: hostility and hate. *Hostility* goes beyond a momentary reaction to a particular aversive situation to infuse relationships in a more lasting way. Someone provokes you, you feel angry, and that's that. When hostility comes into play, you feel antagonistic in a relationship without being provoked at a given moment. A hostile person, for example, may seem generally nasty and ill-tempered. In its extreme form, hostility becomes *hate*—an enduring, intense, passionately embittered attitude that can destroy relationships. Yet even at the level of hate, we should be careful of thinking in absolutes. Contemporary philosopher Claudia Card[162] pointed out that the inability to hate when hatred is earned can be dangerous. She argued, "It can be a sign of progress to hate rather than worship an oppressor or to hate the oppressor rather than oneself" (p. 49). She contended that hate can be energizing rather than all-consuming, and hate can be self-protective by distancing us from what we hate.

As we all know, like hate, power is a double-edged sword. Anger and aggression can fuel a healthy sense of power, but they can also fuel an unhealthy sense of power. When you've been hurt, dominated, or threatened, you may naturally want to turn the tables. Persons who have been traumatized and made to feel helpless and powerless may be loath to give up the feeling of power associated with hostile destructiveness. A man who as a child was made to feel powerless by his intimidating father may relish being able to intimidate others as an adult. Moreover, aggression can often be effective (in the short run) in getting you what you want. By bullying and intimidating others, you can get your way. Thus, destructive aggression can be highly reinforcing. Feeling powerful beats feeling powerless. At worst, passionate aggression can become like an addiction. And, like other addictions, destructiveness can provide immediate gratification—even a feeling of euphoria—but then leave an aftermath of guilt, shame, and self-hatred. Then you're caught in a vicious circle: destructiveness fuels self-hatred, which fuels destructiveness, around and around.

Resentment and Forgiveness

I'd also put resentment, a potentially smoldering form of anger, in the ballpark of hostility and hate. Resentment is a natural response to having been traumatized by deliberate actions, such as assault or abuse, as well as by negligence, such as drunk driving. And it's not just suffering through traumatic events but also the legacy of trauma—ongoing psychological injury and the damage to quality of life—that fuels resentment. Along with its cousins, hostility and hate, resentment spawns a desire for revenge. Yet, as Grayling[157] contended, by contributing to the escalating cycle of violence, revenge always makes bad things worse.

We're accustomed to thinking of resentment as a vice and its antidote, forgiveness, as a virtue. Whereas resentment is conducive to vengefulness and escalating aggression, forgiveness is conducive to reconciliation and peaceful relationships. Plainly, a life consumed by resentment manifests trauma of the worst sort. As my colleague psychoanalyst Leonard Horwitz[164] construed it, forgiveness entails letting go of obsessive rumination about the injury as well as giving up the wish for retribution. Plainly, this letting-go process can be healing, but it may be achieved only by virtue of long and painful psychological work.

Yet philosopher Jeffrie Murphy[165] urged that we should not be too quick to jettison resentment in favor of forgiveness. As a response to wrongdoing, resentment can maintain self-respect, promote self-protection, and reinforce respect for the moral order. From this perspective, we could see outrage as a healthy form of intense resentment. While there's no disputing the benefits of forgiveness, Murphy argues that forgiving too readily may be tantamount to acquiescing to wrongdoing—an extreme case being the battered woman who returns to her batterer, failing to respect and protect herself.

Murphy's perspective jibes with views of traumatized persons in groups I lead. The topic of forgiveness often elicits spirited debate. Some patients say they could heal only after they forgave; others say they cannot imagine forgiving—ever. I agree wholeheartedly with Murphy's view that there are no universal prescriptions, that forgiveness should be given cautiously, and that forgiveness is not easy. These complexities are consistent with research that shows no simple relation between forgiveness (or hatred) and recovery from trauma.[166]

To complicate matters further, I'm not sure we should view forgiveness as a once-and-for-all matter. As events over the lifetime re-evoke trauma, feelings of resentment are likely to resurface. We might view forgiveness as a process or long-range project. Moreover, as Card[162] elucidated, forgiveness has a complex structure and need not be an all-or-nothing act. She delineated several facets of forgiveness: renouncing hostility out of compassionate concern for the offender; acceptance of the offender's contrition; foregoing opportunities to punish; and renewing the relationship (i.e., reconciliation). Writing about forgiveness in the context of extreme wrongdoing—evil deeds—Card echoed Murphy in advocating a cautions approach to forgiveness while taking seriously the idea that some actions may be unforgivable. Card's analysis helpfully allows for many varieties of *partial forgiveness*—for example, renouncing hostility or resentment without renewing the relationship with the offender.

Anger Management

All the strategies of self-regulation (Chapter 12, "Emotion Regulation") and the full range of treatment approaches (Chapter 13, "Treatment Approaches") are pertinent to coping with trauma-related anger. Here I'll describe one specific intervention, anger management. First, however, I'll comment on what I believe to be a misguided approach to dealing with anger: catharsis.

Many persons who have been abused and who struggle with hostile destructiveness think of themselves as *filled* with anger or rage. Perhaps the repeated experience of being provoked to anger and holding it in—stuffing it—time after time makes you feel that you're accumulating it, filling yourself up. But I think this is a harmful illusion. Where *is* all this anger? In the bowels? If you are filled with anger, the solution is to purge it. But endless blowups, in therapy or elsewhere, do not reduce hostile destructiveness. On the contrary, they may even lower your threshold for hostility and rage. Blowing off steam may feel good in the short run, because it relieves tension—although the aftermath of guilt may bring all the tension right back. But endless blowups do no good in the long run. You could even think of blowing off steam as *practicing* anger—strengthening the habit.

You'll have a better chance of dealing with anger constructively if you think of yourself as easy to anger or as having a hot temper instead of as filled with anger. Picture yourself with a short fuse, not as a huge container. Try letting go of the image of yourself as being filled with rage, and think of yourself as being too ready to flare up. You're not filled with a legacy of rage from past trauma; rather, you're sensitized—easily angered by *current provocations* that are reminiscent of the past trauma. Diminishing your anger entails dealing with these current provocations in effective ways—and not contributing to them—so that your anger isn't continually restimulated.

Cognitive therapy is the linchpin in current treatment approaches to anger management. Our angry and hostile reactions are affected by how we appraise and interpret situations. Persons who have been abused had little leeway in how they interpreted the abusive situations; those situations involved extreme provocation and distress. The early feelings, however, continue to be aroused by current situations that are both similar *and different*. Your current reactions may reflect the 90/10 phenomenon—90% of the emotion comes from the past and 10% from the present. These reactions call for reappraisals that better fit current reality.

Decades ago, psychologist Ray Novaco[167] pioneered a comprehensive, multistep approach to anger control that focuses on education, relaxation, and stress management. Applying this intervention to treating combat veterans, Novaco and Chemtob[168] aptly characterized context-inappropriate anger as *survival-mode functioning*. There are several components to this approach. The first step involves learning about anger, as you're doing here. As I've been advocating, to control your anger, you must become *more aware* of it. Blocking your awareness leaves you vulnerable to being blindsided. If you can feel *mild to moderate* levels of anger, then you can identify the problem, and you stand some chance of resolving it before your anger spirals into rage. I encourage traumatized patients to cultivate feelings of frustration and irritation; the sources are endless. Cultivating irritation and anger can help you avoid hostility, hate, and rage. Learn to distinguish between angry feelings and aggressive behavior; you can be angry without necessarily being aggressive.

Anger management also involves learning to relax. Like anxiety, anger and hostility entail high levels of arousal. To lower your level of arousal, any means of inducing relaxation is appropriate. Relaxation is as basic to anger management as it is to anxiety management. If you're in a state of high tension, a minor last straw can tip the balance to rage in a flash. If you feel more relaxed, you'll have more time to avert an explosive buildup of rage.

The cognitive component of anger management entails learning to think about yourself and provocative situations in a way that diminishes anger and hostility rather than fuels them. What you say to yourself in a provocative situation, as well as before and afterward, plays a major part in your emotional reaction and in your ability to handle the situation effectively. Novaco counsels against focusing on the provocations as personal affronts or ego threats; in short, don't take them personally. You will pour kerosene on the fire of your anger by thinking, "He has it in for me." Instead, Novaco recommends a task orientation—that is, focusing on desired outcomes and on behaving in such a way as to produce that outcome. Lerner's book *The Dance of Anger*[160] is full of good examples.

Each individual must become aware of the thoughts that fuel anger and then come up with alternative thoughts that dampen it. Novaco[169] gave many examples of thoughts that can alleviate destructive levels of hostility (p. 150): "This could be a rough situation, but I know how to deal with it"; "You don't need to prove yourself"; "There is no point in getting mad"; "Time to take a deep breath."

Anger management involves not only changing the way you think but also learning new coping skills, including assertiveness. Often, persons who have been traumatized in childhood have not had the opportunity to learn reasonable ways of expressing anger; their models have been extreme and destructive. Many anger management programs involve role-playing effective behavior in provocative situations. Practicing more graded expressions of anger is helpful. I suggest starting with irritation and building up to anger.

Like any skill, learning how to express anger appropriately takes time. It's far more difficult to master than most other skills, however, because problems with anger are embedded in a history of trauma, where feelings run high. Mentalizing emotionally is especially challenging in the context of anger and, like any other high-level skill, requires a great deal of practice. Aristotle, too, viewed anger as good, with a major caveat: we must be angry at the right people for the right reason in the right way.[170] Not easy. Nussbaum[117] thought Aristotle's standards to be perfectionist and downright tyrannical. Few people I know claim expertise in expressing anger, even if they've not had a history of trauma.

Shame and Guilt

A woman in psychotherapy averts her gaze in shame as she tries to talk about her adolescent sexual relationship with her piano teacher, a woman who was 20 years older than she. Orphaned in early childhood, the patient was raised on a farm by an aunt and uncle who did not want her. She keenly felt their resentment and sometimes overheard them talking about ways to get rid of her. At school she was isolated, and after school she had to hurry home to do chores on the farm, so she had little contact with other children. Her only respite from chores was her weekly piano lessons, and playing in recitals and competitions was her whole source of pride. Her piano teacher gave her much-needed encouragement and praise. Gradually, however, her teacher became more physically affectionate, and ultimately seduced her into a sexual relationship. She felt guilty for going along with her teacher's advances, and she felt dirty as well. Now in her 40s and married with children, she has felt ashamed about the relationship for more than two decades. Even looking back, she has little compassion for the lonely girl who seized an opportunity to feel loved and who had little comprehension of the exploitation involved.

Shame and guilt feelings are self-conscious emotions that pertain to conforming to social rules and upholding the moral order.[141] These emotions begin developing in the second year of life, when we become both self-aware and sensitive to the reactions of others.[140] Although they overlap, shame is a feeling of pervasive defectiveness, whereas guilt feelings stem from specific actions that are hurtful to others. Shame also has a more public face, a sense of knowing that someone else knows you've violated a norm or failed to live up to your own or others' ideals. Hence, feeling ashamed, you have the impulse to cover your face, withdraw and hide. In short, shame is a feeling that the core self is bad, whereas guilt is a feeling that specific actions are bad.[141] Because it relates to a more pervasive sense of badness, shame tends to be more destructive than guilt feelings.[117]

Both shame and guilt feelings have an adaptive side. Bearable shame can have a salutary effect if it prompts constructive self-scrutiny and a fair appraisal of our shortcomings, sparking self-improvement. Too, shame can be excruciatingly painful, and this memorable experience can lead us to avoid any recurrence by working on our failings. Bearable guilt feelings also can have beneficial effects. They serve as a brake on actions—including destructive aggression—that may harm persons to whom we are close. And guilt feelings are also positive in motivating reparative behavior, including confession, apology, and atonement. Our inclination to repair wrongs develops early, in the second year of life. But trauma can render shame and guilt feelings unbearable, in which case they may do more harm than good, motivating avoidance rather than self-improvement and reparation, keeping you stuck.

Shame

Damage to any facet of self-worth may contribute to shame and related feelings that range from embarrassment to mortification and humiliation. These instigators include feeling incompetent, stupid, damaged, defective, dirty, exposed, small, weak, out of control, powerless, helpless, unloved, and unlovable. Nussbaum[117] emphasized the cardinal role of neediness and vulnerability, stating that we all must contend with shame, given the importance of attachment relationships and their limitations. She highlighted primitive shame as stemming from the inability to tolerate any lack of control or imperfection. And she noted the sheer pervasiveness of shame, which may "sully the entirety of one's being" (p. 216).

Little wonder that shame is a common facet of trauma.[171] Traumatic events render you helpless—the core of shame. Trauma wounds the self, the sense of competence, and the capacity for mastery. This is true whether the trauma results from a tornado, a car wreck, or an assault. But shame stems most directly from abuse, whether in childhood or adulthood, in a home or a prison camp. Any form of abuse will be demeaning, particularly to the degree that abused persons are made to feel humiliated for their participation in shameful acts. But psychological abuse—deliberate terrorizing and humiliating—is the most direct attack on the self and the most shaming. Nussbaum's view that deep shame sullies the entirety of one's being finds ample support in abused persons' self-concepts, which include not just a sense of helplessness and worthlessness but pervasive self-hate and self-loathing, a sense of being despicable, evil, and unwanted—even invisible.[25]

Although bearable shame can be adaptive, abusive trauma creates unbearable shame, and attempts to escape from shame can lead to additional problems. Psychiatrist Donald Nathanson[172] identified four common escape routes. First, rather than leading to healthy self-examination, shame can prompt *withdrawal*. You can isolate yourself, avoiding any exposure to others. At best, you can lick your wounds and then return to society. Second, shame can prompt *avoidance*. You can try to block out shame with alcohol or other tension-reducing mechanisms. Or you can blot out the self-image associated with shame by creating a false self-image, resorting to arrogance and narcissism, fabricating an unrealistically positive self-image to assuage the pain of failure. Third, you can *attack yourself*. You can avert shame by mobilizing anger against yourself in the form of self-destructive behavior. Finally, you can retaliate by *attacking the other*. Feeling overpowered and ashamed, you can turn shame into destructive aggression. You can attempt to overpower others by humiliating them and exposing *them* to shame. Yet aggression is a particularly dangerous way of coping with shame, not only because of its potentially damaging effects but also because you can become ensnared in a *shame-rage spiral*.[161] Exploding in rage leads to a feeling of being out of control, which itself is humiliating, fueling further shame and rage, a volatile mix that often ignites physical abuse and battering.

The pathway out of shame includes making peace with your dependency and vulnerability, as well as developing a stronger sense of self-worth. As Nathanson[172] argued, *pride* is the antithesis of shame; hence recovering from trauma entails cultivating pride. Alas, I'm now advocating another of the seven deadly sins, this one the greatest of all, as C.S. Lewis[173] proclaimed. But Lewis equated pride with self-conceit and took pains to distinguish it from healthy pleasure in being praised and receiving warm-hearted admiration. A feeling of pride goes with healthy striving and a sense of success and accomplishment. The opposite of shame, pride evokes a wish to be seen and admired by others. Pride is worth cultivating, and I'll discuss it further later (Chapter 12, "Emotion Regulation").

Guilt

To reiterate, guilt feelings stem from a sense of responsibility for having harmed others, that is, having caused suffering, loss, or distress. Overlapping with shame, guilt feelings may also stem from engaging in actions felt to be morally wrong. Guilt feelings can be more or less realistic—when the sense of responsibility or degree of harm is exaggerated, we think of guilt feelings as being unrealistic.

Many persons who've been assaulted and abused not only are ashamed but also feel guilty. They feel responsible for having acted contrary to their values. A woman who is raped may feel that she has acted sinfully, even when a knife was held to her throat. An abused child may desperately try to avoid anything that would arouse the rage of an abusive parent; failing to do so, the child may attribute the parental rage to her own behavior—as if she is the cause of the parent's distress and thereby blameworthy for the abuse. As Nathanson[172] contended, feeling guilty in relation to parental abuse may protect the child's image of the parents as loving; better to feel guilty than to believe ones' parents are incapable of love and protection. In addition, feeling responsible for mistreatment can provide an illusion of control: I could prevent it if only I were good enough. This illusion counters feelings of helplessness, but at a high cost: feelings of guilt and shame.

Guilt feelings are particularly prominent in close relationships, such as attachment relationships, because these relationships entail an especially keen feeling of concern for the other person's welfare.[174] Thus we feel most guilty when we hurt those whom we love, as we will inevitably do. Hence unrealistic guilt feelings are particularly strong in attachment relationships that involve being abused; being abused by no means necessarily undermines loving feelings. Children can feel guilty for enraging their beloved parents.

Trauma-related guilt feelings can be highly destructive, contributing to self-sacrificing and self-punitive behavior. Much of healing from trauma therefore entails rethinking your level of responsibility for traumatic events. Not uncommonly, ongoing shame and guilt feelings stem from seeing the past through the lens of the present. The patient who continued to feel ashamed and guilty for her sexual relationship with her piano teacher not only failed to appreciate the coercive aspect of the relationship—her teacher was a far older person in a position of authority—but also acted as if she should not have compromised her values. She lacked compassion for the intensity and reasonableness of her needs for attention and affection, and she was looking back on herself as if she should have the values, wisdom, and self-control of a woman in her 40s when she was in mid-adolescence.

No doubt, we all have plenty to feel guilty about. Just as we can think about the possibility of overcoming resentment by forgiving those who have done us harm, we can think about the possibility of *self-forgiveness* in relation to the harm we've done to others. Like forgiving others, forgiving oneself is a complex achievement; it requires that you renounce hostility toward yourself, adopting instead a compassionate attitude toward yourself.[162] Moreover, Murphy[165] argued that we should take self-forgiveness no more lightly than forgiving others, lest it become a meaningless act. Making a complete parallel, he questions whether self-forgiveness should occur in the absence of genuine repentance. And self-forgiveness should not necessarily be total; we all must live with some legacy of guilt feelings. Yet for persons who have been traumatized, and especially those who have been abused, the guilt *feelings* far outweigh the actual guilt—the harm done. Thus we must see the trauma for what it was, with an attitude of compassion rather than self-condemnation.

Disgust

Nussbaum[117] construed disgust as a visceral emotion; at its core, disgust entails a feeling of revulsion in relation to the oral incorporation of substances that are contaminated, deteriorated, or spoiled.[126] We associate disgust with a bad taste or feeling sick to the stomach. Objects of disgust usually relate to animals and animal products, as well as our own: mucus, blood, vomit, urine, and feces. By extension, we can be disgusted by objects we take in through other senses: offensive smells and abhorrent sights such as gruesome wounds. Like other basic emotions, disgust is adaptive in motivating us to avoid and expel contaminated substances, such as by vomiting. Disgust also motivates us to maintain personal hygiene and a sanitary environment as well as to engage in purifying acts, such as washing and cleaning.

Many traumas engender intense disgust. Some forms of psychological abuse capitalize on disgust, for example, when children are purposely forced to eat unpalatable foods. Being forced to engage in fellatio and other oral sexual activities also can trigger core disgust. Because of its inherent connection with oral incorporation, trauma-related disgust can play a role in the development of eating disorders.[175]

Disgust develops later than shame and guilt feelings, and it's influenced significantly by social teaching. And oral disgust becomes symbolically extended to interpersonal disgust, which also motivates avoidance and rejection.[141] Ekman[126] added *fed up disgust* to this array. For example, wives commonly become fed up with their husband's stonewalling—angrily clamming up and refusing to deal with the wife's feelings. Fed up disgust does not bode well for marital stability.

We may find a wide range of actions disgusting, and a history of trauma may sensitize a person to disgust. But interpersonal disgust can be perniciously far ranging: targets may come to include persons or groups whom we perceive to be strange, diseased, unfortunate, or morally tainted. In this context, Nussbaum[117] emphasized a potential defensive function of disgust. Mired in shame, we can project our self-disgust onto others, regarding them with contempt.

To reiterate, like other basic emotions, disgust is powerful and self-protective in its origin. Disgust can motivate us to maintain firm boundaries, providing protection from whatever we may find offensive. As Nussbaum articulated, however, we may become haunted by self-disgust and may reject our own humanity and animality. Then we're vulnerable to shame as well as destructive projection. Extending our boundaries too widely abets disgust and contempt toward others and undermines our capacity for tolerance, empathy, and compassion for others.

Sadness

Sadness is an attachment emotion. Prototypically, sadness is a response to loss, and, as Grayling[16] stated, it was to stanch the pain of loss that the Stoics were motivated to counsel us against forming attachments to objects we cannot control—everything beyond the sphere of our own mind (as if we could fully control that!). Grayling well captured the profound impact of loss, which can reshape the world, sometimes with cruel suddenness that undermines confidence and faith.

But our attachments expose us not just to the prospect of permanent loss but also to temporary losses: separations. As Bowlby[176] brought into bold relief, attachment is essential to our survival, and our cries of sadness evolved to beget reunion. These cries not only alert the attachment figure to the offspring's distress and location but also motivate caregiving by evoking contagious distress in the attachment figure.

Bowlby characterized sadness as an emotional *protest* against separation and loss. In the face of devastating losses, such as the sudden death of a child, we need a stronger word. Ekman[126] proposed *agony*. Acute agony may evolve into prolonged sadness. Bowlby observed that prolonged separations lead to a transition from protest to despair; prolonged sadness can bridge into the hopelessness of depression.

Many traumatized persons struggle with agonizing sadness. I've emphasized the core traumatic experience of feeling afraid and alone: endangered and separated. Not just fear—and anger—but also distress, sadness, and crying are inherent to this basic trauma experience. But it's not just acute sadness that is involved; much trauma entails more enduring neglect and deprivation and thus prolonged sadness, longing, and loneliness. And sadness lodges in memory and is easily brought to the fore by reminders of trauma, such as experiences of feeling let down, rejected, abandoned, or isolated.

But trauma unfortunately entails not just repeated separations—temporary losses—but also permanent losses. Some losses like violent deaths can be especially traumatic. But trauma itself, from any source, brings losses. At worst, with a long history of attachment trauma in childhood, survivors may feel as if they've lost the opportunity to be a child or lost their childhood dreams. And, like any other illness, trauma brings a loss of health and loss of functioning. These losses of health and functioning—depression is a prime instance—may precipitate other losses, for example, by damaging relationships, careers, or employment opportunities.

Sadness can be so painful that it's hard to appreciate its adaptive functions, but we must keep these in mind. Cries of sadness and distress evolved in relation to their communicative function—you're suffering, and you need help and comfort.[126] In addition, sadness promotes grieving, because it tends to slow you down and to encourage reflection, evoking memories of whatever you've lost. As we all know, these memories can come unbidden, evoked by far-flung reminders of the loss. As Grayling[16] put it, absence is a large presence; we're attuned to what we are missing. Sadness fosters the painful mental work of remembering and mourning that ultimately enables us to let go. But sadness also enables us to stay connected to what we have treasured, to keep it in mind. Over time, true to its evolved function, sadness can motivate us to form new attachments.

Working With Emotions

Although painful, negative emotions are natural, potentially adaptive responses to aversive situations. Thanks to eons of evolution and a long history of individual social learning, we rapidly make highly sophisticated emotional judgments that organize and motivate us to cope adaptively. But adaptation is imperfect at best, and trauma not only evokes inordinately strong emotions but also may undermine the development of our ability to make use of attachments and self-regulation skills to manage our emotions. Then it's tempting to go the Stoic route, squelching emotions.

Instead, I've advocated cultivating emotion. Thinking in terms of emotional *control* isn't wrong. As Levenson[119] argued, we come equipped with automatic core programs surrounded by various control mechanisms. Yet I find the term, control, a bit iron fisted in its connotations. *Mastering* emotions is more ambitious still. *Working with emotions* seems more modest. To reiterate Nussbaum's[117] view, thinking we should let reason dictate our emotions is downright tyrannical.

We're not finished with emotion; we're just getting started, as all other topics in this book pertain to emotion. I'll consider ways of working with emotion more extensively in the section on healing. Here I want to emphasize the wisdom of prevention. All the things we recommend for dealing with problematic emotional responses are hardest to do when emotion has reached extreme levels of intensity. It's well nigh impossible to relax when you're in the midst of a panic attack, to think reasonably about a situation when you're in a rage, or to do something to cheer yourself up when you're in the depths of despair.

To reiterate, you can exert most influence when your feelings are at mild to moderate levels. To grasp this point, imagine your feelings rising on a curve, as depicted in Figure 3–1. At the lower levels of the curve are more workable feelings. As the curve rises, your feelings become more difficult to regulate. At a certain point on the curve, you've gone beyond the point of no return—your feelings have escalated to the level at which you may feel impelled to resort to emergency measures, such as striking out, running away, using alcohol or drugs, or engaging in self-injurious behavior. At that point, most of the techniques recommended by us therapists are beyond reach.

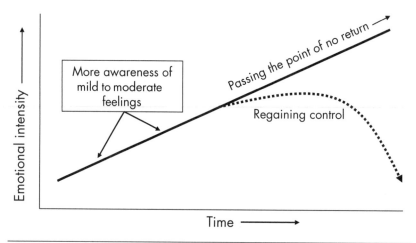

FIGURE 3–1. Emotional control by prevention.

Actually, to refer to the point of *no* return is something of an exaggeration, because you *do* recover from a state of panic or rage, and you *can* pull yourself up from the depths of despair. Yet, when you're in a panic, you may be able to do little more than keep yourself safe and wait it out, perhaps reassuring yourself, "I'll get through it; I have before." Trying to dissuade me from histrionics, my colleagues Kay Kelly and Lisa Lewis recommended substituting the point of *difficult* return for the point of *no* return.[148] Right they are: often *very* difficult.

Certainly, you'll work best with your emotions—seeking comfort from others, using relaxation, or talking yourself through it—when your emotions are at mild to moderate levels. This approach, however, requires more awareness of emotions, *more feeling* rather than less feeling. You're in the best position to mentalize emotionally when you're attuned to mild anxiety, frustration or irritation, or discouragement. Then you can successfully implement coping strategies and, most important, engage in interpersonal problem solving that will resolve the affronting situation. Emotional feelings are signals; we can make use of them, work with them.

```
┌─────────────────────────────────────────────────────┐
│  ┌───────────────────────────────────────────────┐  │
│  │   •    C h a p t e r    4    •                 │  │
│  ├───────────────────────────────────────────────┤  │
│  │                                                 │  │
│  │            MEMORY                               │  │
│  │                                                 │  │
│  └───────────────────────────────────────────────┘  │
└─────────────────────────────────────────────────────┘
```

By definition, traumatic experience overwhelms us when it occurs. Sadly, trauma does not necessarily end when the traumatic situation is long past. Many traumatized persons continue to reexperience the trauma whenever memories of the event are evoked. Along with the memories come painful emotions and the sense of helplessness. This chapter addresses two aspects of traumatic memories. First, you may feel beset by intrusive memories that you can't keep out of mind, and you need to learn how to cope with them. Second, your memories may be clouded and confusing such that you don't remember clearly what happened and you don't know what to believe. At worst, these two problems may go together: you may have an amalgam of too much and too little memory, being bombarded by fragmented traumatic images that make no sense.[177]

You'll be in the best position to cope with these two challenges if you're armed with a bit of knowledge, so I begin this chapter with a primer on memory. Then you'll be in a position to understand intrusive memories and to think about constructing an autobiography that can make remembering traumatic experiences more bearable.

A Primer

As you go about your day, you're remembering continuously. You wake up in the morning and automatically remember where you are. You remember the layout of your home and identify the objects in your environment. You start anticipating what you'll do during the day on the basis of memories of those activities in days past. Where you are, what you do, what you think about—all stimulate elaborate memory networks, and these memory networks guide your actions and thoughts.

Memory networks include sensory, semantic, and emotional aspects. We're highly visual creatures, so much of our *sensory* memory involves picturing events in our mind. But we also have elaborate memory for the full range of sensory experience—sound, smell, taste, touch, and pain. We also remember ideas and retain knowledge—*semantic* memory. Early in life, we naturally learn to translate our sensory-perceptual experience into a verbal narrative, a story, and we use this autobiographical knowledge to communicate our experiences to others.

As we go about our day, continuously remembering, we are feeling. We always remember emotionally. Sometimes the feelings may be subtle, barely noticeable. Sometimes our emotional remembering is so powerful that we can be plummeted into intense emotions—terror, panic, or rage. Intrusive traumatic memories typify this extremely painful remembering. But our well-being depends on remembering emotionally: the emotional component of remembering provides an essential steering function,[118] guiding us toward what has been good for us (rewarding and pleasurable) and away from what has been harmful to us (threatening and painful). When they're overwhelming, traumatic memories block this adaptive process.

Explicit Versus Implicit Memory

In Chapter 2 ("Attachment"), I discussed how we mentalize both explicitly and implicitly; the same goes for remembering (see Table 4–1). If you're asked to talk about a pleasant memory from your high school years, you'll be remembering *explicitly*. The hallmark of remembering explicitly is putting an experience into words, although you can remember explicitly in pictures as well—you could draw something from the memory or just imagine a scene. You remember explicitly when asked for knowledge, for example, when you take a test. Explicit memory is also called *semantic* memory (to the extent you can put it into words) as well as *declarative* memory (you can declare it). Remembering explicitly is a relatively conscious and deliberate process; you're aware of remembering.

But we also remember *implicitly,* without conscious awareness of the events that are associated with the memory network that has been activated. This implicit memory also has been called *procedural* memory; you remember procedures for doing something. We might also call it habit memory or skill memory. When you ride a bicycle, drive a car, or play the piano, you are

TABLE 4–1.	Types and stages of memory

Implicit memory

    Procedural (automatic, habitual responses, e.g., motor skills)

    Conditioned emotional responses (e.g., automatic response to reminders of trauma)

Explicit memory

    Sensory memory (e.g., visual images of past experiences)

    Semantic memory (verbal knowledge, e.g., remembering facts)

    Autobiographical memory

        Personal event memories (memories for specific events)

        Autobiographical narrative (describing one's past in words)

Stages of explicit memory

    Encoding (form a memory, e.g., by paying attention and putting experience into words)

    Consolidation (automatic process that converts short-term to long-term memories)

    Storage (retention of remembered information over time)

    Retrieval (deliberately bringing memory to mind)

relying heavily on implicit, procedural memory. You might conjure up an explicit memory of a time when you were learning to ride the bicycle, but you could hardly use that explicit memory to do the riding!

To a large extent, our emotional remembering is implicit, based on automatic associations between situations and emotional responses. Because emotional remembering is implicit, we may not explicitly remember the basis of the emotional responses. How many times have you had a vague feeling of discomfort, not knowing where it comes from? As discussed in Chapter 3 ("Emotion"), we can think of these reactions as *conditioned emotional responses*, evoked automatically, rapidly, and unconsciously by certain stimuli and situations. Typically, when you become aware of a feeling, you try to think about its basis, and you might come up with an explicit memory: "Now I know why I feel uncomfortable around him; he reminds me of the guy who used to bully me in school!" When these conditioned emotional responses take on traumatic intensity, we refer to the stimuli or situations that evoke them as *triggers*. To reiterate, when an implicit emotional memory has been triggered, you may or may not be able to retrieve an explicit memory that enables you to make sense of your feelings.

Stages of Explicit Memory

Your nervous system is designed to form conditioned memories quickly. You learn immediately not to touch a red-hot burner on the stove and to keep your distance from a person with an angry facial expression. As discussed in Chapter 3, your conditioned emotional responses are fast—you can feel frightened in a small fraction of a second, long before you have a coherent thought about what's disturbing you.

In contrast, we form explicit memories over time in a process that unfolds in stages (see Table 4–1).[178,179] First, to remember something explicitly, we must *encode* it—pay attention, comprehend it, put it into words, mull it over, perhaps talk it over with someone else. Such elaborative encoding is most obvious if you're consciously trying to remember something complicated, such as when you're preparing for an exam, but the same basic processes are involved in anything you remember explicitly. Encoding is followed by *consolidation*, a slow neurobiological process that transforms short-term memories into long-term memories. Encoding and consolidation lead to durable *storage*. A head injury, for example, can block the process of consolidation, such that an event that was encoded is no longer stored. Storage permits *retrieval* or recall, that is, deliberate reactivation of the memory. Memory can be disrupted at any stage. You might fail to encode, consolidate, store, or retrieve events from your past. Of course, encoding, consolidation, and retrieval are a matter of degree, such that much of your recall is partial, as you know all too well from taking tests.

Autobiographical Memory

Few of us have written one, but each of us has an autobiography, and it's an ongoing creation. Unlike a book, our autobiography is fluid, not just always under construction but also undergoing reconstruction—sometimes major revision. And unlike the way we read a book, we don't go through our autobiography from beginning to end; we dip into it at various places—more like a book of poetry or artworks. But it's helpful to think about the process of explicitly remembering our past as an autobiographical work, and the role of memory in constructing an autobiography is less straightforward than you might think—especially if you have a history of trauma.

I think it's helpful to distinguish *autobiographical narrative* from autobiographical memory. Autobiographical narrative is what we say or write about our past. Our autobiographical narratives are based partly on what psychologist David Pillemer[180] helpfully pinpointed as *personal event memories*, that is, explicit memories of past events. A personal event memory is specific to a particular time and place, is detailed in sensory imagery, includes a sense of the surrounding personal circumstances, is believed to be a truthful representation of your history, and is remembered vividly, with a sense of reliving the event.

Typically, on the fly, we construct autobiographical narratives from our personal event memories. Our autobiographical narratives range from telling about events of the day to recounting an amusing childhood story. But remembering personal events is not the only basis of what we believe and what we say about our past.[181] Our autobiographical beliefs and narratives also take into account what we have been told or led to believe about our past by others, such as family members. Many of us take reams of pictures to aid our memory. Our memory is patchy, and we fill in the gaps with plausible ideas, which we associate with sensory images. Our memories can become intermingled with fantasies, daydreams, and even dreams. How often have you wondered: Did it really happen, or did I dream it? And, when in doubt, our memory can be influenced by what we prefer to believe about our past. Nothing is infallible about a written biography or autobiography—and nothing is infallible about our autobiographical narratives, which are based only partly on personal event memories, themselves hardly infallible, albeit usually believable.

Intrusive Memories

Remembering emotionally includes much painful remembering—we feel the sting of shame or embarrassment as we remember our gaffes. Inherent in personal event memories is a feeling of reliving. When the events were traumatic, so can the reliving be, as remembering entails feeling terrified or enraged. Such memories can be intrusive—unbidden, unwanted, and unbearable. Persons who have witnessed violent injuries and death in car crashes, fires, combat, or terrorist attacks may be haunted by vivid, gruesome images—sights, smells, and sounds. Similarly, growing up with violence in the home—or living through it as an adult—may leave a legacy of recurrent images of yelling, screaming, and beatings. Many emotions prompt actions. You may feel like turning your head or running away, or even attacking. It's not unusual to find a traumatized person cowering in a chair or a corner, paralyzed by fear.

Flashbacks

Traumatic memories associated with a feeling of painfully reliving the event are called *flashbacks*, a term that connotes the rapidity with which such memories can be evoked. Many persons are blindsided by flashbacks that have been triggered out of the blue by some reminder of trauma. Not uncommonly, the triggers are hard to identify, compounding fear with bewilderment. Traumatic memories also intrude into sleep in the form of nightmares (see Chapter 9, "Posttraumatic Stress Disorder").

Flashbacks and nightmares can be relatively direct replicas of the traumatic experience. Some traumatic events are remembered and relived with crystal clarity, in full detail, accompanied by a coherent sense of what happened. These are prototypical personal event memories, albeit with a traumatic intensity of emotion. At the other extreme, just as terrifying or even more so, some flashbacks are more like the typical nightmare, a collage of images that defy comprehension. Accordingly, some persons refer to their flashbacks as "daymares." Like other memories, flashbacks vary in historical accuracy and may blend memory, emotion, imagery, and fantasy.[182] At worst, in a full-blown flashback, you may lose contact with current reality, superimposing traumatic images on the current situation. I remember an experience that was as uncanny for me as a therapist as it was terrifying for my patient. In the midst of a session, when we were talking about her relationship with her abusive father, she began seeing me as him: she was looking straight into my eyes, but I was he, and it took a long while for her to become reoriented and see me for who I was. Her current reality had been completely overshadowed by memory, and she only regained a sense of reality with effort.

As all roads lead to Rome, all connections seem to lead to trauma. It's not surprising that thinking and talking about traumatic events, as we do in psychotherapy, can trigger a flashback. But even a small cue can do so—not just external stimuli like sounds and smells but also internal stimuli, like body sensations or physiological arousal. Thus traumatic memory networks have been likened to black holes.[183] Whereas you might strain to remember some things, there seems to be a hotline to traumatic memories—or, as one person with posttraumatic stress disorder put it, a "superhighway to the trauma center." The connections can be very strong, and they may be made more so by recurrent flashbacks. Ironically, the very effort to suppress such memories may keep them active and even bring them to mind—particularly when you are under stress.[184] Also, vulnerability to intrusive memories can be increased by drugs and alcohol and by lack of sleep.[177]

To remember is to recreate previous experience. To remember trauma with its full emotional force is to undergo trauma again, in your mind. Such experience keeps the traumatic memory stirred, and it could become a form of rehearsal; like any other memory, the more the traumatic memory is rehearsed, the more easily it will come to mind. As I'll discuss further in Chapter 7 ("Illness"), repeated exposure to traumatic events may sensitize your nervous system, such that you become more and more reactive to stress. Flashbacks, just like repeated traumatic events, can contribute to this process of sensitization, highlighting the need to do whatever possible to interrupt this process.[185] Hence the most pressing question about flashbacks: how do I stop them?

Stopping Flashbacks

I find it helpful to formulate two goals: first, the short-term goal of learning how to interrupt flashbacks; second, the long-term goal of preventing them. Preventing flashbacks requires the whole of trauma treatment, as will be discussed in Chapter 13 ("Treatment Approaches"). As discussed there, medication can be of help in treating intrusive symptoms, and prompt intervention is important to help avert an escalating spiral of flashbacks, nightmares, panic, and further sensitization of the nervous system.

In the short run, the first step in interrupting flashbacks requires mentalizing. Flashbacks illustrate a glaring failure of mentalizing in the sense that the traumatized person is reliving the trauma as if it were happening all over again in the present, rather than recognizing the traumatic memory for what it is—a *mental state*. Failing to mentalize confuses an internal mental state with external reality. Consider the parallel process of a nightmare: you're dreaming, but the dream seems real. You wake up and feel relieved when you begin mentalizing: it was just a dream.

As I'll discuss further in Chapter 12 ("Emotion Regulation"), mentalizing puts you in a position to regulate your emotional states deliberately and constructively. Specifically, you can employ various means of *grounding* to interrupt flashbacks.[186] Grounding entails becoming reoriented to the present, typically by drawing attention to sensory input. Our first instinct when someone seems out of touch is to call their name, drawing their attention to the present. Often, this intervention does not suffice, and the process of reorientation can take many minutes, or even hours in some instances. There are many forms of grounding, including looking around, naming objects in the room, feeling the weight of your body on the chair, getting up and walking, splashing water on your face, and talking to someone. Some patients find it helpful to squeeze their fist or a rubber ball, chew a strong mint, or even hold crushed ice in their hand. If possible, holding a conversation is best, because conversing forces you to engage with another person in the present and brings the possibility of emotional support. Of course, reorienting yourself to outer reality is easier said than done when you are in the midst of a full-blown flashback. As with controlling extremes of emotion, prevention is the best medicine. Becoming aware of building anxiety that heralds a flashback enables you to implement grounding techniques *before* you begin losing control of your state of mind, at which point grounding yourself becomes far more challenging.

It's worth mentioning here in the context of stopping flashbacks a point I'll reiterate throughout this book: you must pay attention to current relationship patterns that are reminiscent of past traumatic relationships, because these current interactions play a large part in keeping traumatic memories active. To give a blatant example, a woman suffering flashbacks related to her father's beatings would be rowing upstream in trying to stop them in psychotherapy if she's going home every night to an abusive husband. But the process can be subtler. Traumatic memories of an assault by a gang can be evoked by a feeling that your colleagues or friends are ganging up on you. Subtler still, a stressful lifestyle conducive to chronically high levels of tension and anxiety can keep traumatic memories alive—emotional states alone can serve as reminders. I cannot state this point too emphatically: *coping with current life stress and actively resolving relationship conflicts plays a major role in coping with past trauma, flashbacks included.*

The Power of Positive Remembering

As emphasized in cognitive therapy,[187] you can exert some control over your emotional experience by what you think about. This power of thought may be used for good or for ill. The power of *negative* thinking is substantial; negative thinking—and negative remembering—can fuel anxiety or deepen depression. We can spend a lot of what I think of as "mind time" mired in distressing thoughts and memories. It might be a good idea to devote more mind time to positive memories.

The power of positive remembering is worth cultivating. Good memories should be treasured. Good experiences are deserving of our attention, and they're worth adding to our store of good memories. You can learn to draw your attention to a network of good memories associated with positive feelings such as pleasure, comfort, tenderness, safety, peace, and confidence. As an exercise, try to remember an event that goes with each of these positive feelings. By dwelling on these memories, you can more readily call them to mind.

The Accuracy of Autobiographical Memory

A woman in her late 30s entered psychotherapy for the treatment of anxiety and panic attacks. Her psychotherapist had no special interest or expertise in treating the effects of sexual abuse, and she conducted the exploratory therapy in her usual fashion. She prescribed medication for the woman's anxiety symptoms, and she attempted to help the patient appreciate the many current stresses that contributed to the anxiety. Like others who struggle with anxiety, the patient often felt that things were out of her control. In addition to reviewing current problems, the therapist and patient explored childhood experiences that might have laid the foundation for her feelings of being out of control. Several months into psychotherapy, the patient began remembering having been molested by an older man. She had stayed with him occasionally when her mother was working and her usual babysitter was ill or out of town. The patient was chagrined by these memories. They seemed to come from out of the blue, precipitated only by her exploring the feeling of being out of control. Her therapist was also taken aback, having no prior inkling that this childhood sexual abuse might have been a factor contributing to her patient's anxiety.

For a long time, the patient was bewildered by her emerging memories. She didn't know what to make of them. They were spotty and vague. Her memories never did become very clear, although she spoke with family members and confirmed that she had indeed occasionally gone to this man's house when other caregivers were unavailable. Gradually, taking her inner experience seriously, she became convinced that she had been molested. She developed a deeper understanding of the reasons for her extreme anxiety and her feelings of being out of control. She experienced justified outrage and learned more fully to express her anger about what troubled her in the present. In turn, she gained a sense of being more in control. Eventually, months after the traumatic memories first came to mind, she was able to leave them behind, rarely dwelling on them again.

Most persons who have been traumatized remember their traumatic experiences relatively clearly. They've never forgotten them, and they have no doubt about what happened. For others, like the woman whose exploration of her anxiety led to a revelation of childhood sexual molestation, matters are not so clear. These persons may have gone for years—even decades—without remembering various traumatic childhood experiences. Then, seemingly out of nowhere, images suggestive of traumatic experience start coming to mind. These intrusive images may be triggered by new traumatic experiences reminiscent of the earlier trauma. A rape could rekindle memories of incest. But the connection need not be so direct; traumatic memories could be evoked by any stressor—an accident, a move away from home, a loss, or conflict in an intimate relationship. *Anything* that engenders a feeling of extreme helplessness might rekindle traumatic memories. Or, as in the case just described, the memories may resurface in the course of exploratory psychotherapy sought out for other reasons.

The sudden eruption of intrusive memories is terrifying and bewildering. You might agonize, "Did it really happen?" "Am I just imagining it?" "Did I make it all up?" You're in a no-win situation: "If it really happened, it's horrible beyond belief. If I'm making it up, I must *really* be crazy!" If you find yourself in this predicament, you might go back and forth; sometimes you think it's an accurate memory, but at other times you conclude it's just a fantasy. You may take solace in the fact that your own puzzlement is mirrored by a century of professional debate and controversy. If you're reading this chapter to come to grips with cloudy memories, I encourage you to cultivate tolerance for ambiguity and uncertainty. Be prepared to think in shades of gray rather than black and white.

Freud's Quandary

A century ago, Freud[188] labored to understand the causes of debilitating symptoms, including anxiety, depression, suicide attempts, painful physical sensations, and eruptions of intense emotions associated with images of hallucinatory vividness. He had worked with 18 patients with such symptoms and concluded that, in *every instance,* the symptoms were connected with sexual trauma in early childhood. He proposed, "At the bottom of every case ... there are one or more occurrences of premature sexual experience, which occurrences belong to the earliest years of childhood but which can be reproduced through the work of psycho-analysis in spite of the intervening decades" (p. 203).

Freud was prepared for criticism, and he anticipated the charge that his patients were reporting fantasies or imagined events rather than memories of actual trauma. But he found his patients' memories to be highly convincing, and the memories made sense of their symptoms. Once the traumatic experience was known, the symptoms could be understood. The symptoms only *appeared* to be exaggerated reactions. As Freud[188] wrote, "In reality, this reaction is proportionate to the exciting stimulus; thus it is normal and psychologically understandable" (p. 217). Here, in Freud's writings of a century ago, is the thesis I'm reiterating in this book: the reactions are natural and understandable, given the traumatic experience.

Freud anticipated the objection that his patients' memories of trauma were purposely invented fantasies. He argued the contrary: his patients were extremely reluctant to uncover them, and they were loath to believe them once they had uncovered them. Freud[188] considered this point "absolutely decisive," arguing, "Why should patients assure me so emphatically of their unbelief, if what they want to discredit is something which—from whatever motive—they themselves have invented?" (p. 204). Nor did he believe that he had suggested the traumatic experiences to the patients. Moreover, he was impressed by the consistency from one patient to another in the reported traumatic experience. Finally, working through the experience helped the patients to overcome their symptoms. He also reported that, for two of his patients, there was some corroborating evidence of sexual abuse.

In 1896, Freud made a strong and convincing case for believing his patients' memories. By 1897, he'd changed his mind. In a letter to his colleague Wilhelm Fleiss, Freud[189] recounted, "There was the astonishing thing that in every case ... blame was laid on perverse acts by the father" (p. 215). Then he gave a number of reasons for his newfound disbelief—among them that "it was hardly credible that perverted acts against children were so general" (pp. 215–216). This dramatic turnaround is in contrast to what Freud[188] had written a year before: "It is to be expected that increased attention to the subject will very soon confirm the great frequency of sexual experiences and sexual activity in childhood" (p. 207). Looking back on this period many years later, Freud[190] wrote, "Almost all my women patients told me that they had been seduced by their father. I was driven to recognize in the end that these reports were untrue and so came to understand that ... symptoms are derived from phantasies and not from real occurrences" (p. 120). He began to interpret his patients' symptoms as stemming from forbidden childhood sexual desires and conflicts about them rather than from actual traumatic experience. Although Freud never abandoned the trauma theory, his *emphasis* shifted from external reality to internal fantasy.

Yet undeniable traumatic experience wouldn't go away. With each war, psychiatry confronted the potentially devastating psychological and psychiatric consequences of trauma. During World War II, a sophisticated understanding of traumatic neurosis developed.[191,192] In the aftermath of the Vietnam war, *posttraumatic stress disorder* became part of the diagnostic lexicon.[11]

While wars kept trauma in the picture, psychoanalysts did not entirely lose sight of child abuse.[193] Karl Menninger spoke out against child abuse on numerous occasions.[194] Of Freud's about-face, Bowlby[71] wrote, "Ever since Freud made his famous, and in my view disastrous, volte-face in 1897, when he decided that the childhood seductions he had believed to be aetiologically important were nothing more than the products of his patients' imaginations, it has been extremely unfashionable to attribute psychopathology to real-life experiences" (p. 78). Bowlby[71] lamented that "we have been appallingly slow to wake up to the prevalence and far-reaching consequences of violent behaviour between members of a family, and especially the violence of parents" (p. 77). Although Bowlby began by focusing on the traumatic effects of separation and loss, he had no doubt about the prevalence of maltreatment, violence, and abusive experience. He believed that our adult relationships are patterned after our childhood experiences: "The varied expectations of the accessibility and responsiveness of attachment figures that different individuals develop during the years of immaturity are *tolerably accurate* reflections of the experiences these individuals have actually had" (p. 202, italics mine). He counseled therapists accordingly: "I believe patients' accounts are sufficiently trustworthy that a therapist should accept them as being reasonable approximations to the truth; and furthermore that it is anti-therapeutic not to do so" (p. 149).

Although the syndrome of posttraumatic stress disorder was delineated in the aftermath of the Vietnam war, it's just as applicable to childhood trauma. Judith Herman[58] has written about other casualties of violence—women and children. The knowledge gained about posttraumatic stress disorder (PTSD), coupled with the political contribution of the women's movement, has enabled the mental health field to begin confronting the impact of domestic violence.[55] Sadly, we now must apply the same knowledge to understanding sexual abuse of boys by priests.

False Memories

Trauma is now accorded a substantial role in the etiology of psychiatric symptoms, but the memory-versus-fantasy controversy continually recurs. The debate's escalation in recent years was marked by the creation of the False Memory Syndrome Foundation, a large network of parents accused of abusing their own children. The False Memory Syndrome Foundation does not dispute that child abuse is widespread and harmful. Rather, the organization urges caution in accepting all reports of abuse at face value, raising particular concern about the validity of long-forgotten memories recovered in the process of psychotherapy. Members of the organization are especially alarmed about the possibility that inadequately trained or misguided therapists are suggesting or inadvertently engendering false memories in their patients. Accused family members protest that their children, influenced by a therapist, "remembered" events that never occurred. Then—also with encouragement of the therapist—the children cut themselves off from any contact, blocking any hope of reconciliation. As a result, families have been torn apart. Elizabeth Loftus,[195] a cognitive psychologist who has studied memory intensively for many years, put the concern pointedly in acknowledging the justification for women's anger while worrying that the net of rage was cast too widely.

Although there's no reason to confine concerns about false memories to any particular form of trauma, childhood sexual abuse provided the focus for the controversy. Fortunately, clinicians, researchers, and professional organizations have managed to transcend acrimonious debate to arrive at a well-informed middle ground that can guide clinical practice.[196–198] Thanks to ever-expanding research, we now have some solid ground under our feet. There's extensive support for our intuitive sense that emotionally charged events generally are best remembered. Yet *extremely* intense emotional arousal can interfere with the process of encoding explicit memories.[199] Many persons go through long periods of not remembering traumatic events.[200] Moreover, many such persons who remember traumatic events long afterwards are able to corroborate their memories, or there is independent evidence of trauma.[201] Although it's true that psychotherapy is one common context for remembering forgotten traumatic events, most persons first remember trauma in other situations, such as when they are exposed to trauma in the media, in conversation with a family member, or undergoing some related form of stress or traumatic experience.[202]

Factors That Impair Autobiographical Memory for Trauma

Given our common experience of remembering emotional events so vividly,[203] it's difficult for many people to understand how anyone could fail to remember traumatic events. Furthermore, many persons—including psychologists—labor under the misconception that memory is like a video recorder,[204] rather than the result of active construction and reconstruction. To add to the confusion, as discussed earlier, it's not uncommon for a person to be haunted by fragmented images that reflect an excess of implicit emotional memory coupled with a paucity of explicit personal event memory. Thus it's important to understand the wide variety of factors that can impair memory for traumatic events,[205] and I'll enumerate several key factors here.

- Perhaps the greatest enemy of memory is *time*,[206] so it's not surprising that adults forget childhood events.
- In addition, we all go through a period of *infantile amnesia,* that is, remembering very little before age 2 years and relatively little before age 5 years, because the cognitive and social capacities that enable us to construct elaborate personal event memories undergo major developmental changes in these early years.[207] Nevertheless, there are substantial individual differences in extent of early memory.[208]
- Our early memories are also influenced by our *social context.* We learn to talk about and make sense of our experiences—or fail to do so—in our close relationships. Encoding emotional events is part of mentalizing, and mentalizing flourishes in secure attachment relationships. An atmosphere hostile to such conversation, especially when secrecy is enforced, undermines the development and maintenance of personal event memories.[209]
- Some persons cope with isolation, loneliness, and trauma by retreating into fantasy, and, for some particularly *fantasy-prone* individuals, the fantasy world seems more real than reality.[210] For such persons, abetted by trauma, fantasy and reality become intermingled in memory.
- As I'll discuss further in Chapter 10 ("Dissociative Disorders"), *dissociation* is another coping mechanism that can interfere with personal event memory. Although dissociation takes many forms, detachment from outer reality is a common feature. Examples are feeling spacey, far away, unreal, dreamlike, and, at the extreme, "gone." Such dissociative states interfere with attention and thus may block the encoding of personal event memories.[211] In addition, dissociative amnesia can block retrieval of traumatic memories that have been encoded.[212]
- Importantly, *neurobiological* processes associated with trauma may interfere with every stage of memory: encoding, consolidation, storage, and

retrieval. Whereas moderate levels of emotional arousal facilitate memory encoding,[199] extreme levels of arousal can interfere with encoding, storage, and retrieval of explicit traumatic memories.[213] In addition to excess emotional arousal, neurobiological factors such as head trauma and substance abuse contribute to memory impairment, and these factors also may be intertwined with trauma.[214]

- Although the concept is controversial,[215] *repression* can play a role in not remembering traumatic events.[200] When we deliberately avoid trying to think about something—often making matters worse—we are employing *suppression*. In contrast, repression is an automatic, nonconscious process that inhibits emotionally painful thoughts and memories from being elaborated in consciousness.

- Along with using suppression and experiencing repression, many traumatized patients keep the trauma out of mind by *distraction*. They may be engaged in frantic activity—such as being a workaholic or always being on the go in other ways. Unfortunately, this pattern only adds to the pileup of stress, paradoxically increasing the likelihood of depression and posttraumatic symptoms, including the eruption of intrusive memories.

- Finally, efforts to *force the process* of remembering can interfere with remembering events accurately, because of our natural tendency to fill in the gaps.[216] Forcing the process, you run the risk of *confabulating*—making up what you don't know. And when you're confabulating you don't know you're making it up; you believe it.[217] What you recall *spontaneously*—without any particular axe to grind—is most likely to be accurate.

A Spectrum of Accuracy

With all these factors potentially impairing personal event memories, particularly when trauma is part of the history, it's little wonder that autobiographical narratives are patchy and inaccurate to varying degrees. Reading this, you may be protesting, "But I am *certain* that much of what I remember is true!" Plenty of research supports this protest. Even if the details are false, the gist of autobiographical memories is generally true.[218] But you should be aware that the degree of confidence in a memory is unrelated to its accuracy.[219] And there's no litmus test for judging the accuracy of a memory from any of its features; for example, vividness by no means indicates accuracy.

To put all this back into perspective, most traumatized persons remember the traumatic events clearly—all too clearly. But many persons who have undergone extensive trauma in childhood are confused about much of what they remember and, at worst, their implicit emotional responses make no sense in the absence of corresponding explicit personal event memories. I find it helpful to think in terms of a spectrum of accuracy in traumatic memories,[205] ranging from coherent and corroborated memories on one end of the continuum to essentially false and confabulated memories at the other end (see Table 4–2). It's fair to say that, for all of us, our autobiographical narratives are based on many sources, including personal event memories all along the spectrum of accuracy. And I want to emphasize that persons with a history of many forms of childhood trauma are likely to have memories all along the spectrum, from clear and accurate to cloudy and inaccurate, and perhaps some that are both clear and inaccurate.

TABLE 4–2.   Spectrum of accuracy in memory of trauma

1. Continuously/clearly remembered memory with corroboration
2. Delayed/fragmentary memory with corroboration
3. Continuously/clearly remembered memory without corroboration
4. Delayed/fragmentary memory without corroboration
5. Exaggerated/distorted memory
6. False memory—patient constructed
7. False memory—therapist suggested

Implications for Psychotherapy

When you're in the midst of a storm, it's hard to get your bearings. Many persons who are struggling with intrusive memories seek psychotherapy to make sense of this confusing experience and, in the course of therapy, they often remember more traumatic events. To understand the role of psychotherapy in the process of healing, we need to consider the value of remembering trauma, understand the distinction between narrative and historical truth, clarify the role of the therapist, and, not least, appreciate the value of forgetting.

The Value of Remembering

I believe in letting sleeping dogs lie. I see no reason to bring traumatic events to mind just for the sake of remembering or clarifying the past. I do not *assume* that psychiatric symptoms are caused by trauma, and I'm disinclined to go on psychological fishing expeditions looking for trauma just because there's a possibility that trauma plays a contributing role—there's always that possibility. But, what if the dogs are howling and barking? There are two indications that you may need to explore trauma: either you're struggling with intrusive memories, or you're reenacting traumatic events in your behavior.[62]

First, as I'll discuss more fully in Chapter 13 ("Treatment Approaches"), the goal of trauma treatment is not to get rid of traumatic memories. Rather, the goal is to make remembering more meaningful and emotionally bearable. Many persons have the idea that traumatic memories need to be excised by means of gut-wrenching catharsis, and hypnosis sometimes has been used in the service of evoking such catharsis. I think this approach is misguided—especially in the context of extensive trauma with complex and severe symptoms. Just as flashbacks can be retraumatizing, such catharses can be retraumatizing rather than therapeutic.[220] Rather than producing catharsis of extreme emotion, therapy should facilitate control and mastery over the emotion and provide some understanding of the traumatic experience.

As horrendous as intrusive experience is, there can be a positive, constructive side to it. Much of your history may be blocked off or compartmentalized. Pages or chapters of your autobiography may be blank. The reasons for your feelings, behavior, and symptoms may be obscure. The intrusive experiences provide an opportunity for integration and a sense of wholeness that were previously beyond reach.[221]

If you're beginning to grapple with intrusive memories, you might be terrified and bewildered. The process of reconstruction can lead to self-understanding. Even if you haven't struggled with memories for years, you might have contended with various symptoms. Remembering the traumatic experience can help explain these previously incomprehensible symptoms. You can put the experience into words, and you can organize fragments into a more coherent autobiographical memory. Think of autobiographical memory as a container: when you can translate previously fragmented images and feelings into a coherent narrative, you may not be so emotionally reactive to reminders of trauma.[177]

Converting the memory fragments into an organized narrative not only fosters self-understanding but also enables you to talk to others about the traumatic experience. Talking to others will help with the construction of autobiographical memory. As discussed in relation to attachment, the core of trauma is feeling afraid and alone. The lack of opportunity to obtain comforting and make sense of the events is a paramount contribution to traumatic experience. Talking about trauma entails shedding the shackles of secrecy and allowing someone to bear witness. Then you're no longer alone with the experience, and, albeit belatedly, you can experience some understanding, comforting, and reassurance. Thinking and talking about trauma in the context of a secure attachment relationship is the framework for mentalizing, making sense of experience, making the emotion more bearable, and opening up the possibility of healing and a more fulfilling life.

The value of remembering and talking does not stop with self-understanding and being understood. In the process of talking and being understood, you can begin to develop compassion for yourself. In part, this self-compassion can evolve from your sense of others' compassion as they bear witness. And you also might have opportunities to show your compassion for others who have been traumatized. The compassion can even be extended back to yourself. Ultimately, only you can know the true depth of trauma you have undergone; full compassion may only come from within.

Narrative Versus Historical Truth

Healing from trauma entails making sense of what happened. Often enough, especially in the context of extensive childhood trauma, it's not clear just what happened. Understandably, the traumatized person wants to know the truth.

Yet psychotherapy is not designed to provide historical truth. Instead, psychotherapy may provide what has been called *narrative truth*—a coherent view of your past that makes sense of your present experience.[222] When trauma-related confusion reigns and you're not sure what to believe about what's in your mind, you cannot derive historical truth from memory alone, no matter how vivid it may be. Thus traumatized persons who seek historical truth may need to do some detective work to corroborate their memories. Many actively investigate their past, although the feasibility of doing so depends on the availability of informants, such as family members, and their receptiveness to the quest. In endeavoring to find out about the past, persons with confusing memories are in the position of the biographer. Of course, *auto*biographers have the advantages of all the personal event memories at their disposal. Yet personal event memories are only one contributor to autobiographical narratives, and they come with a full spectrum of accuracy.

The Role of the Therapist

Traumatized persons struggling to make sense of confusing intrusive memories are hardly reassured when they seek professional counsel only to discover the furor about false memories. The last thing you want is to encounter skepticism or outright disbelief. In the face of all this controversy, the majority of therapists believe their patients.[195] I am among that majority. I believe my patients who show signs of trauma for the same reason that Freud initially believed his patients: their symptoms are most understandable if some role is accorded to trauma. Therapists today have three advantages over Freud: First, the extent of maltreatment of children has been thoroughly documented. Second, a clearly defined syndrome—PTSD—is similar across a wide range of traumatic experiences. Third, the social climate is increasingly conducive to acknowledging the extent of childhood trauma.

I can believe that *some* of my patients' memories are relatively false, exaggerated, or distorted. But I find it utterly implausible that their PTSD was caused by false memories. I consider it more likely that whatever false memories they may hold in conjunction with a host of more or less accurate memories were created to fill in gaps or to escape from some form of traumatic experience. As psychiatrist Richard Kluft[223] summed it up: *something terrible happened.*

In search of historical truth in psychotherapy, it's not uncommon for traumatized patients to request hypnosis. This request is not unreasonable, because hypnosis has a venerable history in the treatment of trauma as well as in memory enhancement.[197] Misconceptions about hypnosis abound; for example, that you give up control in hypnosis. On the contrary, hypnosis is employed to enhance self-control.

In the realm of memory, another misconception about hypnosis requires correction and explanation. This misconception is tied up with the video recorder image of memory; that is, believing that hypnosis will unlock traumatic memories and that the memories will be accurate. Indeed, hypnosis may enhance memory, in the sense that persons generate more memories. But the fact that memories are generated in hypnosis does not mean that they're necessarily accurate or inaccurate. Like any other means of remembering, hypnosis will yield a *construction*—narrative truth, not necessarily historical truth. Like any other way of evoking memories, the vividness of the construction is no guarantee of accuracy. Thus, when employed as a memory enhancement technique, hypnosis must be conducted with great expertise and proper safeguards, and the patient must be well informed about its benefits and limitations. Many trauma therapists use hypnosis not for memory enhancement or emotional catharsis but rather to foster self-control, relaxation, and containment of intrusive memories.[224]

Whatever the therapeutic technique, patients want to be believed. And, understandably, many patients want their therapist to validate their memories. But psychotherapists cannot be detectives, nor can they take on the role of verifying memories.[225] Your therapist cannot tell you what happened or what to believe. *You* must take on the challenge of deciding what to believe. In the process, however, your therapist can validate the significance of your current experience and your need to make sense of that experience. You may have been accused—or accuse yourself—of "imagining it." Your therapist will take you seriously while providing support by helping you to tolerate the uncertainty and pain of not knowing. Both you and your therapist may need to strive for the right blend of belief and skepticism as you struggle to sort out your experience. I like British psychologist Phil Mollon's[226] advice to therapists: we must tolerate ambiguity and avoid illusions of knowing. The same applies to patients.

The Value of Forgetting

Trauma at any age can derail development. The value of remembering is to get your life back on track, not to remember for the sake of remembering. How much *should* you remember? Most persons who suffer trauma remember the events relatively clearly and have no doubt about what happened. But for those who have undergone many forms of trauma over a prolonged period of life, it's neither possible nor desirable to remember everything. Remembering should not become an end in itself. It's extremely painful. You should not undergo needless torment, endlessly dredging up traumatic memories. You may begin constructing distorted and inaccurate memories—a glaringly counterproductive prospect. You'd do best to remember only as much as is necessary to do the job of healing so that you can get on with your life. When you're no longer plagued by intrusive memories or repeating the traumatic experience in other ways, when your life makes sense and your autobiography is reasonably clear, the job is done. If more needs to be remembered and reconstructed at some later point, your mind will make this known. *There's no reason to push it.*

Then what? How about forgetting? I find Lewis Thomas's[227] heretical advice appealing:

> If after all, as seems to be true, we are endowed with unconscious minds in our brains, these should be regarded as normal structures, installed wherever they are for a purpose. I am not sure what they are built to contain, but as a biologist, impressed by the usefulness of everything alive, I would take it for granted that they are useful, probably indispensable organs of thought. It cannot be a bad thing to own one, but I would no more think of meddling with it than trying to exorcise my liver, an equally mysterious apparatus. Until we know a lot more, it would be wise, as we have learned from other fields in medicine, to let them be, above all not to interfere. Maybe, even—and this is the notion I wish to suggest to my psychiatric friends—to stock them up, put more things into them, make use of them. Forget whatever you feel like forgetting. (pp. 141–142)

Chapter 5

SELF

A woman in her late 20s graduated from law school with honors and was on her way to a successful career. She sought psychotherapy for anxiety and nightmares, and she'd begun sliding into depression. She had a history of significant trauma in childhood, having been left adrift in a chaotic and violent household, often bearing the brunt of her mother's violent rages. She never forgot her tumultuous childhood, but she'd previously been able to keep it out of her mind by immersing herself in school and work. As one would expect in a successful attorney, she was highly verbal and articulate. When she was talking about her legal work or her interactions with others, she was glib. But the moment she was asked to talk about herself or her own feelings, she became dumbfounded. Even the simple question, "How are you?" could prompt a befuddled silence. When she tried to think about her "self," she encountered a void. Gradually, the reason for this void became clear: when she began to accept the idea that she had a "self," she became so filled with self-loathing that she felt overwhelmed.

Trauma—being overpowered and rendered helpless—is an assault on the self. In discussing reactions to prolonged and repeated trauma, Judith Herman[228] concluded: "All the structures of the self—the image of the body, the internalized images of others, and the values and ideals that lend a sense of coherence and purpose—are invaded and systematically broken down.... While the victim of a single acute trauma may say she is 'not herself' since the event, the victim of chronic trauma may lose the sense that she has a self"

(p. 385). Recovering from trauma entails healing the self.

We must understand the self in its social context, as one of two main lines of personality development. The development of the self proceeds in tandem with establishing relationships with others.[229] Self-development emphasizes separation, autonomy, self-definition, individuality, responsibility, initiative, and achievement. Relatedness to others entails attachment, caregiving, intimacy, love, connectedness, and cooperation. Developing the self and developing relatedness are mutually enhancing, not mutually exclusive. The self evolves in attachment relationships; your sense of self gives definition to your relationships with others, and your "self" is inconceivable apart from your surrounding context of relationships. Recognizing their interdependence, I'll focus on the self in this chapter and relationships in the next chapter.

I'll make some key distinctions among different aspects of the self and emphasize three aspects of self-experience directly affected by trauma: self-worth, self-efficacy, and self-continuity. I conclude the chapter with some thoughts about healing the self.

Aspects of the Self

I and Me

Let's start with the most basic distinction, the "I" versus the "me."[230] The "*I*" is the self-as-agent, that is, your subjective self that is active in initiating, organizing, choosing, and interpreting experience. Ideally, as an agent, you have self-efficacy, for example, being able to meet your needs and having an impact. Also, as an efficacious agent, you have a sense of continuity, a cohesive self-feeling, a feeling of being your enduring self. If you find this concept of the "I" difficult to grasp, don't feel badly; the subjective sense of self is among the most elusive phenomena in psychology and philosophy.[231]

In contrast to the "I," the "*me*" is the objective self as seen from the outside. The "me" is the self-as-object, the self as seen by itself. And the objective self is a social construction: your "me" is reflected in your *self-concept*, how you think about your self, and in your *self-worth*, or how you evaluate yourself. Your "me" is greatly influenced by your interactions and relationships with others. How you think and feel about yourself depends a great deal on how others view you, respond to you, and treat you. Ideally, your "me" is associated with a feeling of positive self-worth, derived substantially from caring and affirming relationships.

Here's the puzzling bit: your self is reflexive. The self-as-agent ("I") thinks and feels about itself, creating the self-as-object ("me"). For our purposes, one of the most important activities of the self is creating narratives—

storytelling.[232] Philosopher Daniel Dennett[233] went so far as to characterize the self evocatively as a center of narrative gravity. Among our most important stories are autobiographical sketches—what we think and say about ourselves.

With apologies for twisted grammar, the "me" is the "I's" current autobiographical sketch. Now the most important claim in relation to trauma: your "I"—the kind of active agent you are—is strongly influenced by your "me"—the kind of stories you construct about yourself. Here's the twist in our reflexivity: the narrative ("me") shapes the narrator ("I"). All this can now be made simple: if you think of yourself as helpless, you'll *be* more helpless. If you think of yourself as resilient, you'll *be* more resilient. But just giving yourself pep talks is not what I have in mind here. Changing your self takes a lot of time and effort in close relationships, especially attachment relationships.

Public and Private

It's also helpful to distinguish between the public self and the private self. Your public self is your self as known to others, the image of your self that you project to others. Your public self is the basis of your sense of "me" that is reflected from others—who you are as seen by others. Persons who have a big stake in image management—all of us do to some degree—are buttressing their public self.

Your public self is the outer aspect of your self; your private self is the inner core. Particularly in conjunction with trauma, you might associate the idea of a private self with shame, the need to hide and cover up. True, but a private self is essential to our mental health. Psychoanalyst Arnold Modell[234] characterized the private self as experienced in solitude and composed of experiences that may never be disclosed to others. The private self also can be a refuge in the face of intolerable environments.

Because we construct our self in relationships, I would not take the concept of a private self too far. As I'll discuss at the end of this chapter, the odd thing about us humans is our ability to have a complex relationship with our self—sadly evident in self-loathing and wonderfully evident in self-compassion. So I think of the private self as analogous to relationships with others in which confidences are kept. The private self is the ultimate confidential relationship and, as Modell implies, one to treasure.

Self-Worth

We can best appreciate the impact of trauma on the self from a developmental perspective. Your "me," how you think and feel about your self, is a developmental achievement, and its foundations are laid in childhood. Psychologist Susan Harter[171] researched the development of self-worth and its relation to trauma, and she argued that one important facet of healing from trauma is understanding the origins of low self-worth. Thus her findings merit our attention.

Facets of Self-Worth

The self-concept begins developing in the latter part of the second year, when the toddler begins attaching words to the self. In the third and fourth years, as autobiographical memory takes shape, the child begins developing a narrative self, constructed around stories. Barring maltreatment, young children have a globally positive self-concept. By middle to late childhood, the self-concept becomes increasingly complex. Comparing the self to others, the child becomes more self-critical, contrasts the real self with the ideal self, and develops the capacity for shame and pride in relation to these comparisons. Henceforth, through adolescence and into adulthood, the self-concept becomes increasingly differentiated, such that an ongoing challenge entails integrating discrepancies into a unified self-concept.

The "me" we construct at any given point in time is associated with a relatively stable feeling of *global self-worth*, which takes shape in early relationships. Harter delineated two major contributors to global self-worth: assets in various domains of importance and extent of approval from persons in valued relationships. Important developmental assets are academic achievement, athletic ability, likeability, behavioral conduct, and physical appearance. Reflecting differences in values, different individuals attach different degrees of importance to these various domains. Troublingly, physical appearance, which is somewhat immutable, is the most highly valued domain across age, gender, and nationality. The second major contributor to global self-worth, valued relationships, may include peers, parents, other family members, and other persons in authority. Harter noted that relational self-worth becomes particularly keen in adolescence: how you feel about yourself depends on the relationships you're in.

Harter's research is valuable for its emphasis on the sheer complexity of the self. Your feeling of self-worth will vary, depending on the domain of competence you're focusing on (intellectual, academic, interpersonal) and your sense of connection to other persons at a given point in time (your teacher, boss, romantic partner, or friend). Harter proposed that we have a *baseline* self-concept, associated with global self-worth, and a *barometric* self-concept, which varies depending on our situational context, that is, what competence (or incompetence) we're displaying and who we're with. Thus our sense of self-worth is both stable (baseline) and variable (barometric). It's harder to change the baseline of global self-worth than it is to alter your barometric self-worth. With a foundation in trauma, many persons focus on global and very low self-worth ("I'm worthless"), undermining their self. We can aspire to alter this baseline, very gradually, by taking account of the complexity of the self, paying attention to domains of competence and supportive relationships.

Realism and Self-Worth

Many psychologists, Harter included, argue that your self-concept should be realistic. This is what I've taught students and patients for years: take the bad with the good, mix them together, balance them out, and achieve realistic self-esteem (see Figure 5–1). The few saints among us should feel extremely good about themselves (but wouldn't because of their saintly humility); the true louts should dislike themselves (but wouldn't because they are louts); and the rest of us, with our mixtures of good and bad, should wind up somewhere in the middle. Mental health rests on accurate self-appraisals. There's good evidence to support this view; for example, children with inflated views of themselves who are actually disliked by their peers are at especially high risk for trouble.

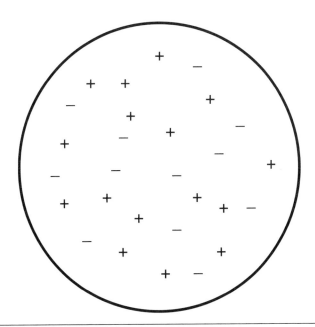

FIGURE 5–1. Positive and negative in the realistic self-concept.

Yet the case for realism is not unassailable. Psychologist Shelley Taylor, in her book *Positive Illusions*,[235] marshaled a great deal of research evidence showing that most persons have overly positive views of themselves and overly optimistic views of their futures. These positive illusions about the self are usually most prominent in childhood and gradually erode with age as we become disillusioned. But even in adulthood, a positive bias remains. Most people see themselves in more flattering terms than they are seen by others. For example, if two individuals complete a joint project and they are asked afterward to indicate the percentage of their individual contributions, the percentage typically will be greater than 100. Ninety percent of automobile drivers consider themselves superior to the average driver. Can they all be right?

Taylor argues not only that most people have unrealistically positive biases about themselves but also that these mildly positive illusions are adaptive and beneficial to mental health. Positive illusions foster positive moods and contentment, and they promote effective behavior. Positive moods can bolster positive attitudes toward others and helpfulness toward them. As I'll discuss in Chapter 14 ("Hope"), optimism about your abilities contributes to motivation and persistence, and thus to higher productivity and achievement. If you're confident about succeeding, you'll work harder, and you'll be more likely to succeed. If you are riddled with self-doubt, you'll be more likely to falter or give up, and you'll be more likely to fail. To reiterate: the "me" influences the "I."

Without reference to illusion, Jon Kabat-Zinn[236] proposed the principle: "As long as you are breathing, there is more right with you than there is wrong, no matter how ill or hopeless you may feel" (p. 2). Accordingly, we're all entitled to a self-concept tilted toward the positive end. If nothing else, we're extremely complicated, and we're entitled to complicated self-concepts. There's ample evidence that focusing on the positive and downplaying the negative—within limits—is adaptive and enhances the self.

Nevertheless, on balance, our self-concepts need to be reasonably accurate. But forming an accurate self-concept is no easy feat. How accurate is your concept of *any* person? Individuals are extraordinarily complex, and any concept you have of other persons, no matter how well you know them, will be incomplete, partial, and to some degree inaccurate. Why should it be different with your self? You have even more information about yourself. But that only adds to the complexity. And you can deceive yourself, just as you can be deceived by others. You can have a distorted view, and others may have a more realistic view of yourself than you do, at least in some domains.

Trauma and Self-Worth

Maltreatment in childhood and in adulthood may lower self-worth in many ways. In childhood and adulthood, the assault on self-worth can be direct.

Antipathy in valued relationships, whether it be in the form of hot or cold rejection, lowers self-worth. And psychological abuse, particularly when it takes the form of deliberate humiliation and degradation, profoundly undermines self-worth. Similarly, self-worth is undermined by pressures of combat that lead to participation in atrocities.

But the attack on self-worth need not be so direct. Those who are traumatized by other persons almost always blame themselves. Abused children feel that they deserved it, that they brought it on—or at least that they should have been able to prevent it, stop it, or minimize it. Battered women try desperately to please and appease their battering partner and blame themselves for failures to do so that precipitate assaults. Taking responsibility can be seen as a last-ditch effort to preserve some sense of control: better to feel blameworthy than helpless. This effort to rescue the core self from a sense of helplessness is laudable; the worst thing for the "I" is helplessness. But the "me" pays a high price: low self-worth. Ironically, low self-worth just renders the "I" more helpless.

Unfortunately, persons who have been traumatized often pile insult on top of injury, compounding their already damaged self-esteem by a sense of blameworthiness for the ensuing effects: "If I were a stronger person, I wouldn't have all of these symptoms and problems." I've addressed this book to this final assault on self-esteem. To the extent that I'm successful, I might deflect this last blow. Self-understanding can lead to more patience, self-tolerance and, ideally, self-compassion.

Self-Efficacy

> A young man in psychotherapy recalled his helpless paralysis in the aftermath of a violent argument between his parents when the three of them were returning home in their car. He was so scared that he huddled in the back seat after they got out. His seeming refusal to get out of the car only infuriated them further. His mother opened one door, and his father opened the other. Both screamed at him to get out. To this day, he remembers feeling frozen with fear, terrified to go one way or the other. Whenever he finds himself faced with a dilemma, having to make any decision that entails choosing between two unpleasant alternatives, he can be riddled with paralyzing anxiety akin to the overwhelming feelings that washed over him as he cowered in the back seat of the car. At such times, he has no idea of what he wants or what to do.

Back to the "I," again, from a developmental perspective. Psychiatrist Daniel Stern[237] made countless observations of babies in their social contexts to formulate a comprehensive theory of the early development of the sense of self. Among the core facets of the self he described is self-agency, being the author of one's own actions. Peter Fonagy and his colleagues[79] detailed a developmental progression in self-agency. Infants first develop physical agency, for example, being able to move their limbs and external objects. Then they develop social agency, for example, being able to evoke their mother's smile. When they come to understand goal-directed behavior—interpreting actions as efficiently achieving goals within the constraints of physical reality—they have arrived at teleological agency. Next, becoming mentalizers, they come to interpret goal-directed actions as intentional, stemming from mental states, such as desires and beliefs. Ultimately, this ability to understand the self and others as mental agents is enriched by narrative capacity: to understand our actions, we create stories with varying degrees of autobiographical richness.

Ideally, this evolving self-agency is associated with *self-efficacy*—a feeling of power and influence, the ability to bring about an intended result. As discussed in Chapter 2 ("Attachment"), George Gergely and colleagues[84,85] have shown that self-agency evolves in interactions with emotionally sensitive caregivers. The infant's emotional expressions elicit social feedback that enables the infant to develop a sense of self. Infants' capacity to elicit responses contingent on their actions is highly rewarding, contributing to self-efficacy. Consistent with this view, secure attachment relationships, which entail a high level of responsiveness, are conducive to self-efficacy in infancy.[87] Hence, as discussed in Chapter 2, secure attachment provides a secure base that allows the child to explore the world confidently, including the world of other persons and the mind. Self-efficacy is thus the basis for developing competencies and relationships, the foundations of self-worth.

The capacity to influence the world—perhaps most importantly, the sense of oneself as a mental agent able to bring about relationships in which the other person has your mind in mind—is at the core of self-efficacy. Being unable to have an influence—especially over other persons—is the core of trauma. I believe trauma revolves around power, be it the power of an earthquake, a terrorist bomb, or a raging parent. To be traumatized is to be overpowered, rendered helpless. Exposed to repeated traumatic events, repeated experiences of being overpowered, a person can *learn* to be helpless,[238] develop a sense of futility, give up, and languish. No wonder that people who've been traumatized often complain that the helplessness they experienced was the hardest thing to endure. Adding insult to injury, posttraumatic intrusive memories can lead you to feel you've lost control over your own mind, abetting your sense of helplessness.

Any form of trauma will engender helplessness—natural disasters, accidents, or being overpowered by an assailant in a robbery or a rape. The most profound experience of helplessness, however, is associated with psychological abuse. Some abusers sadistically enforce a sense of helplessness as a part of the abuse.[58] You may have been physically overpowered, cornered, or trapped. Or you may have been so terrorized psychologically as to be immobilized. Such abuse is likely to occur unpredictably, further increasing the sense of helplessness, given that your sense of control rests strongly on predictability. The loss of predictability and control squelches self-efficacy. The antidote is empowerment in any sphere, but particularly in close relationships.

Self-Continuity

The subjective self, or "I," entails a feeling of being "myself" that is stable across time and space. I feel that I continue to be myself day after day, month after month, year after year. I continue to be myself whether I'm at home, at work, or out on the town. I continue to be myself at different times and in different places, despite the many changes in my self from time to time and place to place.

Continuity in the face of discontinuity is perhaps the essence of the subjective sense of self. I know who I am, and I continue to be who I am. Implied in continuity is a sense of cohesiveness, unity, integrity, wholeness, and identity. Despite differences from time to time and place to place, I am myself. Included in continuity and cohesiveness is a sense of distinctness from others, a sense of individuality, and a sense of separateness. This sense of continuity goes hand in hand with self-agency and self-efficacy.

Self-continuity and self-cohesiveness are ideals—to some degree, illusions.[233] You have a sense of continuity—more or less. You are not born with a sense of subjective self or a sense of continuity. As a newborn, you shifted from one state to another. You went from quiet wakefulness, to distress and crying, to sleeping. You gradually learned that you were "yourself" throughout these changes. Your sense of continuity was a developmental achievement, not a given. Nor is this developmental achievement accomplished once and for all; self-continuity and self-cohesiveness pose a continual challenge.

Long after you attain some sense of continuity in your self-experience, you continue to experience many discontinuities. You may feel the same day after day and month after month—but how about year after year or decade after decade? After how long are you no longer the "same person"? As it has been since infancy, your experience is radically interrupted every day by sleep. Your experience is also continually punctuated with lapses in continuity in the form of forgetting or absentmindedness. You experience gradual or more abrupt changes in mood. You even say "I wasn't myself" after saying or doing something that's out of character.

As with self-worth and self-efficacy, trauma can undermine self-continuity. Radical changes in consciousness associated with dissociative states are profoundly disruptive to the sense of continuity, and I'll discuss these in Chapter 10, "Dissociative Disorders." Here I'll focus on the disruptiveness to self-continuity posed by severe internal conflict and contradictory relationships.

Heightened Internal Conflict

One of Freud's major contributions was his discovery of the power and ramifications of internal conflict in conjunction with unconscious motivation.[239] He believed that instinctual sexual and aggressive drives come into conflict with reality and with morality. Hence these sexual and aggressive drives, which are part of our biological heritage, can be frightening and overwhelming. Specifically, we fear that expressing them will lead to rejection, retaliation, punishment, or loss of love. Accordingly, we try to block them from expression and even from our own awareness.

As discussed in Chapter 3 ("Emotion"), anger and aggression are natural responses to being threatened and hurt. Yet anger in attachment relationships provokes conflict and anxiety, because it threatens the attachment, which provides security. Hence trauma in attachment relationships evokes conflict: the natural instigation toward aggression is inhibited by fear of hurting the attachment figure as well as fear of punishment for the expression of anger. Destructiveness collides with protectiveness, threatening the cohesiveness of the self.

Sexual abuse, too, may evoke extreme conflict. Sadly, sexual abuse of children often takes place in the context of neglect and a longing for comforting touch. The desire for loving touch comes into conflict with the aversion to sexual contact. The natural and healthy desire for touch thus contributes to guilt feelings. And sexual arousal is just as natural and even more abhorrent to the child. As psychologist Darlene Ehrenberg[240] poignantly described, in the midst of feeling helpless, the child may be surprised and horrified by sexual arousal that naturally stems from the sensual and sexual contact. Evoking such conflict will be problematic in any relationship, such as sexual abuse by a neighbor or a member of the clergy. But the conflict will be most intense in attachment relationships, particularly with primary caregivers. For example, a girl who is sometimes a daughter and sometimes a lover in her relationship with her father will be unable to integrate these contradictory aspects of her identity. As Freyd[31] described, such betrayal trauma tends to split the cohesiveness of the self; consciously knowing about the abuse—having it in mind as part of one's identity—is intolerable. Part of her self, the self as father's lover, will be kept separate. Rather than being integrated and cohesive, the self becomes compartmentalized and fragmented.[25]

Contradictory Relationships

As all I've just said about internal conflict attests, severe internal conflict is often embedded in contradictory attachment relationships. Keep in mind how your sense of self develops in close relationships. Thus your sense of continuity and cohesiveness depends on reasonable continuity and unity in your relationships with others. We all adapt our behavior to different relationships, and we behave differently in relation to different people. As long as your various relationships are compatible and the alterations in your experience and behavior are within bounds, your sense of continuity and sameness can be preserved.

Our sense of continuity and integrity is challenged, however, by abusive relationships that repeatedly entail 180-degree shifts. A child may be treated with affection and protection at one time and then be violently castigated or physically beaten at another time. Or the child may be loved at one time and severely neglected at another. A wife may be violently assaulted then showered with flowers. Such shifts may be associated with alcohol or drug abuse. How is one and the same self to reconcile such dramatic contradictions? How can one and the same self be worthy of love and affection and yet also be subjected to beatings and neglect? How is self-continuity possible in such contradictory relationships? These conflicts can tear the self apart. Hence one pathway toward greater self-continuity is more stable and secure attachment relationships.

Self-Healing

In the wake of trauma, developing a greater feeling of self-worth, self-efficacy, and self-cohesiveness is a major undertaking. Understanding yourself better should be of some help. But self-understanding does not necessarily come easily. By blocking your mentalizing capacity, attachment trauma blocks self-understanding. Creating the autobiographical narrative that constitutes your self can require major reconstruction. But the effort is justified. In the process, you can develop some appreciation for the basis of your intense feelings, strong urges, and powerful conflicts, and this appreciation can begin to restore some sense of unity. Ideally, self-understanding will promote self-acceptance and help undo some of the damage to self-worth. Plainly, changing your view of yourself requires much active work.

Steering Past Negative Illusions

Shelley Taylor[235] has shown how people who have been spared severe trauma usually develop positive illusions that sustain a sense of well-being and promote success. The converse is also true. With negative illusions, you can steer yourself right into a pit. You can damage your self; your self can become more and more incapacitated and impaired. How you think of yourself has a major *steering function:* it shapes how you feel, how you behave, indeed, who you *are.* The "me" influences the "I." When defined on the basis of self-hatred, the "me" damages the "I."

It's easy to see the shaping effect of your self-concept on your self by thinking of the negative side. How often do you criticize yourself? Tear yourself down in your own mind? Berate yourself? Express contempt for yourself? Belittle yourself? What's the effect of these negative thoughts on your self-efficacy? Like being abused by others, this self-abuse fuels despair and a sense of helplessness.

If your trauma includes maltreatment in attachment relationships, you may be inclined to insist that you are simply no good, worthless, or a complete failure—at worst, evil beyond description.[25] This negative self-assessment may seem like the unvarnished, immutable truth. Adopting this view, you're not mentalizing, which entails viewing your "self" as a mental representation that you've constructed with the help of others. Mentalizing, you're in a position to deconstruct and reconstruct, shaking yourself loose from such unquestioned convictions. Your self-concept is, *in principle,* extremely complex and flexible. It's not *necessary* to be locked into an unwavering, globally negative view of yourself. On the contrary, in principle, you're free to think what you wish about yourself. I think of it this way: it's a free country in your own mind.

The truth about yourself is extremely complicated, just as the truth about anyone is extremely complicated. Any person is extremely complex. A tremendous amount of *potential* mental freedom comes into play here. No matter what you were told, no matter how you were treated, no matter what you were compelled to do, it's not *necessary* to continue the mistreatment in your own head.

In *principle,* it is possible to be free, flexible, and open in how you see and think about yourself. This essence of mentalizing—adopting an open-minded attitude of interest in present reality—brings a fresh perspective to bear on your experience.[83] While possible in principle, mentalizing can be difficult in practice. Exercising your mental freedom is a long-term project that requires tremendous effort and concentration. But with growing awareness that helps you notice whenever you tear yourself down, you can develop the capacity to step back from those thoughts and feelings and take a more detached perspective. This process involves trying on for size some different ways of thinking about yourself.

Recall Kabat-Zinn's maxim: there is more right with you than wrong with you. Try it on for size. Contemplate it. Unbelievable? There's nothing to stop you from using this concept as a guiding rule in thinking about yourself—in principle. It's not easy to change established patterns; it goes against the grain, requiring resolve and practice. In the long run, however, it's possible, and it steers the self in a better direction.

My work with individuals who have been severely traumatized confirms Kabat-Zinn's view. I'm repeatedly impressed by their strengths—to which they are often inattentive. These strengths are condensed in the term *survivor*—preferable to *victim*. Victim and survivor are vastly different perspectives on the same traumatic reality. *Both* are true. As you construct your narrative autobiography, you can tell yourself victim stories and survivor stories. You can tell yourself failure stories and success stories—all true stories. Where should the focus of your attention be?

In person after person, I see persistence, courage, intelligence, creativity, kindness, compassion for others, openness, and spunk. Interestingly, many traumatized persons come up with positive attributes like these when prompted to think more flexibly. Recall Harter's finding that global self-worth stems from competence in many domains; paying attention to areas of competence contributes to self-worth. You may need encouragement from others to do so. Your self-worth is partly barometric, dependent on your focus of attention at the moment. The reality, the truth, is multifaceted. Mentalizing, you can adopt various perspectives. I'm not suggesting rose-colored glasses; I'm suggesting multi-colored glasses.

I emphasize changing how you think about yourself because, although it is not easy, you have *relatively* good control over what you think. To some degree, you can take charge of what you think, exerting some control over what you feel in the process. The potential to control your thoughts is the rationale behind cognitive therapy.[187] It's not easy, especially if you're depressed; but it's possible. It takes lots of work, like everything else worthwhile. The first step in cognitive therapy is becoming aware of your automatic negative thoughts—and demoralizing stories, I'd add. Perhaps you are only dimly aware of it, but you're telling yourself stories about yourself much of the time. The next step in cognitive therapy is questioning your automatic negative thoughts. Mentalizing, you can start constructing alternative stories.

The Self in Relationships

As stated earlier, the "me" is formed to a substantial extent in relationships. Looking at others is like looking into a mirror. You see the "me" in reflection. How you see yourself reflects how you are seen by others, how you are treated by them, and how you feel in relation to them. Many persons have been told that they are bad in myriad ways. But you need not be told directly; when you're mistreated, you may just infer it.

The antidote to reflections that damage the "me" is healthier relation-ships and better reflections. But the negative illusions are not easily altered. Affirming attitudes of others may not make a dent; positive comments and praise are often discounted. Why is this? Here's what many patients say: They've learned to conceal their angry feelings. They've been hurt or pun-ished even more severely than usual whenever they protested or showed their natural anger. When others tell them they're friendly, kind, considerate, or nice, they protest internally (if not outwardly), "If they really knew how hateful I am inside, they would not think so well of me"; "The fact that they like me just *proves* what a phony I am." Such thinking takes the positive re-gard of others and uses it as fuel to tear yourself down further: "The truth is, I am a phony, a fake." I'd counter with an equally true story: such a kind—and angry—person is making a valiant effort to relate positively against great odds created by internal conflict, distrust, and fear. If both of these are legit-imate perspectives, to which should you pay attention?

To reiterate, Susan Harter noted that different areas of potential self-worth are tied to different areas of competence, and we can enhance our self-worth by paying attention to areas of competence. But she also emphasized relational self-worth, that is, how self-worth varies from one relationship to another. The implication is clear: it's crucial to invest time and energy in those relationships that enhance your self-worth and to minimize contact with persons who diminish it.

But healing relationships are not just the wellspring for improving self-worth; they also provide an opportunity to bolster self-efficacy. When we think about healing the self in relationships, we most often focus on self-acceptance, validation, and affirmation from others. All these are enor-mously important, but I want to draw your attention to a more subtle yet pervasive form of empowerment: being mentalized. Granted, hitting the ten-nis ball, performing the song, and getting the grade, raise, or promotion all contribute to self-efficacy. But such achievements may pale in relation to something potentially far more common: actively expressing yourself in close relationships and evoking understanding in others so that you have a sense that the other person has your mind in mind. And this process goes both ways: mentalizing others so as to evoke a smile or relieve suffering also contributes to self-efficacy—and self-worth.

Your Relationship With Yourself

Persons who've been traumatized in any way, and those who've been abused in particular, have a deep longing for a relationship in which they can feel safe and obtain comfort. As discussed in relation to attachment, they seek a safe haven and a secure base. Establishing secure relationships, however belatedly, is the cornerstone of healing. But think beyond relationships with others; you also need a secure relationship *with yourself*.

You might find it puzzling to think of having a relationship with yourself, but there are parallels to your relationships with others. You have conversations with yourself. Most importantly, you have feelings about yourself. Like your relationships with others, your relationship with yourself is multifaceted; you can be kind to yourself and cruel to yourself. Developing a healthy relationship with yourself is of utmost importance: you're with yourself all the time, and the relationship is lifelong. Think of secure attachment as a model for your relationship with yourself. You could be encouraging, supportive, nurturing—at best, loving—toward yourself. That doesn't mean you won't also be frustrated with yourself and critical of yourself, but a generally benevolent and compassionate relationship with yourself will make your self-criticism more tolerable.

Thinking more flexibly about yourself can be a stepping stone toward a more secure relationship with yourself. With a history of trauma, you might be locked into rigidly negative thinking about yourself. This negative thinking is akin to having an abusive relationship with yourself. Imagine living with an abuser, all the time, throughout the day, in your own brain/mind/head! You need not continue to do so. Just as you should feel an urge to protest being mistreated by others, you should protest being mistreated by yourself. You need not keep putting up with it. But you'll need to *work* at developing a more supportive relationship with yourself. This advice shouldn't be surprising; any good relationship requires work.

Susan Harter noted the problem of depending too much on the views of others for your self-worth. Your feelings about yourself can be buffeted by the ups and downs of your relationships. The barometer can plummet in a stormy relationship. Thus she points to the value of *internalizing* the positive opinions of others, which provides more stability in your self-concept and buffers you in times of stress. In my way of thinking, you can potentially rely on the security of your relationship with yourself for stability in your self-worth.

Think of your relationship with yourself from the perspective of mentalizing. I've emphasized the importance of your sense that another person has your mind in mind. You, too, may have your mind in mind—or fail to do so, in effect, neglecting yourself. We think of mentalizing as a benevolent, compassionate activity.[83] To reiterate, don't think that mentalizing precludes self-criticism; on the contrary, mentalizing makes self-criticism more open-minded, balanced, and productive. You have a complex self, and you have a complex relationship with yourself that should allow for praise and criticism. Again, flexibility is the key.

Mentalizing, you can adopt a benevolent interest in yourself, and then you're in a position to comfort yourself and care for yourself. And, by comforting yourself, I don't mean just talking to yourself in a compassionate way, although I think such conversations can be enormously important. Although it may go against the grain, you also need to take action, doing things for yourself that provide pleasure and comfort. There's a limit to how much you can do by thinking; actions indeed speak louder than words. Don't think you must feel good about yourself before you start doing good things for yourself; feelings often follow actions.

I pointed out at the beginning of this chapter that two major lines of development are self-development and the development of relatedness to others. I also emphasized that these two aspects of development are interdependent. Your relationships with others influence your sense of self and vice versa. Finding relationships in which you are treated with compassion, and allowing yourself to experience and take in that compassion, is a major route to being able to adopt this compassionate attitude toward yourself. Conversely, the more you're able to be compassionate toward yourself, the more open you will be to compassion from others, and the more skilled you'll become at showing compassion for others. The challenge is to get these mutually enhancing cycles going.

C h a p t e r 6

RELATIONSHIPS

Relationships are the single most important source of satisfaction in life while also being the most potent source of human misery.[241] As we've seen, attachment relationships are a mixed blessing—they're essential for developing a sense of self, learning to mentalize, and regulating distress, while also being potentially traumatic. Even under the best of circumstances, forming attachment relationships renders us vulnerable throughout life. As Freud[15] so plainly put it, "We are never so defenceless against suffering as when we love, never so helplessly unhappy as when we have lost our loved object or its love" (p. 33).

There's far more to relationships than attachment, but I emphasize attachment because any threat or trauma powerfully evokes attachment needs. When you're threatened or injured, you feel a need to seek security in the safe haven of attachment. Hence coping with trauma invariably will have a strong impact on attachment relationships, no matter what the source of the trauma. Furthermore, as we've seen, trauma can interfere with your capacity to make use of attachment relationships. Even if you were traumatized by something impersonal, you may lose confidence in the protectiveness of your attachments. Or you may be concerned that your struggles with trauma are burdening your loved ones, and your attachments are thereby threatened. Finally, as described in Chapter 2 ("Attachment"), trauma embedded in close relationships is usually most difficult to bear, especially when the relationship ought to provide a feeling of security.

Given that relationships are central to well-being, we must clarify the potential obstacles you may face in making the best use of relationships. This chapter focuses on relationship patterns stemming from trauma and considers the role of relationships in healing.

Relationship Models

We're great categorizers. We learn patterns. We continually encounter novelty, but we immediately connect whatever situation confronts us at the moment with memories of our past experience. And we're always categorizing ongoing experience in relation to our feelings, our needs, and our safety. Before long, we learn to attach labels to categories. This is "good," that's "bad," this is "scary." We categorize quickly and unconsciously, for example, responding fearfully to a threatening face in well under a tenth of a second.[145] Thus, just as we categorize the inanimate world of chairs, trees, and trains, we categorize relationships with others on the basis of previous patterns—although not so consciously and not with such simple labels.

We all develop *models* of how relationships go, based on recurrent patterns of interactions—father holds comfortingly when child cries; mother beams proudly when child performs; brother retaliates fiercely when sister interferes. As life goes on, our models become increasingly diverse and complex. Yet earlier models always serve as a foundation for later relationships. We repeat. And we're always modifying and shaping old models to new relationships, developing new patterns of relating that we generalize into subsequent relationships. We learn.

Your relationship models not only govern your experience of relationships but also govern your behavior toward other people. If you expect others to mistreat you, you keep them at a distance. In this way, your expectations influence how people respond to you. You tend to shape other people's behavior so as to bring them into conformity with your models. Accuse others of having it in for you—and they will! *You repeat.* Conversely, others influence you to conform to *their* models. *They repeat.* You select partners whose relationship models are compatible or complementary with your own. We all try to work out reasonable matches with each other, for better or for worse.

Relationship models have two parts—self and other. The self is distressed, the other comforts; the self yearns, the other neglects; the self is in pain as the other attacks. These two-part models lend an easy flexibility to your relationships. You can readily switch roles: mother comforts child; child comforts mother. In an abusive relationship, both roles are learned with full force: being injured *and* injuring. Those who have suffered abuse may establish subsequent relationships in which they mistreat others. Or you can play out these two-part models in your relationship with yourself; you can assault yourself in thought and in action.

Secure attachment is a key relationship model. The infant develops the expectation that contact with a caregiver will be soothing: when I feel bad, mother holds me, and I feel better. As development proceeds, and opportunities for contact with others expand, this model of secure attachment is generalized to relationships with others—father, sister, brother, grandmother, and teacher. But secure attachment is never the only model. Frustration is a universal model: sometimes when I feel bad, mother doesn't help. Being injured is a universal model: sometimes contact with mother hurts.

Bowlby[176] proposed the concept of *internal working models* of the self and the attachment figure. These working models shape our expectations and behavior toward others. For example, confidence in the accessibility and responsiveness of the attachment figure hinges on two factors: your expectations about the responsiveness of the attachment figure and your view of yourself as worthy of responsiveness. Bowlby[176] summarized this point:

> An unwanted child is likely not only to feel unwanted by his parents but to believe that he is essentially unwantable, namely unwanted by anyone. Conversely, a much-loved child may grow up to be not only confident of his parents' affection but confident that everyone else will find him lovable too. (pp. 204–205)

Bowlby maintained that our attachment models are reasonably accurate reflections of how we have been treated by parents and caregivers. But this doesn't mean that children play no part in the models that they develop. Children are active interpreters of their caregivers' behavior, constructing models on the basis of their individual perceptions and reactions. The models developed by a more sensitive child will be different from those developed by a more obstreperous child. And the child's behavior and temperament will shape the behavior of the caregivers, thus playing a major role in the models that develop.[242] For example, a hyperactive child is likely to evoke criticism. Whatever our environment, we all have models with our own individual stamps. But we can all be overpowered. In the face of severe trauma and malevolent intent on the part of caregivers or others, there's no avoiding pernicious relationship models.

Bowlby's term, *working model*, emphasizes flexibility. Ideally, you can shift and adapt your models from moment to moment. You can expect to be criticized but be open to praise. You can be angry and frustrated, then forgiving and affectionate. Yet you can be caught in unwitting patterns of repetition. My colleagues Peter Fonagy and Mary Target[243] emphasized that these models are not generally conscious; rather, they are implicit *procedures* for interacting with others. Recovering from trauma often entails becoming more aware of these procedures—mentalizing—so as to better adapt to the reality of the present and to be able to modify these procedures so as to relate more flexibly and adaptively. Of course, as you become more aware of these relationship models, you're likely to remember interactions that may have contributed to their development, memories that are more or less accurate constructions. Yet, as Fonagy and Target point out, it's not recovering memories that's healing but rather learning to mentalize and to develop new procedures that promote more satisfying relationships, less generalized from the past and more responsive to the present.

I routinely observe several common themes in the relationships of persons who have experienced trauma—isolation, yearning, fearfulness, dependency, victimization, controlling, and aggression. These relationship models are universal. Yet they seem to stand out more starkly in those whose relationships have been marred by trauma. This list is hardly exhaustive, but it might prompt you to reflect about some of your own patterns.

Isolation

I think the most natural response to interpersonal trauma—having been hurt by someone more or less deliberately—is to stay away from people. If you've been hurt in close relationships, you'll naturally tend to maintain emotional distance. You may prefer solitary activities or find refuge in fantasy, perhaps also keeping your interactions with others on a superficial level. As described in Chapter 2 ("Attachment"), we see this pattern in infancy: the infant who consistently encounters rejection is likely to develop a pattern of avoidant attachment.

But isolation is not always a choice. Many abusive relationships entail enforced isolation. Abused children and battered spouses are likely to be isolated from their peers. Even if their isolation is not rigidly enforced by an abusive and domineering parent or partner, it's engendered by secrecy and shame, which become internal barriers to intimacy.

To a degree, isolation and avoidance are workable strategies, and many traumatized persons have followed these strategies for years. Ultimately, however, when distress mounts or crises evolve, isolation is no longer an effective strategy. Paradoxically, while you're seeking safety in isolation, you also may feel more vulnerable, having given up the potential safety of secure attachment. Moreover, isolation is depressing.

Yearning

Given the power of attachment needs established by evolution over millennia, isolation is rarely an ideal solution. In my trauma education group, we used to tender the "happy hermit theory" as an alternative to attachment theory. We never had any happy hermits in the room. As group members' experience attested, isolation holds sway by keeping at bay a yearning for closeness, affection, comforting, and protection. A paradox is at work here: the history of trauma abets isolation but also fuels attachment needs. Isolation thus alternates with longing for much-needed caregiving, closeness, and intimacy.

Fearfulness

The inevitable yearning for contact invariably propels traumatized individuals back into relationships. But any closeness or intimacy will be frightening. A slew of working models based on past experience spells all sorts of danger. Distrust may be pervasive. The specific fears will reflect the past traumas. Common fears include being physically injured, exploited, dominated, controlled, trapped, intruded upon, smothered, terrorized, humiliated, degraded, betrayed, and abandoned.

Dependency

No one who has suffered trauma in relationships is doomed to a life of isolation, yearning, and fearfulness. Driven by attachment needs and undaunted by prior injuries, many persons eventually find relationships that provide affection, protection, nurturance, and intimacy. Of course, trust in such relationships is hard won, achieved only over a long period. It's not surprising that, once found, such relationships grow to be profoundly important. Your seemingly overwhelming needs become focused on the one individual who can meet them within a context of safety. Your newfound attachment relationship becomes the only safe haven in a world of danger.

The capacity to depend on others is not a weakness; it's a strength, essential for attachment and well-being more generally.[244] Yet, in excess, dependency paradoxically undermines security. You may have overcome fearfulness only to find that your long-awaited safe haven does not turn out to be an unmitigated blessing. Your fear of being injured may gradually give way, only to be replaced with a fear that the relationship will end, particularly to the degree that you feel you are burdening your partner with your intense needs. To complicate matters further, your dependency and fear of abandonment may engender feelings of resentment and hostility associated with a sense of being trapped and vulnerable. Then your long-awaited safe haven and secure base may not feel so safe and secure after all.

Victimization

At worst, the dependency that naturally evolves in any comforting relationship can contribute to a vulnerability to repeating past trauma. The fear of abandonment may outweigh the pain of further exploitation and injury.

The person who suffers harm is commonly considered a *victim,* and no one working with traumatized persons can doubt the reality—indeed, the tragedy—of victimization. But "victim" has now become a pejorative term: "You're always acting like a victim!" I think such criticism stems partly from the denial that all of us can become victims. It's reassuring to blame the victims. We should keep in mind that the dissociative defenses of detachment and numbing that served to buffer childhood trauma (see Chapter 10, "Dissociative Disorders") can permit the adult to put up with mistreatment that would otherwise be intolerable.[240]

But we should distinguish the reality of victimization from the adoption of a generalized *victim working model* of relationships. In such relationships, the traumatized person gives up power and control, having developed a passive and submissive stance that promotes additional victimization. Of course, this relationship model is often frustrating and annoying to others. And thinking of yourself as a passive victim is damaging because it erodes self-efficacy, being a clear case of the "me" undermining the "I." Accordingly, persons who have been traumatized are often encouraged to think of themselves as *survivors* rather than victims.

Rather than focusing on victimization, Judith Herman[58] emphasized the *failure of self-protection* in relationships that entail repetitions of abuse. For persons who have been abused or traumatized by others, self-protection was not possible initially; they were victims. Failure of self-protection implies an extension of this early model into subsequent relationships in which self-protection is a possibility. In such changed circumstances, to think that you have been victimized again leads nowhere; to think that you have failed to protect yourself implies a solution. Failure of self-protection points the way from the learned helplessness of depression to active coping. For example, a woman who is raped at a party after having become intoxicated may feel guilty and berate herself. She may wrongly blame herself, rather than the rapist, for being raped. But, in this instance, her guilt feelings can serve a useful purpose by motivating her efforts to avoid such vulnerability in the future.

Controlling

The worst aspect of traumatic experience is the sense of helplessness it engenders. Trauma entails feeling out of control and being at the mercy of others. It's little wonder that control becomes a paramount concern. At one level, you may be extremely averse to any interaction that smacks of being out of control. You may find it extremely difficult to comply, to go along, to follow, or to submit to the desires of another person—even when going along entails no danger or harm. Having your own way may seem absolutely necessary. You may find yourself in power struggles. Avoiding being controlled may not be enough; you may feel secure only when you are able to exert active control over another person. Your sense of security may depend on turning the tables, controlling and dominating others rather than being controlled or dominated by them. Of course, this working model works badly, as it only increases the odds of conflict and additional trauma.

Aggression

The tables may be turned even more dramatically when one who has been abused becomes the abuser. Anna Freud[245] recognized this pattern in children, calling it *identification with the aggressor,* a defense by which the individual transforms being threatened into threatening others. Recall that relationship models have two parts, self and other, and both parts invariably are learned. This applies to the comforter and the comforted as well as to the batterer and the battered. Switching roles is common; we learn to comfort by being comforted. Moreover, the role of aggressor appeals to the person who has been threatened because it's associated with a sense of power and control, thus providing an antidote to feelings of weakness and helplessness. Of course, aggression begets aggression; it provides not only a model but also the emotional provocation to go with it: anger. When we feel angry, we naturally want to hurt someone.[158] As noted in Chapter 3 ("Emotion"), beating a child for being aggressive is a futile attempt at control: it makes the child angry, and it provides the child with a model for how to behave when angry—aggressively.

Because those who were mistreated as children tend to mistreat their own children, child abuse is often passed down through generations.[246] This intergenerational transmission of abuse is by no means inevitable, but it's nevertheless common. Importantly, abused children who are most likely to become abusive parents are those who deny that they were abused and idealize their abusive parents. Conversely, facing the reality of the past—mentalizing—prevents such repetitions.[159]

Problematic Cycles

As just described, the self-other structure of your relationship models is conducive to alternating roles. Ideally, you can nurture, and you can allow yourself to be nurtured. You can depend and be depended on. But you can also abuse and be abused. You can abandon and be abandoned. And, as described in Chapter 5 ("Self"), traumatic relationships often entail 180-degree shifts in relationships. These shifts not only undermine self-continuity but also make for stormy relationships, owing to cascading internal working models. Judith Herman[58] painted a vivid portrait:

> The survivor oscillates between intense attachment and terrified withdrawal. She approaches all relationships as though questions of life and death are at stake. She may cling desperately to a person whom she perceives as a rescuer, flee suddenly from a person she suspects to be a perpetrator or accomplice, show great loyalty and devotion to a person she perceives as an ally, and heap wrath and scorn on a person who appears to be a complacent bystander. The roles she assigns to others may change suddenly, as the result of small lapses or disappointments, for no internal representation of another person is any longer secure. (p. 93)

Such sequences do not arise de novo; they are repetitions of alternating hope and disillusionment that were part of the 180-degree shifts in earlier traumatic relationships.

Therapists construe reenactment of traumatic relationships in terms of three roles, each of which has an active and a passive position: rescuing-rescued, abusing-abused, and neglecting-neglected.[247] Individuals who are caught up in reenactments tend to cycle among all these roles. A common pattern, for example, is hoping for rescue, feeling abused, then retreating into isolation, feeling alone and neglected. As I view it, the neglecting-neglected roles are the black hole into which all traumatic interactions tend to spiral.[25]

In Chapter 4 ("Memory"), I described how memories play a key role in traumatic stress. Remember, however, that the reexperiencing of trauma involves implicit, procedural memories as well as explicit personal event memories. Reenactments of trauma, based on these implicit patterns of interacting, play a major role in triggering the reexperiencing of trauma.[25] Most important, attesting to the overgeneralization of relationship patterns, ordinary interactions can spin out into traumatic reenactments. When someone is tactless or rude, you can feel abused; when you snap back in irritation, you can feel you've been abusive. When someone offers help, you can long for rescue; when someone fails to empathize or ignores you, you can feel abandoned and neglected. All this can happen unconsciously, as these ordinary interactions evoke implicit procedures for relating. But the traumatic pattern is badly matched to the current situation, and others are perplexed at the emotional intensity of your 90/10 reaction. Hence we encourage mentalizing, making a conscious effort to separate the traumatic past from the ordinary—if often aggravating—present.

Traumatic Bonding

Most problematic are relationships in which prior trauma is reenacted in full force. It's not uncommon, for example, for a person who has been abused by a parent to choose an abusive mate or to become involved in relationships that carry a high risk for injury or exploitation. Freud[248] called this the *compulsion to repeat* because of the compelling need to repeat the earlier destructive pattern.

Why would anyone compulsively repeat an injurious and painful pattern of behavior? There are many reasons why individuals who have been injured by others express their aggression by directing it back onto themselves. But other persons can be enlisted as accomplices in this scenario. You can attack yourself by provoking or permitting others to attack you.

It's tempting to chalk up such behavior to a naive concept of *masochism*—finding pleasure in pain. In my view, this is a flimsy and harmful explanation (see Chapter 11, "Self-Destructiveness"). Seeing yourself as a masochist, like seeing yourself as a victim, undermines self-efficacy. I have no doubt, however, that many traumatized persons unwittingly perpetuate their suffering for a wide variety of reasons.[25] For example, suffering can stem from a need for punishment, prohibitions against pleasure, an attempt to elicit nurturing, and an effort to take control by inflicting pain actively rather than suffering it passively.[45]

Freud[249] thought that the repetition compulsion might reflect a belated effort at mastery. Trauma stirs up severe conflict and painful emotion. The mind does not sit quietly with a terrifying sense of helplessness. Trauma becomes an unsolved problem in the mind, and unsolved problems press for solution. Traumatized children commonly repeat the trauma in their play, often in relatively undisguised form.[250] Through play, they seem to be attempting to assimilate, digest, and overcome the traumatic experience. Perhaps the same could be said of repetition in adult relationships. A girl who was completely overpowered by an alcoholic father might strive in adulthood to sober up an abusive alcoholic husband. But there's no evidence that repetition of trauma consistently leads to mastery or resolution; on the contrary, it just leads to further suffering.[62]

If not for the sake of suffering or mastery, why repeat? I find it helpful to shift the focus from suffering to learning. The *compulsion to repeat* is one form of the *compulsion to relate*. And we all repeat what we have learned in earlier relationships; we re-create the familiar. We all develop models of relationships, and we're always employing them. When a friend keeps going back to an abusive husband, we think in exasperation, "She'll never learn!" On the contrary, she's merely reenacting what she's learned all too well.

The powerfully destructive attachments that evolve in abusive relation-ships have been called *traumatic bonding*.[251] Although perhaps most dra-matic in cults, kidnappings, and hostage situations,[252] traumatic bonding is far more common in troubled households. How can a child love and even idolize an abusive parent? How can a battered wife love and protect her abu-sive husband?

A patient in group psychotherapy recounted a childhood in which she was continually frightened by her stepfather's violence toward her mother. Her stepfather was a well-respected union leader, and he was accustomed to hav-ing plenty of power. In contrast to his stable image at work, he was intimi-dating and domineering at home. When he was drinking, he would not only scream at his wife but also slap her, shove her, and push her around. In turn, his wife was verbally abusive toward the children, haranguing them for their shortcomings and misbehavior. The stepfather rarely laid a hand on the chil-dren, and he doted on his stepdaughter. He was occasionally intimidating to-ward her but generally loving and attentive.

Partly to get away from home as soon as possible, the patient married im-mediately after she graduated from high school. Her husband was a kind and gentle young man, but he became addicted to drugs and died of an overdose. Heartbroken and feeling abandoned, she quickly married an attractive man she hardly knew. Their relationship rapidly deteriorated. He beat her so fre-quently and so brutally that she feared for her life. She packed her bags when he was away at work, and she left the state. She resolved never to marry again, but she could not tolerate being alone. She moved in with another man, and this relationship was an improvement. He never physically as-saulted her, and he could be loving and affectionate. Yet he was also ex-tremely controlling and intimidating, and she felt as if she continually walked on eggshells. She was reluctant to have children, and she was socially isolated because his possessiveness and belligerence kept all prospective friends away. To the consternation of her friends, her relatives, and even her-self, she stayed in this relationship for many years until he left her abruptly to marry another woman.

To say that this patient was merely repeating what she had learned from observing her parents' marriage does not do justice to the force of the repe-tition compulsion evident in battering relationships. Common sense dictates that someone who has been repeatedly hurt and mistreated in a relationship would do everything possible to flee or at least to maintain distance. Yet we continually observe the opposite. Individuals become locked into traumatic relationships and cannot let go. The abused person may be beaten and tor-mented, and may occasionally attempt to break away, but will repeatedly re-turn to the abusive relationship. Common sense and intuition fail us in understanding such behavior.

Hard as it may be to believe, being abused and mistreated can actually *strengthen* the bond in relationships. And this phenomenon is not unique to humans; maltreatment has been shown to accentuate attachment in a range of mammals.[108] Perhaps it's not so hard to understand why a person would maintain a relationship *despite* abuse; any relationship may be better than none. Moreover, the penchant for denial is all too human, and it's tempting to ignore all prior evidence and believe the abuser's claim that he will not do it again. But how could abuse and maltreatment *increase* attachment? This anomaly is the essence of traumatic bonding: the more you are abused and terrorized, the harder you may cling to the abuser.

To understand the paradox of traumatic bonding, we must first learn to appreciate the social context of the abusive relationship. Two factors are critical. First, *social isolation*, often enforced by possessiveness, precludes other sources of secure attachment.[58] Second, a gross *imbalance of power* in the relationship renders the person increasingly incompetent and helpless, ever more reliant on the person in the position of power.[54] Notably, the power imbalance is only superficial: the controlling behavior masks feelings of weakness, dependency, and a fear of abandonment, all of which fuel the batterer's jealousy and possessiveness.[253]

The combination of attachment needs, isolation, and the imbalance of power conspires to create a situation conducive to traumatic bonding. The abused or terrorized individual feels *completely dependent on the abuser or terrorist*.[254] Abuse in an exclusive relationship with an attachment figure creates an intolerable conflict: the secure base is a source of danger. Traumatic bonding escalates this conflict. The more the individual is injured and terrorized, the stronger his or her need for protection and comforting.

The alternation of distress and relief cements the traumatic bond. As Walker[54] described, any shred of affection, comfort, or even respite from injury and terror will tighten the bond. But intermittent kindness is only one key to traumatic bonding; the bond is also cemented by the individual being spared even more grave harm. Walker found that psychological battering is sustained by the threat of bodily harm, including being killed. Any reprieve from injury and terror and, most important, *the fact of being allowed to live,* evokes enormous gratitude.[252] The terrorist becomes the protector—protector from the terror and injury that *might* be inflicted. The terrorist escalates the need for a safe haven and then gratifies the heightened need that has been created. As Herman[58] explained, the perpetrator becomes the savior. And the worse the injury, the greater the terror, the stronger the need for security, the tighter the bond.

As one such victim of battering told me, it's extremely difficult to leave the relationship by "jumping into the void." Yet, courageously, she did so, and she eventually found other sources of support. Typically, because of the strength of the attachment, letting go is a long and painful process. And, having let go, many persons return, perpetuating the cycle.[255] But many others don't.[251] There are options, including shelters that provide temporary safe haven.[256]

Developing New Models

I've painted a bleak picture with this litany of traumatic relationship models and cycles, culminating in the quicksand of traumatic bonding. Yet, for all its pitfalls, attachment offers a hopeful perspective, as the desire for secure attachment relationships is powerful and persistent.

In our specialized treatment program for women with a history of severe interpersonal trauma,[257] we asked patients to list their current attachment figures and to indicate the degree of security in those relationships.[101] Then we contrasted these findings with those for women in a community sample. Not surprisingly, we found that women in the community listed significantly more secure attachment relationships than those in trauma treatment. More surprisingly, the difference was small. On average, traumatized patients listed four, whereas women in the community listed six. Of course, in both groups there was a lot of variation, and a small number of the traumatized patients listed none. But the vast majority had one or more, and many had a whole network of relatively secure relationships—despite their history of traumatic attachments and a significant level of conflict in some of these relationships. Thus the secure attachment model, established by evolution and by whatever instances of good experience with caregivers occurred, is highly resilient.

Positive Models

Not only does the yearning for secure attachment persist, but also we are always capable of new learning. The very capacity for learning and generalization that perpetuates abusive experience can be the pathway out of destructive relationships. The traumatic models are not dissolved, unlearned, or exorcised. What is learned stays learned. Once a model, always a model. But new models can be learned and generalized, old models supplanted. My advice: put the old models on unemployment, unless you need to spot another abusive person.

How are new models learned? They're learned from and with other people. They're taught, not didactically as in a classroom, but procedurally as in riding a bicycle, through relating and interacting. For good or for ill, others tend to shape us into the molds of their models. Abusive models are taught in relationships and interactions. So are nurturing models. Models of others as reliable and trustworthy are necessarily learned only over a long period of time. You must find good teachers—persons who are kind, trustworthy, and reliable. Abusive relationships set up a vicious cycle: the more you're mistreated, the more you feel devalued, and the more mistreatment you tolerate and feel you deserve. Healthy relationships turn the tide, creating a benign cycle: the more you're treated with kindness and respect, the more you feel confident and worthy, and the more you'll assert your needs and be treated accordingly.

Nothing is foolproof, and this scenario is not flawless. No one is a perfect judge of character; we're all susceptible to being deceived. Self-protection is possible to a degree, but anyone can be overpowered. Rescue is illusory; all helpful relationships are flawed, limited, and disappointing to a degree. Conflicts wax and wane; closeness and distance ebb and flow. Healthy development just requires a good-enough mother.[94] We need not just good-enough parents, but also good-enough companions, friends, mates, and therapists.

And we should not associate traumatic relationships exclusively with problematic models. In addition to hindering development, trauma and suffering can promote growth.[258] I've worked with many persons who credit their deep capacity for caring, empathy, and compassion to their traumatic experience. Thus trauma often promotes a profound concern for the welfare of others, which is arguably one of the most fundamental dimensions of close relationships.[174] Hence, ironically, trauma may promote models of secure attachment in the form of an exceptional ability to provide comforting, nurturing, protecting, soothing, and caregiving to others. As discussed in Chapter 5 ("Self"), extending the compassion to the self is an important challenge.

Although I find it hard to overemphasize attachment, it's important to recognize many other aspects of relationships that go beyond attachment, although there may be areas of overlap. There are models for making connections: communicating, accepting, affirming, and empathizing. There are models for intimacy: loving, being affectionate, and confiding. There are models for cooperation: helping, teaching, supporting, collaborating, sharing, giving, working together, and complying. There are models for resolving controversy: confronting, challenging, contesting, and asserting. Not least important are models for just plain having fun—often not so easy for traumatized persons.

The possibilities for benign relationships are limitless and well worth contemplating. Seeking pleasure of any sort, including in relationships, requires an active effort. You may benefit from taking an inventory of your own relationship models. Which models do you most frequently employ? Which models should you put on unemployment? Which models should you develop and cultivate? What persons in your life go with which models? What are the patterns and sequences of interactions that characterize your relationships? How stable and steady are your interactions? How changeable and stormy?

Networks

For persons who have been extremely isolated, it can be a monumental challenge to develop a single close relationship, much less a network of relationships. Yet, as discussed earlier, many severely traumatized persons are able to develop small networks, although they may need considerable help and support in doing so. The reasons for going beyond a single relationship are plain: your lone close relationship can become unduly burdened with strong attachment needs, then infused with anxiety and hostility. Ordinary conflicts can spiral into traumatic reenactments and posttraumatic reexperiencing symptoms.

In thinking about the importance of networks, psychologist Helen Stein and I developed a relationship education course,[259] based on an assessment of healthy adult functioning by Jonathan Hill and his colleagues.[260] We distinguish several potential domains of support, which vary in level of closeness and intimacy. We emphasize flexibility and diversity in ways of meeting attachment needs. We also emphasize the benefits of having relationships at different levels of closeness. We distinguish several *domains* of relationships.

Social contacts are limited to a particular circumstance, such as playing in a band or on a sports team, meeting at your child's preschool, congregating at church, hanging out with a few regulars at the coffee shop, greeting your favorite clerk at the grocery store checkout counter, or chatting with a fellow passenger on an airplane. Social contacts are built on small talk, which is an important skill, notwithstanding the disdain that many persons have for it (possibly because they're not very good at it). Although social contacts are not confiding or intimate relationships, we should not minimize their importance. They foster a sense of belonging, countering feelings of isolation and alienation, thus providing a sense of familiarity and safety in the world. They afford an opportunity for pleasurable social contact, also an antidepressant. And, crucially, they serve as a gateway to deeper relationships.

Friendships are founded in shared circumstances and interests, but, as the relationship develops, friends make special arrangements to get together in a variety of circumstances. Friendships are not exclusive and tend to be relatively free of conflict; often they involve a considerable degree of confiding and hence may meet attachment needs as well as many other needs. Importantly, friendships require active maintenance and reciprocity, without which they are likely to founder. In contrast to other kinds of relationships, friendships are noteworthy for their potential stability, and they often provide an optimal combination of emotional support and practical help.

Romantic relationships involve love and sexual affection. They're generally exclusive, or, when they're not exclusive, there's a very high potential for conflict. For many persons, romantic relationships are primary attachment relationships, although, like friendships, they meet many relationship needs beyond attachment. Of course, with greater closeness and intimacy—not to mention living together—romantic relationships entail considerable conflict and place a premium on negotiation and conflict resolution. Negativity in close relationships tends to escalate as one partner responds negatively to aversive behavior of the other; hence a hallmark of stable romantic relationships is accommodation, that is, responding constructively to the partner's bad behavior.[241] As one of our educational group members said wisely, it's important to know when to hold your tongue.

Family relationships are diverse, including everyone from extended family in the family of origin to in-laws and children in the family of marriage. Hence few generalizations are possible in this broad domain. We do not choose our family of origin. Importantly, except for in-laws, family members share not just history but genes. Like romantic relationships, owing to their closeness—and living together—family relationships have the potential to provide enormous satisfaction as well as to engender extreme conflicts. To reiterate Freud's sage words, we are never so defenseless against suffering as when we love; this pertains to many family relationships as well as to romantic relationships. For all their potential problems, families provide the widest ready-made network of support.

Work and school relationships resemble social contacts in being confined to circumstances. Also, like social contacts, work relationships may develop into friendships or romantic relationships—notwithstanding that blurring these boundaries can be enormously problematic. Many work relationships go beyond social contacts, however, in the sheer amount of closeness and contact. Not rarely, persons may spend more time with colleagues at work than with spouses and children. Hence work relationships may provide substantial opportunities for social support, and many persons who work alone feel a lack in this regard. Of course, work and school relationships offer many opportunities for conflict, such as competition with coworkers and authority problems with supervisors and teachers. Hence interpersonal skills play a huge part in occupational success.

Relationships with professionals, for example, members of the clergy or psychotherapists, provide an important source of support for many traumatized persons. I'll discuss psychotherapy more in Chapter 13 ("Treatment Approaches"), but note here that the boundaries and contractual nature of the relationship—although frustrating and confusing in some respects—provide a much-needed sense of safety and predictability. For persons who have been hurt and betrayed, these safeguards foster confidence and trust. Like any attachment relationship, psychotherapy also fosters dependency. Yet the professional relationship should not become an end in itself, but rather a bridge to other close relationships.[25]

We could carve up the pie of relationships in many different ways, and the topic of relationships fills many books. And we don't minimize the importance of relationships with animals (see Chapter 2, "Attachment"). I've highlighted some key domains here only to emphasize the wide range of opportunities for support. I want to emphasize the sheer variety of ways in which different individuals can form healthy networks of relationships along with the potential for creativity in meeting attachment needs.

Self-Dependence

To reiterate, development of the self and development of relationships are intertwined over the lifetime. We must all find a balance between self-development and relatedness, closeness and distance, openness and privacy, togetherness and solitude. Each individual must find the optimal blend; no ideal suits everyone.

In thinking about a healthy balance between self-development and relationships with others, I find psychoanalyst Joseph Lichtenberg's[105] concept of *self-dependence* to be most useful. Since its inception, American society has placed great value on independence. But aspiring to independence can be problematic, particularly for individuals who have been traumatized. For many, independence comes to connote not needing anyone—what we call *counterdependence*—and, as such, becomes confused with isolation. Attachment needs are lifelong, and isolation is not viable in reality. Lichtenberg defines self-dependence in a way that balances autonomy and attachment. To be self-dependent requires that you be able to have a sense of continuity in your relationships. You must be able to remember and imagine your relationships with those to whom you are securely attached. Once you develop this capacity, you do not need to be in the continuous presence of the other person to feel secure. The gist of self-dependence is the capacity to bridge the gap between separation and reunion (see Figure 6–1). Ways of bridging the gap include self-regulation of emotional distress (see Chapter 13, "Treatment Approaches") and reaching out to other persons in your support network. When you've bridged the gap, the reunion then serves to renew, refuel, and maintain the sense of secure attachment while fostering autonomy and self-development.

Becoming self-dependent is easier said than done, and, as with attachment, we spend a lifetime working on it. Self-dependence requires mentalizing; bridging the gap entails being able to have a comforting attachment relationship in mind during times of separation. Having a comforting relationship in mind may sound easy, but it's not. When attachment relation-

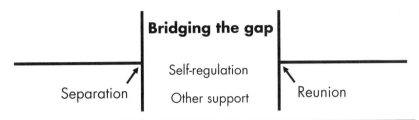

FIGURE 6–1. Self-dependence.

ships have been fraught with conflict, having your attachment relationship in mind may evoke conflict—pleasurable feelings of being comforted may become intermingled with painful feelings such as anxiety, fear of abandonment, resentment, and hostility.

Thus self-dependence requires strengthening your capacity for secure attachment in current relationships. And security in current relationships has a dual benefit. Not only are you sustained in the presence of the relationship but also you have a better capacity to internalize the relationship; you can carry it with you in your mind, bringing it to mind when needed. Then you also have a secure base. Yet, as Lichtenberg declared, self-dependence requires reunions. Bowlby's colleague, Mary Ainsworth,[104] put it well, "The attachment is not worthy of the name if [individuals] do not want to spend a substantial amount of time with their attachment figures—that is to say, in proximity and interaction with them" (p. 14).

Chapter 7

ILLNESS

Exposure to acute stress generates physiological changes throughout the brain and body, adaptations designed to facilitate coping. These adaptive responses to acute stress also set in motion automatic mechanisms designed to shut down the stress response. Yet exposure to extreme stress, particularly when the stress is repeated, can result in persistent and maladaptive physiological changes. Then the stress response creates physical illness.

Psychiatrist Douglas Bremner,[261] a leading researcher in the neurobiology of trauma, laid the cards on the table: "Stress-induced brain damage underlies and is responsible for the development of a spectrum of trauma-related psychiatric disorders, making these psychiatric disorders, in effect, the result of neurological damage" (p. 4). This concept is crucial: psychological stress can result in physical illness. I realize that this assertion rubs salt in the wound; it's bad enough to feel damaged psychologically and even worse to contemplate being injured physiologically. As I'll argue shortly, however, it's worse yet to deny that trauma entails physical illness, because such denial is even more demoralizing. Not understanding your illness, you can blame yourself for your inability to recover quickly. Self-understanding is essential for self-care. If you're diabetic, you need to know it, so you can manage the illness and take proper care of yourself.

We're walking a tightrope in applying the concept of physical illness to trauma. On the one hand, we must face the seriousness of trauma-related disorders. On the other hand, reading that you may be dealing with "stress-induced brain damage" is alarming. Keep in mind that the body has marvelous means of healing its wounds. We break bones; they're damaged, and they heal. Unfortunately, in the field of stress, we know more about the processes of injury than the processes of repair. Until recently, we thought that the brain does not generate new neurons; you could only lose them over your lifetime. Now we know otherwise. More generally, researchers continue to learn about the enormous plasticity of the nervous system—its ongoing capacity for change, growth, and repair. We're beginning to learn about the *reversibility* of brain changes wrought by stress and how treatment with medication and psychotherapy contributes to healing at the neurobiological level.[262,263] Thus it's important not to fall off the tightrope; we must balance the concepts of illness and neurological damage with the concepts of healing, plasticity, and reversibility. The nervous system is designed first and foremost for adaptation and learning, and the reversibility of stress-induced brain changes is an area of active research.[264]

This chapter illustrates how psychological symptoms of trauma relate to physical illness. Some parts are relatively technical, and, if you're not interested in the physiological details, you should feel free to skim. Yet several general concepts are essential and not difficult to understand: illness, hyper-responsiveness, sensitization, and ill health. After considering illness as a social role, I distinguish among several biologically adaptive responses to threat, describe some persistent alterations in the stress response that result from trauma, review ill health, and conclude with some thoughts about caring for your nervous system.

The Illness Perspective

In thinking about depression as a physical illness,[265] I've found it helpful to focus on a dilemma depressed persons face: they're between a rock and a hard place. The rock: "It's not that serious, and I should be able to just snap out of it." The hard place: "I'm seriously ill, and there's no way I can snap out of it."

Traumatized persons, many of whom suffer from depression, face this same dilemma. It's tempting to sit on the rock, which minimizes the seriousness of the illness. But it's crazy-making. You should be able to snap out of it, but there's no way you can do so. You may blame yourself for being a wimp or weak-willed. I think the hard place is a more hopeful stance, because it's more realistic: recovery is possible, but it's long and difficult. If you stay on the rock, you can impede the process of recovery by berating yourself for not recovering more easily. As we'll glimpse in this chapter, research shows that trauma results in physical illness. This isn't good news, but it fits the experience of many traumatized persons who struggle valiantly to get better and encounter many obstacles and much frustration in doing so.

Decades ago, sociologist Talcott Parsons[266] usefully viewed illness as a social role. Being ill, you're exempted from performing normal social obligations, such as working, taking care of the household, and socializing. You have a legitimate excuse; you're entitled to some slack. Moreover, you're exempted from responsibility for your ill state; it's not your fault that you're ill. Most important in my view, Parsons asserted that the ill person "cannot reasonably be expected to 'pull himself together' by a mere act of will, and thus to decide to be all right" (p. 456). This might be the single most important idea for you and your loved ones to understand. Being ill, you cannot just put the past behind you, move on, or snap out of it by *a mere act of will*. Recovery takes *many* acts of will over a long period of time—such as just getting out of bed day after day when you're profoundly depressed. And it takes considerable help from others.

Parsons went on to add that being ill frees you from some obligations but imposes others. To remain legitimately excused, you're obligated to do something about your illness: to seek help, to cooperate with treatment, and to get well as soon as possible. Learning about your illness, as you're doing here, is a good example of fulfilling this obligation. Of course participating actively in treatment is no small challenge, especially to the extent that you're depressed and demoralized. And the idea of getting well as soon as possible sounds much more straightforward than it is: just how soon is "as soon as possible" for the traumatized person? For many, recovery is a slow process with many ups and downs, and the course of illness is not easily predictable. Understanding trauma from the perspective of physical illness helps you to understand why this is so.

Adaptive Responses to Threat

We can understand the stress response best from the perspective of evolution. Species that survive have stood the test of time by developing robust ways of coping with challenges, danger being paramount among them. Adaptive responses to threat must be both fast and flexible. We humans share basic adaptations to threat with all our mammalian kin; hence scientists have learned a tremendous amount about stress and trauma from studying other mammals, from mice to nonhuman primates. The perspective of evolutionary biology can help us understand some of our most fundamental responses to threat as well as some of the ways we can be traumatized by extreme stress.

We mammals are prepared by evolution to respond immediately and vigorously to any dire threat. Walter Cannon,[267] who pioneered stress research in the first half of this century, proposed that we have two basic choices: fight or flight. He made no bones about the significance of the fight-or-flight response: "The strength of the feelings and the quickness of the response measure the chances of survival in a struggle where the issue may be life or death" (p. 377–378). Hence Cannon emphasized the physiological similarities between fear and rage, pointing out that, regardless of whether the organism fights or flees, the bodily needs are similar. Fight and flight call for equally vigorous action, and Cannon and others began elucidating the physiological basis of this stress response.

Thanks to Cannon's many successors, we now understand the fundamental mammalian reactions to threat in a more refined way.[264] Each of these reactions, including fight and flight, involves a complex profile of physiological arousal that supports a particular behavioral demand. These various patterns allow us mammals to respond flexibly to threat; our behavior and corresponding physiology can shift rapidly, depending on the nature of the threat and the best means of coping at the moment.

Taking an evolutionary perspective, we can put our patterns of coping with threat into bold relief by considering how mammals respond to predators.[124,268] Sadly, confrontation with a predator is not a far-fetched analogy to those forms of interpersonal trauma in which we're endangered by other persons.[25] Let's take it in steps, based on the degree to which the attack is imminent (see Table 7–1). First, an animal will show *vigilance* in situations where a predator is likely to be in the vicinity. Second, when an animal detects the presence of a predator in the vicinity, its initial response is to *freeze* so as to minimize its chances of being detected. The freeze response is a state of high alert or vigilance. Third, if the animal is detected and threatened directly, the *defense* response comes into play, with the options of flight or, if the animal is cornered, fight. Fourth, if the animal is caught, a playing-dead reaction response may ensue; the animal goes into a state of *tonic immobility*. When the animal goes limp, the predator may let go, and the animal might then escape through flight. Finally, when the defense response is prolonged, and the animal cannot escape, a *defeat* reaction may take place: the animal gives up and goes into a state that resembles depression. The enormous flexibility of these response patterns is worth underscoring. We can switch rapidly from freezing to fighting to fleeing then back to freezing. Correspondingly, our emotions switch rapidly from fear to anger, and these emotions also can become intermingled.

All these patterns of responding to various degrees of threat are hardwired in the sense that they evolved over eons and do not require elaborate thought. And these patterns of coping are highly sophisticated packages of responses; a specific pattern of physiological arousal supports each form of

TABLE 7–1. Stages of predatory imminence

Adaptation	Nature of threat
Vigilance	Predator in vicinity
Freezing	Sighting of predator
Flight	Sighted by predator
Fight	Cornered by predator
Tonic immobility	Pinned by predator

emotional behavior. The physiological responses involve coordination of the *central nervous system,* which consists of the brain and spinal cord, and the *peripheral nervous system,* which consists of the nerves connecting the spinal cord to the sensory receptors, muscles, and internal organs. The peripheral nervous system is divided into the *somatic* (sensory and motor) nervous system and the *autonomic* nervous system.

The autonomic nervous system merits particular attention in relation to the stress response. The autonomic nervous system, coordinated by the brain, regulates all the internal organs, adjusting their functioning to behavioral demands. For example, your heart rate and blood pressure increase to support running. There are two branches of the autonomic nervous system: the *sympathetic* and the *parasympathetic,* both of which are activated in a highly coordinated way to support these different patterns of coping. Owing to the integration of the central nervous system and the autonomic nervous system, stress-related changes may occur not only in the brain but also in all other organ systems in the body, including the cardiovascular, respiratory, gastrointestinal, reproductive, and immune systems.[124]

From Adaptation to Illness

We all know that stress can make you sick, and traumatic stress is extreme. But our common sense knowledge conceals a puzzle: why would this adaptive and protective response to threat result in illness?[264] It's as if our protective reactions turn against us. The simplest answer is that these responses were designed to cope with time-limited threats like a charging bear. We quickly appraise a situation as dangerous and become appropriately aroused. Our physiology automatically rises to the occasion to support vigorous action, such as fleeing, as well as rapid changes in action plans, such as switching from freezing to fleeing. When the threat is terminated and we are safe, our arousal decreases as our physiology returns to normal.

These marvelously adaptive responses are designed for acute danger, but they become strained under prolonged or repeated threat, such as occurs in

combat and abusive relationships. Being constantly on guard and continually injured puts an enormous load on your body as well as your mind. And
severe assaults, such as being raped or being held at gunpoint for hours, also
may have persistent effects on your physiology. You cannot fully adapt to
such extreme stress; it leads to wear and tear on your brain and the rest of
your body, eroding your ability to adapt to subsequent stress.

Hyperresponsiveness

Two persistent effects of repeated stress are hyperarousal and hyperresponsiveness. Hyper*arousal* is evident in relatively prolonged states of distress,
for example, a high level of anxiety or irritability. Hyper*responsiveness* is evident in high reactivity to stressors, for example, unusually intense startle reactions. Of course, these two are related: if you're in a state of hyperarousal
(fearful), you're likely also to be more hyperresponsive (easily startled).
Thus lowering your general level of arousal, for example, by routine exercise
and relaxation, is one way to decrease your hyperresponsiveness (see Chapter 12, "Emotion Regulation").

Many traumatized persons are understandably distressed by their hyperresponsiveness, particularly when others criticize them for "overreacting" or
"making mountains out of molehills." Thus we need to think clearly about
this problem. If a child were frozen in a state of extreme anxiety in the face
of a raging parent, we wouldn't think he is overreacting but rather that he's
reacting naturally. Yet, if an adult with this history becomes frozen in a state
of panic when his boss is irritable, we'd think of him as overreacting, that is,
hyperresponsive to threat. But nothing is intrinsically wrong with the intense response; it's one of those natural patterns that evolved over eons. As
discussed in Chapter 3 ("Emotion"), you might think of it this way: a perfectly normal response is occurring in the wrong situational context. To reiterate, we call this context-inappropriate response the 90/10 reaction: 90%
of the emotion comes from the past and 10% from the present.

When you've been traumatized, you do yourself a disservice in thinking
that your hyperresponsiveness—context-inappropriate responding—is the
reflection of a personal failure, such as being a wimp. The concept of illness
helps here: your nervous system has been affected by trauma, persistently
changing your reactivity to stress and to cues associated with trauma. Your
nervous system has adapted. If you're in a situation where danger is ever
present, you need to be on guard and prepared to respond quickly. Your nervous system learns. I think of the criticism that you're "making a mountain
out of a molehill" this way: there's a real mountain in the past if only a molehill in the present. Your nervous system has adapted to that real mountain.

Thanks to neurobiological research on trauma and posttraumatic stress disorder (PTSD), we're now in a position to understand some of these persistent alterations in the functioning of the nervous system and the body's other organ systems. Remember that I'm encouraging you to move from the rock to the hard place, considering the possibility that trauma has resulted in physical illness, such that your emotional reactivity has been changed persistently. Keep in mind that, even if this is so, you can learn to manage this illness and reverse some of these physiological effects.

Sensitization

Recall the central point Talcott Parsons made about illness: you cannot recover by a mere act of will. Here's a way to think about why this is so when you've suffered psychological trauma: your nervous system has become *sensitized* to stress.[269] You might best understand sensitization by thinking of its opposite, desensitization. Often we become *desensitized* by repeated exposure to a stressful situation. If you're inexperienced and anxious about speaking in public, you can become less anxious over time with repeated practice, provided that your experience with speaking turns out to be reasonably positive. Often, we desensitize ourselves by approaching stressful situations gradually—speaking to smaller audiences at first and larger audiences later on. Your nervous system gradually adapts to the stress; technically speaking, you *habituate* through repeated exposure, just as you habituate to repeated sounds in your environment. After a while, you're no longer conscious of the clock ticking.

Unfortunately, traumatic stress does not offer the opportunity for desensitization; your exposure is not gradual and manageable but sudden and overwhelming. Then the opposite reaction can occur; your nervous system becomes sensitized, *more reactive* to stress over time rather than less so. Stress accumulates rather than dissipating. You might think of sensitization as akin to the last-straw effect. After a series of hassles during the day that leave your nervous system keyed up, you blow up at a minor frustration that you'd ordinarily take in stride. Sensitized, your nervous system automatically makes mountains out of molehills. Keep in mind that your nervous system can begin responding fearfully to a threatening face in less than a tenth of a second. When your nervous system is sensitized, your reaction is not just fast, it's intense. We now know that trauma may sensitize many aspects of your nervous system's functioning, a few of which I'll consider next.

The Brain's Trauma Center

A little bundle of neurons in the brain stem called the *locus coeruleus* has been dubbed the trauma center of the brain.[270] This little protein factory manufactures norepinephrine, a form of adrenaline. Norepinephrine, one of the neurotransmitters that convey signals between neurons, plays a key role in the regulation of anxiety and mood. When a novel stimulus activates the locus coeruleus, norepinephrine activates widespread areas of the brain. Because of these widespread effects, norepinephrine is also considered a neuromodulator. Other neurotransmitters of interest in psychiatry, most prominently dopamine and serotonin, are also considered neuromodulators, because they regulate brain functioning in a similarly broad manner.

The locus coeruleus–norepinephrine component of the stress response system serves an alerting function, interrupting your ongoing behavior and focusing your attention on high-priority stimuli.[271] When this brain circuitry is activated, your level of arousal goes up; you may become anxious and vigilant. The sympathetic branch of the autonomic nervous system is activated in tandem with the locus coeruleus–norepinephrine circuit, in preparation for the fight-or-flight response. Thus sensitization of the locus coeruleus–norepinephrine circuitry by exposure to repeated stress contributes to hyperresponsiveness to unexpected stimuli, as you are more readily put on guard—as you become *hyper*vigilant.

Fear and the Amygdala

Higher up in the brain is another alarm center that interacts with the locus coeruleus. The *amygdala*, an almond-shaped structure deep in the temporal lobe of the brain, has garnered a lot of attention in relation to trauma.[213] The amygdala quickly detects danger, for example, showing a high level of activation in response to a threatening face.[127] In addition to its role as a threat detector, the amygdala immediately orchestrates central components of the fear response, including the necessary autonomic nervous system responses. To reiterate, this process is so fast that it's unconscious; you can be afraid without knowing why. Thanks to these hardwired responses, when you're endangered, with the help of the locus coeruleus and amygdala, you become alert, focused on the threat, and afraid, with all your body's organ systems geared for action.

The amygdala not only detects danger and organizes the fear response but also plays a key role in learning cues associated with danger, that is, in fear conditioning.[272] As discussed in Chapter 3 ("Emotion"), in the process of fear conditioning, a previously neutral conditioned stimulus comes to evoke fear when it is paired with an inherently noxious unconditioned stimulus. The smell of alcohol can become a conditioned stimulus for being hit. This learning is highly adaptive because, after you've become conditioned, you can anticipate and better avoid danger. Yet these conditioned responses also need to be tempered by additional learning mediated by higher brain centers. The smell of alcohol leads to being hit only in certain contexts; you learn that you're more likely to be hit at home than in a restaurant.

Back to the theme of illness. With the advent of neuroimaging, neuroscientists are able to study the brain in action, for example, observing changes in patterns of blood flow in different parts of the brain in response to various tasks or challenges. Making a significant contribution to our clinical knowledge, a number of traumatized persons have agreed to have their brain activity studied when their posttraumatic symptoms have been evoked experimentally by reminders of trauma. These studies have shown that exposure to trauma-related cues elicits a high level of activity in the amygdala.[273] These reminders are conditioned stimuli, and the amygdala orchestrates the conditioned response: fear. An overactive amygdala, especially when it is unrestrained by higher brain centers, is another manifestation of sensitization that contributes to hyperresponsiveness.

Arousal and the Biochemical Switch

I've been emphasizing the adaptiveness of hardwired responses. In a flash, we become alert and afraid; in a state of high arousal, we begin running. Adaptive as they may be, these hardwired responses are comparatively rigid reaction patterns, and typically we must supplement them with restraint and reasoning. We must strike a balance between action and thought, and high levels of arousal can tip the balance. We all know the experience of being so anxious or agitated we can't think straight. Sadly, for traumatized persons, this experience may become all too common.

Recent research is pinpointing how traumatic stress may create problems in using reasoning to regulate arousal. The *prefrontal cortex* plays a central role in executive functions, that is, planning and sequencing your actions in situations that call for flexibility.[274] Just think of times when you've needed to juggle a bunch of activities under time pressure—making a grocery list while your children are demanding attention and the telephone's ringing. As you can appreciate, keeping your emotional reactions in check plays an important part in such flexible responding. And these executive capacities are crucial not only for complex problem solving but also for social interactions, such as holding a lively conversation while keeping track of the other person's point of view and emotional state—mentalizing.

As arousal escalates, increasing levels of the neurotransmitters norepinephrine and dopamine shift the balance of control between prefrontal cortex and lower brain centers. Mild-to-moderate levels of arousal promote optimal prefrontal cortical functioning, and more extreme levels of arousal trigger a neurochemical switch that takes the prefrontal cortex offline. Then the more automatic patterns, including the freeze and fight-or-flight responses, take over.[275,276]

This switch in behavioral control is adaptive in the context of danger situations that require automatic responding. We don't want to be contemplating what to do when the bear is charging. We must respond immediately to threat, and the locus coeruleus–amygdala system mediates that response. But we also need to be able quickly to reappraise the situation to determine whether fear is justified and what coping strategy is best. For this more sophisticated and deliberate reappraisal, we need our higher cortical functions that, in effect, put the brakes on action prompted by amygdala activation. Indeed, most of the time when we are anxious, we're struggling with something far more complex, albeit less physically dangerous, than a charging bear. We need to be flexible and creative. Unfortunately, owing to sensitization, a history of stressful and traumatic experiences may impair your capacity to regulate arousal, lowering the threshold for this switch process. Then when you become anxious or irritated, you may too quickly switch into the fight-or-flight mode, be unable to think clearly, and respond too rigidly.

I noted that neuroimaging studies of brain activity of persons in the throes of posttraumatic symptoms show high levels of amygdala activity consistent with fear. These studies also show a decrease in cortical functioning consistent with the idea of the neurochemical switch. Neuroimaging of traumatized persons has shown that, coupled with an increase in amygdala activation, is a decrease in higher cortical activity, including activity in the prefrontal cortex.[261,273] Particularly noteworthy is decreased activation of the speech center in the left-frontal cortex (Broca's area). Such findings led trauma specialist Bessel van der Kolk and colleagues[277] to comment that, when they are recalling traumatic events, individuals are in a state of speechless terror.

Like complex problem solving more generally, mentalizing also requires optimal functioning of the prefrontal cortex. Mentalizing emotionally—being able to feel and think about feeling at the same time—is especially demanding of prefrontal functioning. Such mentalized affectivity is crucial for resolving interpersonal conflicts on the fly; you need to be able to think clearly when you're confronting someone who's made you angry. If you switch prematurely into the fight-or-flight mode, rather than getting the conflict resolved, you might escalate the conflict into an argument or fight. With a sensitized nervous system, you'll need to work harder at mentalizing (see Chapter 12, "Emotion Regulation").

Prolonged Stress and the HPA Axis

The physiology of the stress response is magnificently complex, including not just the virtually instantaneous processes of neuron-to-neuron signaling that can bolt us into action but also somewhat slower and more prolonged neuroendocrine processes that regulate the level of hormones circulating in the blood stream and thereby adapt various organ systems to the stressful situation over somewhat longer periods of time. Most pertinent to trauma is the hypothalamic-pituitary-adrenal (HPA) axis,[264] the core components of which are depicted in Figure 7–1. The hypothalamus, buried deep in the brain, plays a major role in orchestrating the autonomic aspects of emotions. The hypothalamus, along with the locus coeruleus and the amygdala, secretes corticotropin-releasing factor (CRF), which contributes to anxiety. CRF secreted by the hypothalamus activates the pituitary gland which, in turn, secretes adrenocorticotropic hormone (ACTH), stimulating the adrenal cortex to secrete cortisol, a major stress hormone. Cortisol plays a dual role in stress, both facilitating coping (e.g., by increasing available energy) and shutting down the stress response. Given its cardinal role in damping stress, cortisol also can be regarded as an *anti*-stress hormone.[278]

As I'll discuss further in the next chapter, depression is a high-stress state, and one of the most consistent biological findings in severe depression is elevations in cortisol levels.[279] We might expect that cortisol would be even more highly elevated in posttraumatic stress disorder, but the reverse is true.[278] Yet, coupled with lower baseline cortisol levels is very high reactivity of the HPA axis, consistent with bursts of cortisol secretion. This is yet another example of trauma-related hyperresponsiveness at the physiological level.

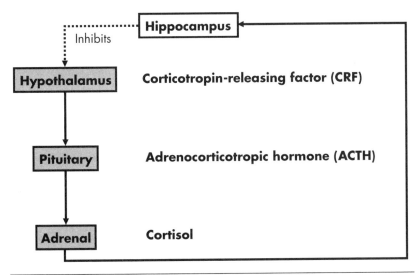

FIGURE 7–1. Overview of the hypothalamic-pituitary-adrenal (HPA) axis.

One of the more disquieting biological findings in the trauma literature concerns another brain structure that plays a significant role in emotion and memory: the *hippocampus*, a seahorse-shaped structure deep in the temporal lobe. The hippocampus plays a major role in the process of encoding and consolidating explicit memories—both personal event memories and semantic memory, the latter handy for passing exams.[178] Part of the its role in memory entails associating events with a situational context. For example, if a rat receives a shock in a certain part of a maze, the rat then becomes conditioned to fear in that particular area of the maze. With a well-functioning hippocampus, the rat will be afraid in that part of the maze—and not in other parts.

Extensive research has shown that PTSD is associated with reduced size of the hippocampus, partly related to the shrinking of neurons in this brain structure.[280] In addition, it has been demonstrated that excess levels of cortisol contribute to this shrinking of neurons.[281] Thus an important part of the wear and tear in the nervous system associated with prolonged and repeated stress is hyperactivity (and hyperresponsiveness) of the HPA axis. Whereas cortisol helps contain the acute stress response, excess cortisol may damage the hippocampus, the very structure that uses cortisol to turn off the stress response.[264]

In part, this stress-related shrinking of hippocampal neurons may protect neurons from excess stimulation that might damage them permanently. Yet cell death also does occur and contributes to reduced hippocampal volume. But don't lose sight of neural plasticity: hippocampal neurons can be rejuvenated, and, moreover, the hippocampus is capable of generating new neurons. Hence all is not lost.

These findings regarding excess HPA-axis activity and hippocampal damage link the physiology of trauma to memory problems. A poorly functioning hippocampus contributes to general problems with explicit memories and to problems in remembering traumatic events in particular.[261] The hippocampus also plays a central role in creating personal event memories. More specifically, the hippocampus actively relates the various facets of an experience to each other to form an organized whole—including relating events to a specific context.[178] Thanks to your hippocampus, you can remember the specific day and the particular stage you were on when you happened to flub your lines!

Consider that trauma may result in an overactive amygdala that fires off conditioned fear responses and an impaired hippocampus that fails to encode the environmental context of frightening events. This combination may well contribute to the context-inappropriate responding—the 90/10 reaction—that so troubles traumatized persons in situations where minimal current danger activates the fear response.

Stress-Induced Analgesia

You've probably had the experience of injuring yourself in the midst of an activity, such as playing a sport, and not being aware of pain until later. This common phenomenon is called *stress-induced analgesia,* and its adaptive function is plain: in the midst of coping with a stressful situation, it's best not to feel pain so that you can keep going. The pain reaction sets in later, forcing you into inactivity so you don't do further damage and you can care for your wounds.

This analgesia is mediated in part by your body's *endogenous opioids—* self-produced narcotics.[282] Traumatic stress can enhance this opioid response, which is another facet of the sensitization process. Research has demonstrated, for example, that persons with PTSD can withstand higher levels of pain.[283] In addition, we know that some persons with a history of trauma cope by deliberate self-injury, for example, cutting or burning themselves (see Chapter 11, "Self-Destructiveness"). Many persons who injure themselves deliberately do not feel pain; rather, they may feel a soothing sensation of warmth, owing to the sensitization of their opioid system.

Genetic Contributions

We know that individual differences in genetic makeup play a contributing role in vulnerability to a wide range of psychiatric disorders, including depression, anxiety disorders, and substance abuse. You might not expect genetic factors to play a major role in PTSD, because this disorder is caused by environmental factors: traumatic stress.

Yet when we consider all the organ systems involved in the stress response, it shouldn't be surprising that genetic factors play a huge role in individual differences in vulnerability to stress. Genes orchestrate development of the body, and gene expression—whether genes are turned on or off at any given moment—continues to play a role in regulating all physiological activity throughout life.[284] Thus genetic makeup plays an ongoing role in stress regulation.

PTSD is one of the anxiety disorders, and we know that genetic factors play a significant role in proneness to distress.[129] Hence, genetically based proneness to anxiety and depression has been shown to increase the risk of developing posttraumatic stress disorder in the wake of stressful events.[285] But there's another facet to genetic vulnerability: genetic factors also play a significant role in whether a person is *exposed* to stress.[286] How could this be? Consider that genetic factors contribute to individual differences in personality, and personality factors influence stress exposure. For example, some persons are more inclined to be very active and to engage in risky or even reckless behaviors. These inclinations are partly rooted in genetically based personality differences. Such persons are more likely to get themselves into traumatic situations by virtue of their risk-taking behavior. Drunk driving can lead to accidents. Drug dealing can lead to shootouts. Hence genetic factors contribute to the likelihood of exposure to traumatic stress *and* to the likelihood of developing a psychiatric disorder in the wake of stress.

Ill Health

We can view trauma-related psychiatric disorders as physical illnesses that, like other chronic medical conditions, tend to wax and wane over time, particularly in conjunction with stress. But many traumatized persons are also ill in the more ordinary sense of having chronic aches and pains along with various general medical symptoms.

You're probably well aware that many physical symptoms and illnesses are related to stress. And ample research shows that chronic stress can compromise the functioning of the immune system.[287] Yet we should remain mindful that the body is designed to cope with stress and to rebound from it. Fortunately, chronic stress does not typically result in diagnosable disease. However, there's a downside: you might seek medical help for physical symptoms only to be frustrated when no clear diagnosis and treatment results. While you're better off not having a diagnosable disease, you can be irked when you get the message that your symptoms are all in your head.

Psychiatrist Herbert Weiner[288] proposed an extremely useful concept for stress-related physical symptoms that can take so many forms: *ill health*. Stress-related symptoms of ill health associated with childhood trauma, for example, include pain in the back, chest, face, pelvis, genitalia, breasts, abdomen, and stomach; headaches; bruising; problems with urination; diarrhea and constipation; appetite disturbance; choking sensations; and shortness of breath.[289] PTSD also has been related to a wide range of physical symptoms.[290]

The greatest danger of concluding that it's all in your head is failing to obtain adequate medical care. Then you will not receive proper care if some treatable disease process does develop. Treating trauma-related physical symptoms in primary care requires exceptional sensitivity and expertise.[291] It's important to find a primary care physician who takes your symptoms seriously, provides whatever palliative care may be available, and monitors your physical condition over time so that you can be assured that disease processes will be addressed if they arise. Above all, *you* must take your physical symptoms seriously, and you must find a physician who will do so as well. The physical symptoms are real, as evidenced by burgeoning research on the physiology of the stress response. Yet there may not be any curative medical intervention, and you may need to rely mainly on stress management and psychiatric treatment.

You must also consider another major contributor to ill health that's intertwined with trauma: your *health-related behavior,* such as alcohol use, cigarette smoking, eating and sleeping habits, and exercise.[292] You may be contending with two overlapping vicious circles.[287] First, chronic stress produces wear and tear on your nervous system and other organ systems that, in turn, compromises your ability to adapt to subsequent stress. Second, stress may fuel behaviors like substance abuse, overeating, and a sedentary lifestyle that add to the wear and tear, further compromising your health and resilience. Hence, in addition to stress management, coping with trauma-related ill health entails engaging routinely in health-promoting behavior.

Sexual Dysfunction

As just discussed, traumatic experience may have an impact on all organ systems, and disturbance of sexual functioning may be one aspect of the physiological consequences of trauma. Sexual arousal is mediated by the autonomic nervous system. As discussed earlier in this chapter, the autonomic nervous system is conventionally divided into the sympathetic and the parasympathetic branches. These two branches are somewhat reciprocal; activating one tends to deactivate the other. The sympathetic branch mediates the fight-or-flight response. Sexual responsiveness, on the other hand, depends on parasympathetic activation. Like your mind, your nervous system has a hard time being prepared for fight or flight and being sexually responsive at the same time.

To the degree that sexual responsiveness and fight-or-flight preparedness are incompatible, it's hardly surprising that traumatic experience interferes with sexuality. The hyperarousal that characterizes anxiety and PTSD may interfere with sexuality, even when the trauma was not specifically sexual. To the extent that sexual responsiveness depends on a sense of safety and relaxation, any resurgence of trauma takes its toll. And it's not just the hyperarousal that interferes; so do depression, numbing, and dissociation. Sexual pleasure depends on being actively engaged, tuned in, and fully aware of the here and now. Detachment diminishes the sense of relatedness, as well as the sensory aspects of sexuality.

Sexual responsiveness involves a gradual sequence of arousal that can be interrupted at any point by depression, anxiety, distress, shame, anger, or intrusive memories. Sexual dysfunctions are diagnosed on the basis of the stage of the arousal sequence at which the interruption occurs. At worst, numbing may be associated with a lack of desire or interest in sex or complete aversion and avoidance of all sexual contact. Or, even when there is desire and interest, trauma may interfere with sexual excitement—for example, trauma may be manifested in an inability to attain or maintain lubrication in the female or erection in the male. Or the interruption may occur at the final stage in the sequence, such that the individual is sexually excited but unable to achieve orgasm.

Sexual trauma, such as rape, interferes more directly with sexual arousal and pleasure.[293] Because of its similarity to the earlier trauma, sexual contact—or even the *anticipation* of sex—may trigger not only anxiety and fear but also intrusive memories or flashbacks. At worst, some individuals who have been sexually traumatized may relive the trauma in the context of the sexual relationship, for example, seeing the assailant's face instead of the spouse's face when having intercourse. Given the frequency of sexual assaults and their potentially traumatizing impact, clinicians have developed effective treatment for rape-related trauma,[17] such that persistent sexual difficulties need not be inevitable.

It is hardly surprising that childhood sexual abuse may interfere with sexual functioning. Psychologist Elaine Westerlund[294] studied a group of women with a history of incest to illuminate their subjective experience of sexuality. She employed a comprehensive questionnaire combined with in-depth interviews of incest survivors. The effects of incest on sexual functioning vary greatly but share many common themes. Importantly, ongoing self-blame contributed significantly to problems with sexual adjustment.

Westerlund discovered several common problem areas associated with a history of incest: negative body perceptions (seeing the body as dirty, bad, out of control; feeling betrayed by the body's arousal); problems with reproduction (apprehension about becoming a parent, reawakening of traumatic memories in conjunction with giving birth and nursing); and guilt feelings about sexual fantasy (especially fantasy involving violence, force, humiliation, or pain, as well as fantasy involving the offender). Westerlund found that a majority of women reported difficulties with sexual arousal. For many, sexual arousal and sexual pleasure were followed by shame and guilt. Inability to achieve orgasm was rare, but some women experienced orgasm in the absence of arousal or pleasure. Orgasm was associated with a sense of vulnerability and of being out of control. Westerlund also observed a frequent split between sexual arousal and emotional attachment. A number of women were able to experience sexual arousal only in the absence of intimacy, associating emotional intimacy with vulnerability to reexperiencing the incestuous relationship.

There's no evidence that incest directly affects sexual preference, but Westerlund found confusion over sexual preference to be common. Many women *believed* that their sexual preference was connected to the incest. Like anyone else, women with an incest history may be celibate, lesbian, bisexual, or heterosexual.

Just as there are a variety of sexual preferences, there are also a variety of sexual lifestyles. A minority of Westerlund's subjects had developed a pattern of aversion—that is, revulsion associated with avoidance of sex—fueled by fear and anger. Many reported inhibition, and many had undergone a period of celibacy. Some engaged in compulsive sexual behavior, and a temporary period of promiscuity (in adolescence or early adulthood) was common. Promiscuity occasionally included a period of prostitution. Compulsive sexual behavior was often associated with a desire for power and control, as well as being a vehicle for expressing anger toward the partner and toward the self. Inhibition was more common than compulsion, and it was common for lifestyles to alternate or to change over time.

You should not infer from Westerlund's findings that incest destroys any opportunity for healthy sexual functioning. Notwithstanding the many problems, the majority of sexually active respondents were more satisfied than dissatisfied during sex. Although Westerlund's respondents were somewhat unusual in being members of self-help groups, it was obvious that they were generally struggling—with considerable success—to improve their sexual experience and functioning. Many women in Westerlund's group were able to regain a sense of bodily control through exercise and fitness training.

A range of treatment approaches has been developed to help incest survivors with sexual dysfunction. These treatment approaches build on a substantial history of successful treatment of sexual dysfunction.[295] Current treatment approaches include education as well as individual and group therapy.[296] As in the treatment of sexual dysfunction with other origins, sexual partners are actively involved in the healing process.

Implications for Self-Care

It's not good news that exposure to extreme stress can lead to physical illness, but the evidence continues to mount. You cannot snap out of it by an act of will, any more than you could snap out of having an ulcer or diabetes by an act of will. To summarize, trauma can sensitize your nervous system, such that you become hyperresponsive to stress or reminders of trauma. The chronic stress associated with trauma and posttraumatic symptoms can put you into a state of ill health, perhaps made worse by unhealthy behaviors you're employing to cope with your distress.

The moral is this: rather than criticizing yourself for the difficulty you're having, you can understand yourself and, ideally, feel more compassion for yourself. You'll need an attitude of concern and compassion toward yourself, because you'll need to take care of yourself over the long haul. Self-care can be undermined by self-criticism or by just chalking up your problems to being a wimp or crazy—as if the problems were just all in your head, not throughout your nervous system and the rest of your body.

I'll discuss emotion regulation and treatment later (Chapters 12 and 13, "Emotion Regulation" and "Treatment Approaches," respectively), but I want to reiterate an important point here. Owing to your amazingly fast responses to threat, you can become afraid before you know what hit you. Thus you can't prevent yourself from reacting, and you're saddled with having to cope with your strong emotional responses after the fact. The situation is not hopeless, because emotional responses are designed to be extremely flexible. Having been stirred up emotionally, we continually reappraise the situation to see how our initial responses are justified and to gauge our prospects for coping.[133] You cannot help responding, and you should not berate yourself for that. But you can adjust your response after you do have some time to think. You can realize, it was not a mortar shell; it was a car backfiring. It's not my father; it's my boss. Perhaps most important: I couldn't protect myself then, but I can protect myself now. Mentalizing in the face of high emotional arousal may be difficult, but it's not impossible.

And you're likely to need help. One of the most significant problems with trauma in early attachment relationships is the combination of high levels of emotional and physiological arousal coupled with a lack of opportunities for comforting. The feeling of security associated with attachment plays a major role in our learning automatically to regulate our state of emotional and physiological arousal.[76] Again, we can find hope in the flexibility of attachment, because it's possible to develop more secure attachment relationships that help regulate emotion. In addition, becoming more skilled at self-regulation techniques can lower your general level of emotional distress and thereby diminish your hyperresponsiveness.

It's important to remember that, above all, the mammalian nervous system—and the human nervous system most of all—was designed for flexibility and learning. But your nervous system, and the rest of your body for that matter, requires care. You must take special care when you're physically ill, particularly when you have potentially recurrent illnesses that reflect stress vulnerability. Then minimizing stress to the extent humanly possible, learning to cope more effectively with stress, and looking out for your physical health more generally become especially important. Stress researcher Bruce McEwen[264] observed that many of the things we do to decrease stress—overeating, drinking too much alcohol, smoking, cutting corners with sleep—undermine our physiological resilience to stress. Such behaviors just increase the wear and tear wrought by stress. As I'm reiterating throughout this book, healthy behaviors—eating properly, sleeping well, refraining from substance abuse, exercising, and maintaining supportive relationships—are essential in coping with trauma.

Part III

TRAUMA-RELATED PSYCHIATRIC DISORDERS

```
  ┌─────────────────────────────────────────────────────────┐
  │ ┌─────────────────────────────────────────────────────┐ │
  │ │    •      C h a p t e r      8      •                │ │
  │ ├─────────────────────────────────────────────────────┤ │
  │ │                                                     │ │
  │ │              DEPRESSION                             │ │
  │ │                                                     │ │
  │ └─────────────────────────────────────────────────────┘ │
  └─────────────────────────────────────────────────────────┘
```

The preceding chapters have described the complex effects of trauma on attachment, emotion, memory, the self, relationships, and physiology. The next few chapters examine the effects of traumatic experience from a somewhat different perspective—through the lens of psychiatric diagnosis. That is, when the biological, psychological, and social effects of trauma are sufficiently severe as to cause marked distress or to impair your social and occupational functioning, you're considered to have a psychiatric disorder. If you're in treatment for trauma-related problems, I think you should learn what your diagnosis is, and you should know something about it. A psychiatric diagnosis, like any other medical diagnosis, is made on the basis of a group of symptoms that tend to cluster together in a *syndrome*. These syndromes are delineated in the *Diagnostic and Statistical Manual of Mental Disorders*, now in its fourth edition, DSM-IV-TR.[2] I start this section with depression, because it's the most frequent disorder we encounter in conjunction with severe trauma.[257]

Depression results from sustained, unresolvable stress.[297] Little wonder, then, that depression is commonly associated with traumatic stress. Darwin[116] made the connection plain in characterizing fear as "the most depressing of all the emotions" (p. 81).

As described in Chapter 7 ("Illness"), repeated stress can result in sensitization, such that you react more strongly to subsequent stress rather than less so. Sensitization might take the form of fearfulness, irritability, and intensified reactions to stressful events. Sensitization to stress might also take the form of depression,[298] and the stress pileup concept is especially helpful in understanding depression.[265] I'm making a potentially confusing point, because we tend to think of depression as shutting down into a state of relative inactivity. Yet depression is also a high-stress state. Hence you can be inactive *and* internally agitated when you're in a state of depression.

There are many pathways to depression; trauma is only one of them, but it's a common contributor. When trauma plays a significant role in the development of depression, we can think in terms of posttraumatic depression,[25] a state of depression intertwined with fearfulness, anxiety, and a high level of reactivity. In understanding posttraumatic depression, it's helpful to reiterate the distinction between depression and anxiety (see Chapter 3, "Emotion"): depression is the absence of positive emotion, and anxiety is the presence of negative emotion. Writer Andrew Solomon[299] likened depression and anxiety to fraternal twins. This analogy is nowhere more true than for persons who are struggling with posttraumatic depression, who know all too well the truth of Darwin's point that fear is the most depressing of the emotions.

In all that follows, I'm not using the term *depression* to refer to the normal blue feeling that most people have from time to time but rather to refer to psychiatric illness. Yet, even within the realm of illness, depression varies in severity and duration. The prototype of severe depression is a *major depressive episode*, which typically results in significant impairment in ability to function. Depressed mood is accompanied by physical symptoms such as problems with eating and sleeping as well as negative thinking and feelings of low self-worth. By definition, an episode of major depression must last at least 2 weeks,[2] although such episodes typically last much longer. *Dysthymia* is a prolonged episode of depressed mood—at least 2 years—with symptoms similar to major depression but less severe, resulting in less obvious impairment of functioning. Not uncommonly, more acute episodes of major depression are superimposed on more chronic periods of dysthymia, a combination characterized as *double depression*.[300] In addition, *depressive personality disorder* does not represent a distinct change in mood but rather a personality disposition characterized by general gloominess, pessimism, feelings of inadequacy, and guilt feelings.[301]

In this chapter, I'll first describe how a pileup of stress over the course of development contributes to a vulnerability to depression. Plainly, a history of traumatic stress and posttraumatic symptoms plays a major role in stress pileup. Second, I'll link trauma to depression through the concept of oppression. Finally, I'll review the challenges in coping with depression, construed as the catch-22s of depression, the gist of which is this: all the things you need to do to recover from depression are made difficult—but not impossible—by the symptoms of depression.

Developmental Perspective

We can best appreciate the potential role of stress pileup in depression by taking a developmental perspective (see Figure 8–1). Unfortunately, the stress sensitization process can start at the beginning of life and continue throughout. Fortunately, resilience, the capacity to cope with stress, also develops throughout life. Of course, in the face of excess stress pileup, we must make an active effort to enhance our resilience.

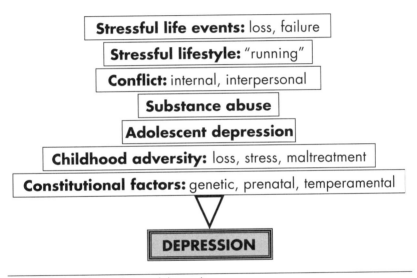

FIGURE 8–1. Stress pileup and depression.

This section lists a number of potential contributors to stress pileup, including genetic vulnerability to stress. But you should not infer that all these factors are required for depression to develop, nor should you infer that these are the only pathways to depression. Most important, whether or not you've experienced trauma or other forms of severe stress, you should not overlook the possibility that your depression is associated with another physical condition. Depression may be associated with Parkinson's disease or Alzheimer's disease, thyroid disease, heart disease, HIV and other infections, certain cancers, and multiple sclerosis, just to give a few examples. And depression also can be secondary to use of certain medications as well as to alcohol and drug abuse. Hence, even when stress is conspicuous, it's crucial to be evaluated and treated for potentially related general medical conditions.

Constitutional Factors

As in other major psychiatric illnesses, genetic makeup makes a substantial contribution to vulnerability to depression.[302] Of course, genes are not destiny; it's the interaction between genetic makeup and experience that determines developmental outcomes.[284] Not only do genetic factors influence the risk of responding to stressful life events with depression, but also, as described in the previous chapter, genetic factors contribute to individual differences in personality (such as risk-taking propensity) that play a role in our likelihood of exposing ourselves to stress and trauma.

As discussed in Chapter 3 ("Emotion"), we can construe these biologically based personality characteristics as *temperament* which, like all else in our genetic makeup, is influenced by our experience over a lifetime. Although nowhere near as well established as anxious temperament,[129] the concept of depressive temperament merits our consideration. Psychiatrist Hagop Akiskal[303] characterized persons with depressive temperament as humorless, pessimistic, introverted, preoccupied with inadequacy, overcritical, and self-critical. He also noted some positive features: depressive persons are reliable, dependable, and devoted, as evident, for example, in their penchant for hard work.

I mention temperament only to underscore that a developmental approach to understanding depression should include individual differences in genetically based biological constitution. Of course, as we've seen in Chapter 7 ("Illness"), experience substantially shapes our biological constitution from the outset, and stress interacts with genetic makeup from the beginning of life.

Mother-Infant Depression

We all know that depression, like other emotions, seems contagious.[304] Not surprisingly, infants of depressed mothers are likely to show signs of depression. More surprising, this process of transmission may precede birth; the pregnant woman's physiological stress can have an impact on the developing fetus,[305] such that infant depression is evident immediately after birth.[306] These infants' depression is evident not just in their unresponsive behavior but also in their physiology. For example, the infants' and mothers' matching biochemical profiles show elevated stress hormones. Maternal depression is also associated with fetal hyperactivity in the second trimester of pregnancy, interpreted as showing a heightened need for self-stimulation in response to the mother's relative inactivity. This research shows that wear and tear on the nervous system can start from the inception of life, perhaps sowing the seeds of sensitization. To reiterate a central point of Chapter 7, however, keep in mind that these physiological effects, along with depressed behaviors, are potentially reversible.

While the prenatal exposure to stress is a relatively new area of research, research on postnatal influences of maternal depression is more extensive.[307] Evidence suggests a matching process in which infants of depressed mothers also show depressed behavior: they're less active and less responsive; they vocalize and smile less; and they show more negative emotions, such as crying and other forms of irritability. These depressed mother-infant pairs engage in fewer positive, playful interactions, as well as in more negative interactions. In addition, a wide range of neurobiological measures reveals high levels of physiological stress coupled with impairment in capacities to regulate distress. Stress pileup may begin early in life.

Also consider the attachment context of maternal depression. Secure attachment and the capacity to mentalize stem from the attachment figure's responsiveness to the infant's emotional states. Depression entails diminished responsiveness. Persistent parental depression can result in unwitting emotional neglect. But attachment is highly flexible. An infant will form a secure attachment with a responsive parent and an insecure attachment with an unresponsive parent. The same holds for infant depression. Infants who behave in a depressed fashion with their depressed mother will perk up and become more engaged and responsive in interactions with a nondepressed father[308] or nursery teacher.[309]

Thus depressed interaction, like attachment behavior, is an adaptation to a particular relationship. Other caregivers can serve as a buffer. Nonetheless, if the maternal depression is persistent, longer-term effects on children are evident. These research findings underscore the need for intervention in maternal depression, particularly in light of the finding that postpartum depression may affect as many as 10%–15% of women.[310] And persistent maternal depression is associated with adverse impact on subsequent childhood development, whereas the effects are reversible when the mother's depression is relatively brief—less than 6 months' duration. Not only standard treatments for depression but also specific interventions for infants and their mothers as well as interventions that enhance mother-infant interaction have been shown to be beneficial.[306] For example, massage reduced depressed mood and physiological stress in mothers, and, when adolescent mothers were taught to massage their infants, the infants showed less emotional stress—both behaviorally and physiologically.

Childhood Trauma

Early stress can produce physiological changes that increase your vulnerability to later stress. Hence biologically oriented researchers are now concluding that Freud started in the right place by emphasizing the role of early adverse experience in vulnerability to psychiatric disorders.[311] We must be concerned about the full range of traumatic experiences that can befall infants and children, but we have particular reason to be concerned about attachment trauma.

Ample research has shown that multiple forms of childhood maltreatment contribute to the risk for adult depression.[25] I described Antonia Bifulco's method for classifying childhood maltreatment in Chapter 1 ("Trauma"), and her work stemmed from an interest in determining what made women particularly vulnerable to depression in the wake of stressful life events in adulthood.[23] As other researchers have done,[312] she found that all forms of childhood trauma—antipathy, physical abuse, sexual abuse, psychological abuse, and neglect—increased the risk of depression in adulthood.

Adolescent Depression

Unfortunately, trauma of any sort may take place at any point in the lifetime, from infancy to old age. And, at worst, trauma in attachment relationships may span much of childhood, persist into adolescence, and even be reenacted in adulthood relationships. Also, whether or not in conjunction with trauma, depression may emerge at any point, ranging from infancy to old age. I want to highlight adolescent depression in the context of stress pileup, however, because trauma is an important contributor to adolescent depression,[313] and there's reason to be concerned that adolescent depression is on the rise.[314]

As would be true at any age, depression in adolescence is both a result of stress pileup and a contributor to additional stress pileup. Given that adolescence is a pivotal point in development, however, adolescent depression merits special attention. Adolescent depression impedes development in many ways, as is evident in findings that young adults who have recovered from depression in adolescence suffer a wide range of adversities, including lower educational and employment levels, less social support, higher rates of child bearing, greater risk of stressful life events, and lower self-esteem, and—notwithstanding their recovery from severe depression—they continue to show low-level depressive symptoms.[315] Moreover, depression itself is a major stressor, and a history of adolescent depression raises the risk of further episodes in adulthood. The finding that persons with a history of adolescent depression are likely to continue to experience low-level symptoms is of considerable concern, because such ongoing depressive symptoms are the most powerful predictor of subsequent depressive episodes.[316]

Adulthood Life Events

Extensive research shows that stressful life events and difficulties play a major role in precipitating episodes of depression in adulthood.[317,318] Hence it shouldn't be surprising that depression is a common problem in the aftermath of adulthood trauma, such as assaults and rape, combat, and battering relationships. In addition, posttraumatic stress disorder (PTSD) and depression commonly occur together in adults with a history of trauma.[319] To reiterate Darwin's prophetic point, fear is depressing, and PTSD entails repeated experiences of fear. Quite often, stressful events in adulthood will be the last straw that brings on an episode of depression, with posttraumatic reexperiencing symptoms following in its wake.[25]

Unfortunately, traumatic stress of all sorts bridges the whole lifespan. Research on elder abuse and neglect is beginning to accumulate,[320] and its effects include not only emotional distress, physical injury, and financial loss, but also increased risk of mortality.[321] Moreover, given the multiple stressors of old age, not least those involving loss and isolation, it's not surprising that symptoms of earlier trauma can emerge for the first time in this period of life.[322]

Stress Pileup: Summing Up

The foregoing sketch illustrates how we must view trauma from a lifespan perspective, with special attention to the cumulative effects of stress that may produce an escalating spiral of both psychological and physiological vulnerability. Yet stressful events aren't the only contributor to stress pileup. Two other trauma-related forms of stress play an important part: a stressful lifestyle and internal stress.

In talking with traumatized persons about stressors that precipitated an episode of severe depression, I became increasingly impressed not just with the pileup of events—an accident, a breakup in a relationship, an illness, a burglary—but also with the chronically stressful lifestyle that went along with them.[25] Many persons who became depressed were constantly on the go, whether their activities involved caring for children or aging parents, working, community service, or all of the above. In part, I came to think of this hyperactivity as a defensive process. As long as they were constantly busy, they were not thinking about the trauma and related problems. Of course, distraction is one of our most basic means of coping with distress,[323] and it serves to keep the mind off past traumas.

But this form of distraction has its price. My colleagues, Lisa Lewis and Kay Kelly, call this the *run-run-run-go-go-go pattern*.[148] I've come to believe that this pattern makes a major contribution to stress pileup and the wear and tear on the body that renders persons more vulnerable to depression and other psychiatric disorders. And many persons seeking treatment ambitiously wish to return to their prior functioning. To me, the handwriting is on the wall: the high-stress lifestyle contributed to depression in the past, and if this lifestyle is continued, it's likely to do so in the future. A major part of recovering from depression and staying well is reducing stress to the extent humanly possible. Doing so isn't an easy task, and the trauma sufferer who is trying to minimize depression will face a dilemma—giving up valued activities for the sake of reducing stress brings about further losses.

Contributors to stress pileup need not be as visible as running around continually or having a car wreck. Much severe stress can also go on in the privacy of your own mind. Frightening intrusive memories of trauma or just repeated bursts of anxiety, fear, or panic are examples. But internal conflicts also play an important role in ongoing stress. One of the most unfortunate legacies of trauma in attachment relationships is a harsh relationship with yourself (as discussed in Chapter 5, "Self"). Continually condemning or berating yourself is akin to being in a psychologically abusive relationship with another person—in some ways worse, because you cannot get away from yourself. Pervasive feelings of guilt and shame are also another form of stress. Some persons have coped with childhood trauma, including chaotic environments, by adopting perfectionistic standards.[324] Perfectionism adds fuel to anxiety and depression, as the perfectionist feels constantly subject to criticism, never measuring up, always raising the bar after every success.

Many other kinds of internal conflicts contribute to stress pileup. As we've seen, traumatic relationships often involve a kind of push-pull conflict, especially when these relationships involve attachment needs. The abused child, for example, is torn between the need for security and fear of the caregiver, what attachment researcher Mary Main[102] called fright without solution. These same conflicts about closeness can persist into adulthood. You can have a strong desire for touch and an aversion to being touched or a strong desire for sexual contact and a strong aversion to sex. You can compromise, putting up with sex just to satisfy your desire for affectionate touch. Struggling with such interpersonal conflicts and trying to find compromises is highly stressful, and, as I'm emphasizing here, struggling with your own conflicting desires and inhibitions is also highly stressful.

Conflict about anger also warrants emphasis in the pileup of stress. As discussed in Chapter 3 ("Emotion"), anger is a natural response to being threatened; just as we need to be able to feel afraid so we can flee, we need to be able to feel angry so we can stand up for ourselves or even fight if need be. But traumatized persons are often afraid of anger, because they have been traumatized in the context of being threatened by anger. If they expressed anger, they may have been hurt worse. Hence they learn to avoid expressing anger and may even suppress their awareness of their own angry feelings. Moreover, in attachment relationships, it's common to feel guilty about feeling anger and the associated aggressive impulses or fantasies; these feelings come into conflict with loyalty and protectiveness toward the attachment figure. But struggling to contain anger is a significant source of stress on the mind and on the body, contributing to the wear and tear discussed in Chapter 7 ("Illness"). Thus learning to express anger effectively so as to confront and resolve current interpersonal conflicts as well as possible is an important part of relieving stress.

Oppression and Depression

As discussed in Chapter 3 ("Emotion"), we readily understand the adaptive functions of many emotions. Fear motivates us to avoid danger; anger motivates us to confront obstacles; guilt feelings motivate us to make reparation; excitement motivates us to seek rewards. The adaptive function of depression isn't so easy to discern.[325]

One intuitively appealing theory about the adaptive function of depression is the *conservation-withdrawal* hypothesis, that is, that depression involves withdrawal from high-stress situations in order to conserve energy and resources.[326] In effect, you get depressed as you're becoming increasingly worn out from stress, and depression prevents you from becoming totally exhausted. By forcing you into withdrawal, depression serves a protective function by lessening the strain of stress. If depression enabled you to rest, this conservation-withdrawal reaction might work. Yet depression is a high-stress state that hardly provides an opportunity for rest and recuperation. You can't even sleep well.

A more recent theory proposes that depression evolved in mammals as a response to being overpowered.[327] We know that, when flight is not an option, fighting back is a natural alternative. Yet, for persons who are overpowered, fight is not an option either. To repeat, fighting back against a more powerful person can lead to dangerous confrontations in which you're liable to get hurt worse. From this viewpoint, depression is an *involuntary subordination strategy:* it forces you into submission and retreat, preventing you from expressing anger and aggression that would only put you in greater danger. Note that depression is an *involuntary* reaction, not a deliberate strategy that requires conscious reasoning. Mice do it.[328] On the other hand, giving in voluntarily is not inherently depressing.

In Chapter 7 ("Illness"), I noted that one of the major ways we mammals have developed to cope with threat is the defeat response, which takes over when fight and flight are not feasible. As the involuntary subordination strategy theory holds, the defeat response may protect us from dangerous confrontations. Yet, like the conservation-withdrawal reaction, the defeat response is an adaptation gone awry. Decades ago, psychologist Martin Seligman[238] linked trauma to depression in his research on *learned helpless-*

ness. He observed that many animals that were placed in a situation of uncontrollable and inescapable shock seemed depressed; they became lethargic and gave up. Moreover, when the experimental situation was changed such that they could escape the shock, they made no attempt to do so. They had *learned* to be helpless, even when the environmental conditions had changed for the better. Thus the persistence of the defeat response, when it becomes generalized into a global sense of futility, profoundly undermines coping. Being involuntary, this response is not easy to change, but recognizing it as such—mentalizing—is one pathway to change.

With these theories in mind, I find it helpful to think of depression as a *response to oppression.* Often, the oppression takes the form of a power imbalance in a relationship. Thus I think of depression as reflecting an *interpersonal imbalance* as well as a chemical imbalance.[25] This interpersonal imbalance is one way to make sense of the popular idea that depression is anger turned inward. Depression arises in relationships in which anger and aggression must be suppressed. Yet I find that many traumatized persons who are suppressing their anger and aggression struggle consciously with chronic resentment that not only contributes to internal stress but also stokes relationship conflicts that fuel external stress. And, like fear, resentment is depressing, reinforcing the one-down position.

Although oppression is most evident in abusive interpersonal relationships, an extraordinary pileup of stress can also become oppressive, triggering a response of defeat. We can easily feel trapped in inescapable situations, not just physically but also psychologically. And posttraumatic intrusive symptoms—painful memories and strong emotions—also can contribute to the sense of oppression. These symptoms might be akin to the inescapable shock in the learned helplessness research. In addition, it's possible to have an oppressive relationship with yourself, perhaps as a legacy of earlier oppressive relationships that involved harsh or relentless criticism. Ironically, you may become the target of your own anger, criticism, and demands, adopting a defeated and resentful stance toward *yourself.*

From this viewpoint, the way out of depression is through empowerment, regaining a sense of self-efficacy. As discussed in Chapter 3 ("Emotion"), anger can be a source of power when used effectively in the service of self-protection and self-assertion. Anger can be a source of healthy protest. Indeed, if you're heaping anger on your own head, you might see if you can find a way of turning that anger around, *protesting your mistreatment of yourself.* You could become fed up or even outraged at the internal abuse and stop putting up with it, moving out of the defeat response. As I noted in Chapter 5 ("Self"), this process is an important step toward developing a healthier relationship with yourself.

Although depression has an adaptive function, it can turn into an illness that renders you helpless and hopeless, at which point you must seek help. Then, ideally, the illness can be turned to advantage if it prompts you to improve your circumstances and take better care of yourself. But you should not expect to rid yourself entirely of feelings of depression. Like other feelings—fear, anger, and guilt feelings—feelings of depression can prompt you to take stock of your situation and to cope more actively when you're feeling oppressed. Thus it's important to learn to tolerate feelings of depression so that you can use them as a signal of a problem that needs attention and resolution.[329] Not heeding *feelings* of depression, like not heeding physical pain, can put you into the *illness* of depression.

Coping With the Catch-22s

Partly owing to the widespread use of antidepressant medication, many persons who are suffering face the stereotype of depression as an acute illness from which they are expected to recover quickly—within a matter of weeks. But quick recovery is not the norm. A careful longitudinal study of persons admitted to major medical centers for treatment of major depression showed that the median time to recovery (i.e., the time by which half the patients had recovered) was 5 months.[330,331] A substantial minority required a year to recover, and some required 2 years or more. While the vast majority do recover, many recover slowly.

Underscoring the seriousness of depression, a World Health Organization study of the extent of disability associated with a wide range of general medical and psychiatric illnesses[332] revealed depression to be the fourth most disabling disease worldwide in 1990 and anticipated that depression will become the second most disabling disease—following heart disease—by 2020. The Medical Outcome Study,[333] designed to reveal patterns of disability associated with chronic illness, showed that depression generally equaled or exceeded several general medical conditions—hypertension, diabetes, heart disease, arthritis, lung disease—in number of days spent in bed, extent of physical pain, and impairment of functioning. These studies of disability reflect both the typical severity and duration of depressive episodes. While taking heart in the fact that people do recover, we might wonder, why is it so difficult to recover quickly from depression?

I find it helpful to think about the challenges in recovering from depression in terms of a set of catch-22s, the ways in which symptoms of depression interfere with your efforts toward recovery. Table 8–1 lists several examples. Take a prime example: to recover from depression, you must feel hopeful, but hopelessness is a common symptom of depression. So, being depressed, you're likely to receive much good advice: "Just get out and enjoy yourself!" But this advice overlooks a cardinal symptom: inability to feel pleasure. Such catch-22s make it difficult to recover from depression. Moreover, with posttraumatic depression, you struggle not just with depressed mood but also with high levels of fear and anxiety, which also interfere with recovery from depression. Keep in mind that, while it's difficult, it's not impossible to recover from depression; the vast majority do—slowly.

TABLE 8–1.   Some catch-22s of depression

"If you'd just…"	Depressive symptoms that interfere
Sleep well	Insomnia
Eat properly	Poor appetite
Exercise	Lethargy
Enjoy yourself	Erosion of pleasure
Be reasonable	Global negative thinking
Stop wallowing	Tendency to ruminate
Stop isolating yourself	Social withdrawal
Be hopeful	Hopelessness

I'll review the major domains of catch-22s: physical health, pleasure, thinking, and relationships. There's a limit to how much you can tackle at once, and you may not know where to start. With severe depression, I'd place the highest priority on physical health, which is a precondition for all else. Medication is likely to provide benefit not just in relation to physical health but also in all other domains. Specific therapies have been devised for the domains of pleasure (behavior therapy), thinking (cognitive therapy), and relationships (interpersonal therapy). Most depressed persons struggle with all domains, so I'll say a bit about each one here and will amplify some of these points in the last section of this book (Part IV, "Healing").

Keep in mind that, if you're depressed, your symptoms will hamper your efforts in one or more of these domains. The best approach is to set modest goals and try to remain content with small steps, as well as recognizing that temporary setbacks are not uncommon. Recognize another catch-22: slow progress toward goals can be depressing,[334] so it's best to keep realistic short-term goals in the forefront of your mind. Also keep in mind that the various strategies highlighted here are hardest to implement when you're trying to recover from depression; they're best used as preventive measures. Ironically, you can best follow all this good advice when you're not depressed, minimizing the risk of recurrence of depressive episodes.

Physical Health

Given that depression is a sign of severe psychological and physiological stress, we can think of depression as one manifestation of ill health. In discussing this topic in my educational group on depression,[265] I routinely ask how many patients feel physically unwell—virtually all hands go up.

Three cornerstones of good physical health are adequate sleep, good nutrition, and physical fitness. Chronically high levels of stress hormones associated with depression can interfere with all three,[279] contributing to problems with sleep, appetite, and energy.

While antidepressant medication may help alter these stress-induced physiological changes, you also can do your part to help the medication do its work. Conversely, you can impede the medication's effectiveness by perpetuating stress. Consider an analogy: imagine a migraine sufferer whose headaches are triggered by a combination of fatigue and stressful mental work. Facing a deadline, she's working hard on a difficult project late in the evening, forcing herself to concentrate when she's already tired. And she hasn't been sleeping well in general. She feels a headache coming on, takes medication, and keeps on working. She'd be wiser to relax after taking the medication. Of course, in the throes of stress pileup, she's trying to meet the deadline, so she's in a bind.

Let's start with sleep. Sleep disturbance isn't just a symptom of depression; it's a potential cause of depression.[335] Moreover, anxiety also conspires with depression to impede sleep.[336] And sleep disturbance plays a major role in stress pileup as people struggle with the slide into depression. Most sleep disturbance in depression takes the form of sleeping too little (insomnia), although some depressed persons sleep too much (hypersomnia), perhaps in part to compensate for a lack of restful sleep. The catch-22: given that depression entails being overloaded with stress, you need rest to recover from depression; yet you need to recover from depression so you can sleep! Perhaps with the assistance of medication, you'll do best by maintaining adequate sleep hygiene (see Chapter 12, "Emotion Regulation").

Major depression is typically associated with a decrease in appetite and weight loss, and poor nutrition further undermines your general health and energy level. Many depressed persons must force themselves to eat. Fortunately, some find that, although they have no appetite or interest in food, when they start to eat, their appetite gets sparked. This effect is a form of the salted-peanut phenomenon: eating one stimulates the desire to eat more.[337]

Stress—and sometimes severe depression—also can be associated with an *increase* in appetite and overeating. We know that overeating—typically foods high in sugar and fat—is a common way of attempting to cope with stress, but it also undermines resilience to stress in the long run.[264] Mood researcher Robert Thayer[338] observed that stressed persons are most likely to binge in a state of *tense tiredness,* especially in the late afternoon and evening. High-sugar, high-fat foods are both calming and energizing in the short run, a setup for an addictive pattern of eating. Yet this pattern can backfire in many ways, in part because an immediate burst of energy may be followed by lowered energy an hour later. Of course, weight gain contributes to depression and a range of health problems, including the stress-related wear and tear on physiology that is part and parcel of the state of ill health related to trauma and depression.

The benefits of exercise for anxiety and mood are widely touted, and rightly so. Thayer's research shows that a brisk, ten-minute walk is an ideal alternative to binge eating as a route to a state of calm energy. Of course, when you're depressed, exercising is difficult, because fatigue and lack of energy are so common in depression. No wonder eating is so appealing. But the beauty of exercise is that it readily lends itself to very gradual increases. You may need to start at the beginning, not with exercise but with more basic activity. If you're severely depressed, getting out of bed can be a major challenge— even sitting up in bed or putting your feet over the edge of the bed may be significant steps. Taking a shower and getting dressed can be a monumental task for severely depressed persons. Getting up and going from one room to another or taking a trip to the mailbox can be significant steps. You might build up to longer walks. Ideally, when you're doing relatively well, you might engage in regular aerobic exercise: 30 minutes of aerobic exercise three times weekly can have a significant antidepressant effect.[339] To reiterate, you can think of exercise not just as a way of facilitating recovery from depression after you're out of the deepest phase but also as a way of maintaining positive mood and preventing recurrence. Moreover, exercise is among the best ways to reverse and prevent the stress-related wear and tear on the body that contributes to depression and other forms of ill health.[264]

Pleasure

Here's some irritating advice for the depressed person: "Quit moping around and go out and have some fun!" Keep in mind the idea of depression as a lack of cerebral joy juice; the pleasure circuits aren't working.[340] Chances are, if you could really have fun, you wouldn't be severely depressed. I think you can force yourself to be active, but I don't think you can force yourself to feel pleasure. The best you can do when you're depressed is try to be active in general and to engage in activities that might provide an *opportunity* to feel pleasure. Gradually, as you become more active, you'll find that pleasure begins to return, if only faintly and fleetingly at first.

Psychologist Peter Lewinsohn,[341] well aware of this catch-22, spent decades developing ways depressed persons can gradually increase their participation in pleasant events and improve their mood. The broad strategy is straightforward: you take stock of the range of activities that might provide pleasure, keep a record of the relation between engaging in those activities and your mood, and gradually increase activities that boost your mood. At the very least, engaging in activities may take your mind off your suffering for a time. Eventually, you're likely to notice the return of pleasure, although you should anticipate that it might not last. Improvement is gradual. I think it's important to pay attention to subtle feelings that might herald the return of pleasure, even moments of interest in something. Thus I'm advocating mentalizing emotionally in relation to enjoyable emotions as well as distressing emotions. A bit of caution: some persons recovering from depression hit on something they enjoy, then they overdo it. I worked with a woman who discovered that flower arranging boosted her mood, then she got so carried away with it that she burned herself out on it. Let pleasure return slowly; it's best not to try to force it.

Thinking

Cognitive therapy is the most widely researched form of psychotherapy for depression, and its effectiveness is well demonstrated.[342] Cognitive therapy targets the negative thoughts that go with depression. Taking the perspective of Chapter 5 ("Self"), because cognitive therapy alters your undeservedly negative thinking about yourself, you might think of it as one practical way of improving your relationship with yourself.

I don't believe that negative thinking *causes* depression; I believe that your depressed mood has your thinking by the tail.[343] Regardless of which is the chicken and which is the egg—thinking or mood—there's no doubt that, when you're becoming depressed, you can drag yourself right into the bottom of the pit with negative thinking.[344] As the saying goes, when you're in a hole, the first thing to do is stop digging!

Intuitively aware of the catch-22s, many people have an adverse reaction to the idea of cognitive therapy, associating it with the power of positive thinking. Like having fun, if you could think positively, chances are you wouldn't be depressed. Psychiatrist Aaron Beck, who pioneered cognitive therapy,[187] stated emphatically that he was not advocating positive thinking but rather advocating thinking that was more realistic. Alternatively, cognitive therapy may hinge on the power of nonnegative thinking.[345] Of course, in the context of stressful life events and difficulties as well as seriously troubled relationships, much of the negative thinking depressed persons engage in is *not* unrealistic or distorted;[346] bad things really have happened, they do have negative implications, and that's a major reason for depressed mood.

Yet the *meaning* you give to stressful events plays an important role in the evolution of depression. Viewing yourself as helpless, trapped, a failure, or worthless can make a bad situation worse. As cognitive therapy emphasizes, depression stems from a particular *style* of negative thinking, namely, *global* negative thinking. Instead of thinking specifically and realistically, "I really screwed that up," the depressed person thinks, "I'm completely worthless, always have been, and always will be." When things go badly, the challenge is to avoid getting *stuck* in such negative thinking. Ruminating about negative thoughts—often with the *illusion* that you're engaging in problem solving—is a major contributor to depression.[347]

Positive thinking is certainly helpful if you can do it but, when you're depressed, you might better aim for more refined negative thinking. If you fail a test and think, "I'm a total loser," you're stuck. If you think, "I need to start studying sooner," you have a constructive direction, moving from ruminating to problem solving. More broadly, I'd emphasize the need to *question* your global negative thinking—take issue with it—and to think more *flexibly*, trying to see the stressful situation from more than one point of view. "I looked like a fool," *and* "Nobody will hold it against me." The catch-22: it's hard to think flexibly when you're severely depressed, in part because the areas of the brain that support flexible thinking may be compromised by depression.[348,349] Thus, when you're depressed, you need the support of others to help you think more realistically and flexibly.

Mentalizing in the midst of depression exemplifies needed flexibility. You can learn to identify depressed mood as a state of mind and recognize that your negative thinking does not reflect the absolute truth. You may have heard—and have been irritated by—the admonition, "That's just your depression talking!" You might feel that such statements minimize your plight. But one highly effective treatment for depression—mindfulness-based cognitive therapy for depression—helps patients recognize the impact of depressed mood on their thinking, take a somewhat detached stance from it, and avoid succumbing to ruminating themselves into severely depressed states.[350] Incorporating mindfulness meditation (see Chapter 12, "Emotion Regulation"), this treatment enhances patients' awareness of their mental states and the influence of their feelings on their thinking. Respecting the catch-22s, the treatment is employed with patients who have substantially recovered from depression and is intended to prevent recurrence of additional episodes.

Relationships

Separation, loss, and social isolation are major stressors and the most obvious precipitants of depression. No wonder that depressed persons are encouraged to socialize. The catch-22: social withdrawal is a common symptom of depression. Interacting with other persons—particularly maintaining a cheerful front—takes a great deal of concentration, effort, and energy.

No doubt, feelings of low self-worth and negative thinking can sensitize you to feeling rejected by others when you're depressed. Yet extensive research has borne out what every depressed person knows from experience: depression often does elicit social rejection. Several features of depressed behavior make it difficult for others to stay positively engaged. Depressed persons tend to avoid eye contact; they do not smile much; their faces are relatively unexpressive; they talk slowly and don't say much; and they tend not to show ordinary politeness, for example, not taking an interest in other persons.[351] Thus depression, like many other emotions, tends to be contagious.[304] In addition, depressed persons often seek criticism to reaffirm their negative self-concept, and, plagued by negative thinking and ruminations, many depressed persons repeatedly seek and reject reassurance, which can be irritating to others.[352] Hence depressed persons are apt to behave in ways that undermine what they most need, as others are inclined to withdraw. Being aware of these depressed behaviors may help you counter this process.

But others' withdrawal is not the only problem. Owing to their mood and behavior, many depressed persons encounter active criticism, especially in their close relationships.[353] In turn, although they generally direct their anger toward themselves, many depressed persons feel chronically resentful and periodically lose their cool, erupting in anger at others, perpetuating the arguments and criticism. Then interpersonal conflict and social withdrawal alternate, each adding fuel to depression.

I think the relationship domain of catch-22s is by far the most complicated. Couples and marital therapy may be essential to help with the struggles in close relationships. Although it is challenging to do so, it's important to appreciate the plight of those who care about you: your withdrawal and irritability may frustrate their compassionate efforts to provide support, and they may feel helpless when their efforts fail. Caregivers walk a tightrope and easily fall off, at worst, alternating between critically pressuring you to do all the things your symptoms make difficult and then giving up and withdrawing when their efforts fail or backfire (see Figure 8–2). Staying on the tightrope entails providing steadfast encouragement and availability, but it's not easy to maintain this middle ground. Often caregivers need coaching. They might benefit, for example, from being reminded that you don't need them to *do* anything to fix you, but rather just listening and being available may suffice. They may feel they must do more than this. Also, making use of other forms of help, such as medication and psychotherapy, may relieve caregivers of some of the burden, taking some of the pressure off them.

As with all else, in socializing you must go slowly. It's easy to overdose

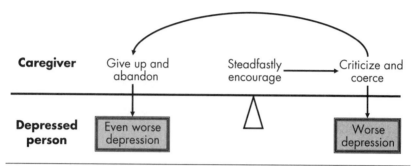

FIGURE 8–2. The caregiver's tightrope.

by going to a lively party where everyone seems to be having fun; then you may feel only more isolated and alienated. Participating in activities in which the demands for conversation are minimal, such as going to a movie or a concert, may be a good first step. Also it's easiest to interact with persons who are relatively tolerant of depression—not uncommonly persons who have struggled with it themselves.

Difficult Versus Impossible

In closing, I want to reiterate the important fact that the vast majority of persons recover from episodes of major depression. The many catch-22s are daunting, and it's therefore little wonder that it can take so long to recover. You can facilitate recovery by seeking help. Although you may want to be alone, when you're severely depressed you may not be able to recover without help. At worst, the catch-22s can make it *impossible* to recover *without help*. With help, you can gradually overcome them.

Appreciating that depression is a serious physical illness that impedes all you need to do to recover from it may help you be more compassionate with yourself as you aspire to take small steps toward realistic goals that will gradually move you along the path to recovery. Remember, you can't recover from an illness by a mere act of will. Not one act of will but many acts of will are needed. Moving forward on the path, some persons manage to kindle a fighting spirit that helps carry them further. Just as there are many vicious circles, there are also benign circles. As your depression lifts, you're increasingly able to do all you need to do to recover, and you can also make increasing use of others' support. Ultimately, you'll be in a nondepressed state, and then you can more easily follow all this good advice so as to stay well.

Chapter 9

POSTTRAUMATIC STRESS DISORDER

Posttraumatic stress disorder (PTSD) is aptly named; it's a disorder that develops *after* traumatic stress. It's a cruel illness, adding insult to injury. Experiencing extremely stressful events induces an illness that renders sufferers vulnerable to continually reliving those experiences in their mind afterward, in the form of flashbacks or nightmares. As psychoanalyst Jonathan Lear[3] put it, having been traumatized by real events, the mind further traumatizes itself. Naturally, PTSD sufferers attempt to avoid stirring up these painful traumatic memories, but they remain highly anxious, and their avoidance blocks the possibility of coming to terms with the trauma. Healing entails mentalizing, making these memories emotionally bearable.

PTSD is one of several anxiety disorders. Because anxiety is a prominent emotional reaction to traumatic experience, the full range of anxiety disorders may stem from trauma. For a long while after traumatic events, *generalized anxiety* may be the tip of the iceberg. The symptoms of hyperarousal may occur without any connection to memories of traumatic experience. Trauma may also contribute to *panic attacks*—abrupt onsets of intense fear with prominent physical symptoms including palpitations, pounding heart, or accelerated heart rate; sweating; trembling or shaking; sensations of shortness of breath or smothering; a feeling of choking; chest pain or discomfort; nausea or abdominal distress; feeling dizzy, unsteady, lightheaded, or faint; feelings of unreality or detachment from oneself; fear of losing control or going crazy; fear of dying; numbness or tingling sensations; and chills or hot flushes.[2] Furthermore, it's not uncommon for persons who have had an isolated traumatic experience to develop *phobias* in relation to the traumatizing situation. For example, an individual who has been in an automobile accident may develop a driving phobia. Children who have been severely bitten by a dog may develop phobias in relation to dogs or other pets. Such reactions could be construed as posttraumatic simple phobias.[354]

Although trauma may contribute to a wide range of psychiatric disorders, including generalized anxiety, panic, and phobias, PTSD is the only diagnosis that *requires* a history of exposure to potentially traumatic events. PTSD entails experiencing anxiety in conjunction with traumatic memories. The psychiatric diagnostic manual[2] spells out the traumatic basis of PTSD as follows: "The person experienced, witnessed, or was confronted with an event or events that involved actual or threatened death or serious injury, or a threat to the physical integrity of self or others"; and "The person's response involved intense fear, helplessness, or horror" (p. 467). As detailed in Chapter 1 ("Trauma"), such experiences are not rare; they're an enduring part of our human condition.

A Capsule History

Although the scope of traumatic events is vast, and the psychological sequelae of trauma have been appreciated for centuries,[355] our modern concept of PTSD has its origins in combat-related trauma. In World War I, the term *shell shock* was employed to implicate subtle brain damage associated with exposure to explosions. In World War II, the term *combat fatigue* continued to imply that physical reactions were at the root of the disabling symptoms.

The concept of PTSD was introduced into the diagnostic nomenclature in 1980 after extensive experience in treating Vietnam veterans.[11] By that time, it was possible to formulate the diagnostic criteria on the basis of extensive research. Decades after the war, the devastating psychological effects of the Vietnam War continued to come to light. Although the majority of veterans successfully readjusted, the National Vietnam Veterans Readjustment Study[356] found the lifetime prevalence of PTSD to be nearly one-third for men and more than one-fourth for women who had served in the Vietnam theater. Moreover, nearly two decades after the war, 15% of the men and

8% of the women continued to suffer from PTSD.

Whereas combat trauma has been in the forefront of PTSD concepts, various kinds of disasters also have long been recognized as leading to psychological disturbance. In 1944, psychiatrist Erich Lindemann[357] described acute grief reactions stemming from traumatic events, including the disastrous Cocoanut Grove fire in Boston. He observed several characteristic reactions in those who lost loved ones in the fire: waves of physical discomfort triggered by thoughts of the deceased, a sense of unreality and detachment, feelings of guilt and hostility, agitation and restlessness, and social isolation. Lindemann noted that the grief reaction might be delayed for weeks or even years, owing to the natural tendency to avoid experiencing and expressing the painful emotions associated with grief. Now, after the events of September 11, 2001, and the ensuing violence, we're more keenly aware of the potential for traumatic grief, as our routine television fare includes countless deaths of civilians in combat and terrorist actions.

Soon after the diagnosis of PTSD was introduced, clinicians began appreciating its widespread applicability to psychiatric disturbances shown by women who had been subjected to childhood sexual abuse, rape, and battering.[29] Then researchers began exploring more systematically the potentially traumatic impact of the full spectrum of childhood maltreatment for both sexes. Although the adverse impact of sexual abuse of boys has long been recognized,[358] the scandal in the Catholic Church finally brought this problem into the public spotlight. As Lindemann observed in conjunction with disasters, the symptoms of PTSD associated with child abuse can be delayed for years, and the traumatic experience itself may be kept out of mind for much of the person's life.

Trauma is ubiquitous. How common is PTSD? Fortunately, most persons who are exposed to potentially traumatic events *do not* develop PTSD. Psychologist Naomi Breslau and her colleagues[359] conducted a comprehensive study of exposure to potentially traumatic events and PTSD in a sample of more than 2,000 adults in the Detroit metropolitan area. Whereas nearly 90% of the respondents had been exposed to a potentially traumatic event, and the majority of those exposed to traumatic events reported more than one trauma in their lifetime, fewer than 10% gave a history of PTSD. Yet the likelihood of developing PTSD varied greatly depending on the type of potentially traumatic event, ranging from nearly 50% following rape to less than 1% after learning of the serious injury of a close friend or relative.

Of course PTSD is not limited to adults; symptoms akin to PTSD have been observed in infants and toddlers who have been exposed to overwhelming experiences.[360] Like adults, traumatized infants show symptoms of sleep disturbance, nightmares, hyperarousal, intrusive memories, and personality changes. PTSD is also common among older children exposed to traumatic events such as war, crime, injury, and accidents, as well as mal-treatment.

The range of traumatic experience is virtually limitless, and there's no doubt that the specific manifestations of PTSD differ according to the type, severity, and duration of the traumatic events. Yet there's also a striking commonality in responses that justifies the diagnosis. These responses fall into three major clusters of symptoms—reexperiencing, hyperarousal, and avoidance/numbing. Just as troubling, although not part of the diagnostic criteria, is the common tendency to reenact traumatic experiences in relationships, which only adds fuel to the fire of PTSD.

Reexperiencing

Reexperiencing the traumatic event is the hallmark of PTSD. Reexperiencing symptoms encompass recurrent and intrusive distressing recollections of the event, including images, thoughts, or perceptions; recurrent distressing dreams of the event; acting or feeling as if the traumatic event were recurring, including a sense of reliving the experience, illusions, hallucinations, and dissociative flashback episodes; intense psychological distress at exposure to internal or external cues that symbolize or resemble an aspect of the traumatic event; and physiological reactivity on exposure to internal or external cues that symbolize or resemble an aspect of the traumatic event.[2]

Traumatic memories are easily stimulated, and they can be evoked unconsciously, in a fraction of a second. Flashbacks are the most vivid form of reexperiencing. To reiterate a point emphasized in Chapter 4 ("Memory"), flashbacks are not necessarily identical replays of traumatic events; like any other memories, they are reconstructions that correspond to the original experience in varying degrees.[182] Flashbacks typically involve extremely vivid visualization and other sensations, along with a feeling of being back in the midst of the traumatic situation. In addition to visual hallucinatory experiences, flashbacks may involve perceptual distortions or illusions, smells, and painful bodily sensations associated with the original trauma. Often dominated by isolated sensory images, flashbacks may make little autobiographical sense.[361]

Long-forgotten memories can *gradually* be activated outside our awareness by escalating stress and accumulating reminders of trauma. With sufficient activation, these recollections break into consciousness in the form of intrusive memories and flashbacks. This gradual priming process, which has been likened to *kindling*,[269] may explain the delayed onset of PTSD. Kindling provides some insight into how persons who had functioned relatively well for years develop PTSD after an accumulation of stressful experiences. The precipitating stressor for PTSD may have been the last straw in pushing the emotion-memory network over the threshold. Two examples in the literature[362] are instructive. An aircraft mechanic spent many hours guarding a helicopter crash site while the bodies of several of his acquaintances were removed. He did not experience any symptoms at the time. Eighteen months later, he developed symptoms of PTSD after *hearing about* another helicopter crash. Although he didn't witness the second crash, he was involved in the preflight inspection of the craft, and he was to have been one of the passengers. Evidently, the mechanic was sensitized by the first crash, and the second crash was the last straw. An analogous example involved a woman who developed PTSD only after being in the *fourth* of a series of automobile accidents: being struck broadside, being forced off the road, backing into an expensive sports car, and finally being struck from the rear.

The process of sensitization from an accumulation of stressors often goes back to childhood:

> A woman in psychotherapy described a childhood filled with violence, illness, and neglect. Perhaps owing in part to having learned to do battle, she became a successful labor negotiator. Yet the high stress of her job took its toll, continually kindling memories of family battles. Against this backdrop of arousal—circulating stress hormones and active memory networks—a new trauma began to incubate. On her way home from work, she was nearly raped but was spared by her combativeness and a police siren that fortuitously sounded in the vicinity. Within a few days of this incident, she had a nightmare in which her grandfather molested her. Then, a couple of days after the nightmare, she began having flashbacks of childhood sexual abuse.

Sleep Disturbance

As this example illustrates, sleep doesn't necessarily afford respite from traumatic memories. As already noted, the reexperiencing symptoms of PTSD include recurrent distressing dreams. Like flashbacks, nightmares may be relatively direct replicas of traumatic experiences. Yet nightmares also may express the emotional impact of traumatic events metaphorically rather than being a literal replay.[363] Because both nightmares and flashbacks keep traumatic memory networks primed, they may escalate each other in a vicious circle.[364] In addition, the hyperarousal symptoms of PTSD are associated with a state of high anxiety that may interfere with going to sleep. Furthermore, many persons with PTSD show a pattern of abnormal movements during sleep, for example, thrashing around and finding their bedcovers askew when they awaken.[365] Of course, sleep-disordered breathing and sleep movement disorders may also contribute to sleep disturbance in persons with PTSD.[366]

Although nightmares are diagnostic of PTSD, trauma may interfere with sleep in other ways as well. Sleep disturbance is a cardinal symptom of depression. Typically, depression results in insomnia, waking up in the middle of the night or early in the morning and being unable to go back to sleep. But trauma-related sleep disturbance, which may compound the sleep-robbing effects of depression, results from anxiety and fear intruding on sleep. I find it useful to distinguish between intrusive and phobic aspects of sleep disturbance.[336] Intrusive aspects include nightmares, which may reflect efforts to process traumatic memories during sleep. But fear intrudes on sleep in other ways as well. You may awaken in a state of fear or in the midst of a panic attack without being aware of any dream or nightmare;[367] nocturnal panic is common among persons with a history of trauma.[154]

Sleep phobias also contribute to insomnia. Anticipating nightmares, you might be afraid to sleep. Persons who have been sexually assaulted may develop phobic reactions to sleeping in bed or sleeping at night. Some sleep fully clothed, on top of the covers. At worst, these different forms of sleep disturbance can fuel each other in vicious circles. Hyperarousal and phobias create anxiety that can increase the likelihood of nightmares and nocturnal panic. The resulting insomnia lowers your resilience, thereby increasing your vulnerability to anxiety and intrusive symptoms. Hence improving your sleep must be a high priority (see Chapter 12, "Emotion Regulation").

Notably, one promising technique for helping trauma survivors with nightmares is *imagery rehearsal*.[368] The technique involves writing down a disturbing dream and changing the nightmare any way you wish, then writing down the new version. Then you engage in repeated mental rehearsals of the new dream. In conjunction with a cognitive-behavioral group treatment approach in which participants rehearsed new versions of their nightmares for 5–20 minutes daily over a 3-week period, the technique was shown to be effective in decreasing the frequency of nightmares as well as improving symptoms of PTSD more generally.

Reexperiencing Neglect

When we think of reexperiencing trauma, we're likely to focus on the frightening aspects of traumatic events. Yet I've emphasized that the essence of much trauma is feeling afraid *and alone*.[25] In the context of trauma, feeling alone can be excruciatingly painful—most conspicuously, in the context of emotional neglect in childhood. Many persons with a history of prolonged childhood maltreatment struggle with intense fears of abandonment. In the context of such trauma, they're prone to reexperiencing feelings of neglect. Like other intrusive traumatic memories, the reexperiencing of neglect is triggered by reminders, which may include separations, miscommunications, lack of attunement, or feeling ignored.

The 90/10 Reaction

Traumatic memories are intrusive in two senses: they reflect an unwanted intrusion of memory into consciousness, and they reflect an intrusion of the past into the present. Quite often, the reexperiencing of trauma is triggered by a present event that serves as a reminder of a past traumatic event. In itself, the reminder may be a mildly stressful event—hearing a backfire, being slighted, or watching a parent angrily scolding a child. Reexperiencing trauma in the context of such a relatively innocuous event, the trauma survivor is likely to be chastised for "overreacting." As I noted in Chapters 3 and 7 ("Emotion" and "Illness," respectively), patients in our educational groups find it helpful to keep the concept of the 90/10 reaction in mind: 90% of the emotion coming from the past and 10% from the present. In the throes of intense emotions—or in their aftermath—you can consider whether you're in the grip of a 90/10 reaction.

As described in Chapter 7, one contributor to the 90/10 response is a nervous system that has been sensitized by virtue of repeated exposure to extreme and uncontrollable stress. As I noted in Chapter 3, this is called context-inappropriate responding. The emotional response is not inappropriate—the fear circuitry is working as it should be—but it's not occurring in the proper environmental context. Consider the child who learns that an angry scowl precedes a beating. This angry scowl is part of a larger context: father comes home from work stressed out and intoxicated then scowls angrily in response to fighting among the children. In this context, the scowl heralds trauma. Outside this broader context—witnessing a father scowling at his child who's clamoring for a toy in a grocery store—an intense fear reaction isn't warranted. Such 90/10 reactions call for mentalizing—distinguishing the current response as a mental state related to past trauma—and mentalizing sets the stage for emotion regulation, for example, such as by grounding techniques that direct attention to the present.

Hyperarousal

Symptoms of hyperarousal include difficulty falling or staying asleep; irritability or outbursts of anger; difficulty concentrating; hypervigilance; and an exaggerated startle response.[2] These hyperarousal symptoms are characteristic of anxiety.

Hyperarousal and hyperresponsiveness are a reaction to threat. Keep in mind that the fight-or-flight response includes anger as well as fear—hence the hyperarousal symptoms include irritability and angry outbursts, which are one manifestation of a sensitized nervous system. With fear and anger easily evoked, it's little wonder that dozens of physiological reactions potentially are associated with PTSD, expressed in many bodily systems:[369] neuropsychological (e.g., dizziness, blurred vision, altered consciousness); circulatory (pounding heart and irregular or rapid heartbeat); neuromuscular (tremor, various pains, headache, weakness); digestive (nausea, vomiting, abdominal pain, diarrhea, difficulty swallowing); respiratory (breathlessness, irregular breathing, hyperventilation); and others (urge to urinate, perspiration, fever).

Unfortunately, anxious persons are inclined to devote an inordinate amount of attention to potentially threatening aspects of situations,[149] which fuels their hyperarousal. The anticipation of intrusive memories also contributes to hyperarousal. Like persons with panic attacks, those with PTSD show a high level of *anxiety sensitivity* (see Chapter 3, "Emotion"). They fear potentially grave consequences of their anxiety:[156] "What if I have a flashback or panic attack?" This fear of fear can contribute to escalating anxiety in response to ordinary stressors. Hence trauma treatment aims to increase your *anxiety tolerance,* lessening the fear of fear, thereby diminishing hypervigilance and hyperarousal.

Avoidance and Numbing

Intrusive symptoms and hyperresponsiveness assault the mind, which quite naturally tries to shut off the overwhelming stimulation. This self-protective response is the third component of the diagnostic criteria for PTSD: the persistent avoidance of stimuli associated with the trauma and the numbing of general responsiveness.[2] This symptom cluster includes efforts to avoid thoughts, feelings, or conversations associated with the trauma; efforts to avoid activities, places, or people that arouse recollections of the trauma; inability to recall an important aspect of the trauma; markedly diminished interest or participation in significant activities; feeling detachment or estrangement from others; a restricted range of affect (e.g., inability to have loving feelings); and a sense of a foreshortened future (e.g., not expecting to have a career, marriage, children, or a normal life span).

Avoidance

Fearful of anything that might rekindle the trauma, you may have learned what to do to avoid triggering a panic or a rage. You may avoid thinking about trauma as well as talking about it, and you may attempt to avoid any situation that might remind you of traumatic events. If PTSD becomes chronic, your life can become increasingly limited and constricted. A prime example is social isolation resulting from being traumatized by other persons. With a history of attachment trauma, you may be afraid to establish close relationships, not just fearing injury but also anticipating the prospect of rejection and abandonment, which can rekindle traumatic memories of neglect.

As I'll elaborate in Chapter 11 ("Self-Destructiveness"), many persons with PTSD have problems with substance abuse. Substance abuse could be considered one of the avoidance symptoms inasmuch as substances blunt the anxiety and anger associated with PTSD.[370] Little wonder, then, that many persons with PTSD resort to abusing antianxiety medication, alcohol, or drugs such as marijuana and narcotics. All these substances blunt arousal.

Avoiding frightening experience is generally adaptive, and avoiding flashbacks and panic is self-protective; reexperiencing symptoms can contribute to further sensitization of your nervous system.[269] Yet excessive avoidance can be problematic. In addition to constricting your activities and limiting your relationships, avoidance may block the processing that enables you to come to terms with trauma. Then you become stuck, alternating between intrusive memories and avoidance.[371] Moreover, even if you succeed in blocking the intrusive symptoms of PTSD, avoidance may contribute to other psychiatric symptoms, such as depression and ill health, as well as leaving you vulnerable to being blindsided by traumatic memories.[361]

Numbing

Parallel to actively avoiding reminders of trauma in an attempt to block intrusive memories, a more automatic process, numbing of emotional responsiveness, may serve to counteract hyperarousal.[372] As noted in Chapter 7 ("Illness"), one neurobiological contribution to numbing is stress-induced analgesia, a narcotic-like process in which endogenous opioids, including endorphins, block pain.[282] Also potentially contributing to blunted emotional responsiveness are dissociative detachment (see Chapter 10, "Dissociative Disorders"), depression, and substance abuse.

Thus, along with the alternation between intrusive symptoms and avoidance, the combination of hyperarousal and numbing gives an all-or-nothing quality to emotionality in PTSD. Individuals with PTSD may seem emotionally remote, detached, cut off, and unresponsive; then, in a 90/10 reaction, a seemingly minor stressor launches them into a panic or a rage. Hence it would be misleading to propose that persons with PTSD show generalized numbing; reminders of trauma easily evoke intense emotional distress. More specifically, persons with PTSD are likely to have particular difficulty experiencing enjoyable emotions, requiring exceptionally high levels of positive stimulation to do so.[373]

Reenactments

As discussed in Chapter 6 ("Relationships"), it's not uncommon for individuals who have undergone trauma in earlier relationships to recreate it unwittingly in later relationships.[62] Sometimes such reenactments are relatively transparent, as when a woman who was abused in childhood enters into battering relationships in adulthood. Somewhat less obviously, a history of childhood abuse substantially increases the risk of being assaulted in adulthood.[374] Conversely, some persons who have been abused end up abusing others; in this fashion, abuse can be passed on through the generations.[159] In persons who have been abused, *self*-injurious behavior (see Chapter 11, "Self-Destructiveness") also can be viewed as a form of reenactment. Plainly, the last thing a person with PTSD needs is exposure to additional traumatic events; thus increasing awareness of reenactment should be a primary focus of trauma treatment.[375]

Persons with a history of trauma who develop symptoms after functioning well for many years invariably wonder, "Why now?" Current stressors are reminders that activate PTSD symptoms, and *reenactments in current relationships may be the main factor that keeps PTSD active.* Thus, as emphasized in Chapter 6 ("Relationships"), resolving relationship conflicts and finding ways of maximizing security in current attachment relationships is a mainstay of trauma treatment.

Variations in Course

The course of an illness, like the course of a voyage, is its trajectory across time. Psychiatric disorders, like other medical illnesses, have a wide variety of courses.[376] As described earlier, PTSD might have a period of incubation. Symptoms of many medical illnesses wax and wane; so do those of PTSD. Illnesses may go into periods of remission followed by recurrence; so might PTSD. Stress is the culprit: extreme stress precipitates PTSD, and subsequent stress affects the course of PTSD, such that minimizing stress and learning to cope with stress better are key to preventing exacerbations of the illness.

Posttraumatic symptoms may become evident at any time after exposure to the precipitating events (see Table 9–1). *Peritraumatic* symptoms[377] are commonly experienced right around the time of the traumatic events. These symptoms may range from shock, disorientation, and detachment to fear, paranoia, and aggressiveness.[378] A diagnosis of *acute stress disorder* is made when peritraumatic symptoms are sufficiently severe as to lead to marked distress or a significant impairment in functioning that lasts a minimum of 2 days and a maximum of 1 month.[2] The symptoms of acute stress disorder include dissociative disturbance (see Chapter 10, "Dissociative Disorders") along with PTSD symptoms.

TABLE 9–1. Time course of posttraumatic symptoms and disorders

Symptom/disorder	Time frame of symptoms
Peritraumatic symptoms	During and immediately after traumatic event
Acute stress disorder	From 2 days to 1 month after event
Acute PTSD	From 1 to 3 months after event
Chronic PTSD	For 3 months or longer after event
Delayed PTSD	Begin at least 6 months after event

Acute PTSD is diagnosed when symptoms persist from 1 to 3 months, and *chronic* PTSD is diagnosed when the duration of the symptoms extends beyond 3 months.[2] Thus peritraumatic symptoms may evolve into acute stress disorder, acute stress disorder into acute PTSD, and acute PTSD into chronic PTSD. These diagnostic distinctions have some value in forecasting the course of PTSD.[379] Yet arbitrarily drawing sharp temporal boundaries that imply discrete disorders[380] goes contrary to research showing a *gradual* decline in the prevalence of PTSD symptoms over the course of several years after the traumatic events, with the steepest decline in symptoms over the first year.[381]

A diagnosis of PTSD *with delayed onset* is made when the symptoms emerge 6 months or longer after the traumatic events.[2] To the chagrin of many persons who have struggled successfully to overcome a history of trauma, the delay goes far beyond 6 months; symptoms may emerge years or even decades after the trauma, when sensitization and stress pileup have taken their toll in wear and tear on the body.

Complex PTSD

To recapitulate, PTSD is defined on the basis of three main symptom clusters: reexperiencing, hyperarousal, and avoidance/numbing. I've discussed these facets of traumatic responses in terms of emotion and memory. But severe trauma goes beyond these three domains. We've seen that traumatic experience may also have profound effects on attachment, sense of self, and relationships.

Consistent with this broader view, several authors have described trauma syndromes that go far beyond the confines of PTSD, both in children[4] and adults.[382] Severe trauma, including attachment trauma, may affect the whole personality. Judith Herman proposed the concept of *complex PTSD*[228] to characterize trauma that includes not only problems in regulating emotion but also disturbance in identity and relationships along with a propensity to experience harm and injury at the hands of oneself and others. I'd add *existential* trauma that damages systems of meaning and alters one's faith, at worst leading to hopelessness and despair. Complex PTSD was not included in the diagnostic manual, which instead lists a wide range of potential associated features that may occur in conjunction with forms of trauma such as abuse, battering, incarceration, and torture.[2]

What Causes PTSD?

On the face of it, the question "What causes PTSD?" seems hardly worth asking. The answer is obvious: traumatic events. But most individuals do not develop PTSD after a traumatic experience,[359] and some individuals develop PTSD after stressful experience that falls short of a narrowly defined traumatic event.[60]

Thus traumatic experience is the key factor in the etiology of PTSD, but it's not the *only* factor. There's a well-established dose-response relationship between stress and its effects: the more severe the stress, the more severe the symptoms. Although there are exceptions to this rule,[64] the more severe the stress, the higher the likelihood of PTSD.[60] At a sufficiently high level of stress—such as Herman described in the etiology of complex PTSD—virtually anyone is liable to succumb.[191] Intermediate levels of stress leave room for many other factors to play a role. In this section, I examine genetic and developmental factors that predispose individuals to PTSD and then review factors subsequent to the trauma that affect the course of PTSD. I conclude with some comments about resilience.

Genetic Factors

I've emphasized the central role of neurophysiology in trauma throughout this book. Genes play a paramount role in the development and ongoing operation of the nervous system, so it should not be surprising that genetic factors play a role in response to potentially traumatic events. The influence of genetic factors on physiological responses to stress has long been established in animal research.[288] Given that PTSD is an anxiety disorder, it's not unreasonable to suspect that a constitutional predisposition to fearfulness makes for vulnerability to PTSD. As discussed in Chapter 7 ("Illness"), proneness to anxiety is a well-established dimension of temperament with roots in genetic factors.

A comparison of identical and fraternal male twin pairs among Vietnam veterans demonstrated a significant genetic contribution to the risk of PTSD.[383] There was not only a genetic influence on PTSD in combat veterans but also a genetic influence on PTSD in those who did not serve in Southeast Asia, suggesting that the findings can be generalized beyond combat-related trauma. Genetic factors also contributed to the likelihood of *participating* in combat. Thus, genetic factors may play a dual role: first, in predisposing some individuals to wind up in traumatic situations, and second, by influencing their responses to traumatic events.

Developmental Factors

I've described how trauma is intertwined with disruptions in attachment, so it shouldn't be surprising that premature separations are a predisposing factor to stress vulnerability in animals[305] and to PTSD in humans.[384] It also shouldn't be surprising that a history of anxiety problems in the individual or the family contributes to vulnerability to PTSD.[384] Vulnerability to PTSD also has been associated with a wide range of other psychiatric and substance abuse disorders in the family or the individual, as well as with a history of behavioral, conduct, and personality problems.[385] Moreover, responses to traumatic events are cumulative; exposure to childhood trauma may increase the risk of PTSD after adult trauma. A study of Vietnam veterans, for example, found that those with a history of childhood physical and sexual abuse were more likely than those without such a history to develop PTSD after combat exposure.[386]

It's also important to note that developmental factors, like genes, may predispose an individual to encountering traumatic events. For example, whereas participation in atrocities and abusive violence in Vietnam increased the risk of PTSD,[387] the presence of personality and behavioral disturbances before military service predisposed individuals to engage in such behavior while they were in combat.[388] More generally, exposure to trauma has been associated with the same factors that predispose individuals to PTSD, including childhood behavior problems and family history of psychiatric disorder and substance abuse.

Posttrauma Factors

The concept of stress pileup underscores the fact that PTSD often develops in the wake of exposure to a multitude of stressful events. Thus the likelihood of developing PTSD after a potentially traumatic event depends on the extent of subsequent stress. A worst-case scenario: a rape may be followed by an antagonistic encounter with police, an unsympathetic medical examination, and an adversarial trial in which the victim's character is attacked. Fortunately, early mental health intervention can ameliorate such stress after rape.[389] But additional stress is not the only problem. Many ways of coping with stress, such as substance abuse and overeating, backfire by undermining the body's capacity to adapt to stress,[264] further increasing the vulnerability to PTSD.

Availability of social support and the capacity to make use of it can protect traumatized persons from developing PTSD. Conversely, lack of social support—or worse, hostile rejection—serves to exacerbate or to maintain PTSD in those who have undergone trauma.[387] And social isolation can be part of another catch-22, as traumatic experience in relationships, as well as chronic PTSD, may undermine the capacity to make use of the social support needed to alleviate the disorder.

Resilience

It stands to reason that factors such as anxiety proneness, psychiatric disorders, and personality characteristics will affect your capacity to cope with stressful events, as well as your ability to deal with their aftermath. As with everything else, there are wide variations among individuals in coping with illness—physical or psychiatric. Looking at the positive side of the ledger, psychiatrist Frederic Flach has discussed the phenomenon of *resilience* in relation to combat trauma,[390] proposing that we should not wonder why some soldiers fall apart but rather why they *all* don't fall apart.

Flach listed several aspects of psychological resilience: insight into oneself and others, high self-esteem, the ability to learn from experience, a high tolerance for distress, open-mindedness, courage, personal discipline, creativity, integrity, a keen sense of humor, a constructive philosophy that gives life meaning, and hope. Consistent with our focus on mentalizing, he observed that those who coped best with traumatic experiences "were those with insight into the emotional impact of what they had just been through and who were able to express their feelings to another immediately following the event" (p. 42).

Reading through Flach's list of resilience factors leaves little doubt that not only innate factors such as temperament but also early life experience contribute to one's vulnerability or resistance to stress. This list also underscores the potentially pernicious impact of prolonged trauma early in life. The consequences of prolonged early trauma are precisely those that are likely to interfere with the development of resilience as Flach defined it. No wonder that coping with complex PTSD poses such an extraordinary challenge. Several decades ago, Karl Menninger[391] proposed the ideal of becoming "weller than well" (p. 406). The illness is the crisis that brings with it the opportunity to develop new ways of coping and more resilience. Difficult but not impossible.

Prevention

We could best prevent PTSD by eliminating traumatic events. A good start would be eradicating poverty, inequality, and intolerance—wellsprings of violence. Mankind has a dismal record by any account; we might have a better shot by putting womankind in charge. And even if our utopian dreams of minimizing interpersonal trauma could be realized, we'd still have to contend with our wily planet. We once thought developing scientific knowledge could help us control natural disasters, but the twentieth century brought us face to face with the most menacing of our technological creations, weapons of mass destruction that can be employed to turn nature against us. Meanwhile, we can only do our best to avoid more of the same by minimizing reenactments and staying out of harm's way—no small accomplishment in itself.

The next best thing to preventing traumatic events is intervening immediately thereafter to decrease the risk of developing PTSD. But the extent of our capacity to block the development of PTSD, and the best means of doing so, is by no means clear.[392] Crisis intervention in the aftermath of disasters often involves group debriefing methods that encourage participants to talk about their distressing experience and educate them about trauma in a way that normalizes their responses.[393] Yet most research to date does not support the effectiveness of group debriefing in diminishing the likelihood of PTSD, and such debriefings may even be harmful for some participants.[394] As with any intervention, the form of help provided must be tailored to the needs of the individual.

In 1941, in his classic book on war neuroses,[192] psychiatrist Abram Kardiner urged haste in working with combat trauma, counseling that "one can … come none too abruptly to the question, 'What happened?'" His goals for treatment were straightforward, if not easily achieved: "No opportunity should be lost to show the patient 1) that these reactions are appropriate defenses, 2) that the world is no longer hostile, and 3) that his powers to master it are growing" (pp. 220–221).

In the absence of systematic research support for any particular interventions, Kardiner's goals remain sound. To reiterate, from the perspective of attachment, I've emphasized that the core of trauma is feeling afraid and *alone*. Hence mobilizing natural social support systems—relatives, friends, and members of the community—plays a major role in early intervention.[395] As Kardiner advised, encouraging the survivor to tell the story combats the feeling of isolation as well as provides an opportunity to make whatever sense can be made of the experience. Although psychiatric medications employed in the immediate aftermath of exposure to traumatic events may be important in managing symptoms, finding medication that will prevent the development of PTSD remains an unfulfilled aspiration.[392]

Prevention strategies being devised to avert the development of PTSD are best suited to public events. The more severe, complex, and chronic forms of PTSD are often associated with traumatic experiences that are not easily discussible, for example, because of secrecy in the family. In such instances, intervention frequently cannot occur in the immediate aftermath of the traumatic experience. The opportunity to answer the question "What happened?" may only come years—or even decades—after the fact. And the question may refer to much of childhood, permitting no brief answer. Given the fallibility of memory in conjunction with trauma, the answer to "What happened?" may be extraordinarily difficult to reconstruct.

Kardiner noted that the treatment of war-related trauma requires first and foremost the provision of security and support. In effect, the first message conveyed to the survivor must be "You're safe now." For anyone who has spent much of a lifetime endangered, however, establishing this sense of safety is no mean feat. For many, the feeling, "I'm safe now," will not be the beginning of treatment but rather the end result.

Chapter 10

DISSOCIATIVE DISORDERS

Dissociation involves altered states of consciousness in the face of over-whelming stress. Psychiatrist Richard Kluft captured its self-protective func-tion well in proposing that dissociation is a form of mental flight when physical flight is impossible.[396] Dissociative alterations of consciousness take many forms, ranging from feeling spacey, unreal, or even outside your body, to periods of amnesia or "lost time" along with abrupt shifts in identity. We have a correspondingly wide range of dissociative disorders, including depersonal-ization, amnesia, fugue, and dissociative identity disorder (formerly multiple personality disorder). Put technically,[2] common to all the dissociative disor-ders is "a disruption in the usually integrative functions of consciousness, memory, identity, or perception" (p. 519). Think of disrupted integration as *dis-association*—perhaps with a feeling of coming "unglued"—when being fully aware of emotions is unbearably painful.

Dissociative disorders overlap with posttraumatic stress disorder (PTSD) in a number of ways. The harbinger of PTSD, acute stress disorder, includes dissociative symptoms along with intrusive and avoidant symptoms. In ad-dition, flashbacks are dissociative states[397] that involve alterations in consciousness, memory, identity, and perception as the past intrudes into the present and memory takes over consciousness. Given this overlap, it's not surprising that many persons who receive a diagnosis of PTSD are also given a diagnosis of a dissociative disorder and vice versa.[398]

We all experience alterations of consciousness on a daily basis, cycling between alert wakefulness, drowsiness, and sleep. Many of us have been delirious with fever or intoxicated to varying degrees with alcohol and drugs. Similarly, when the mind and brain are put under extreme stress, dramatic shifts in consciousness may occur automatically. These dissociative alterations of consciousness can be extremely frightening, and they often make people feel crazy. But dissociative experiences—although seeming bizarre— are quite common in conjunction with stress. For example, 80% of the population reports having felt depersonalized—extremely detached from oneself, as if in a dream, a common concomitant of anxiety and panic.[399]

Because dissociative experiences can be so confusing, educating yourself about them is particularly important. For this reason, psychiatrist Marlene Steinberg, who developed the most refined way to evaluate dissociative disorders,[212] wrote *Stranger in the Mirror* (with Maxine Schnall) to educate traumatized persons about the wide range of dissociative experiences.[400] With similar intent, this chapter first describes how dissociative symptoms arise in conjunction with traumatic events and then groups dissociative experiences into two categories, detachment and compartmentalization. Paralleling the discussion of PTSD, I'll consider some factors beyond trauma that render persons vulnerable to dissociative disorder. The chapter concludes by pointing out that dissociation is a blessing and a curse and considers strategies for overcoming dissociative defenses.

Peritraumatic Dissociation

As discussed in the context of PTSD, peritraumatic symptoms occur right around the time of traumatic events.[401] In the midst of traumatic events, we're liable to go into psychological shock, our sense of reality abruptly altered. Peritraumatic symptoms, occurring during and immediately after the events, may include being in a daze, feeling disoriented, staring blankly into space, feeling numb, being on automatic pilot, feeling like a spectator, experiencing your surroundings as unreal, feeling as if you're in a dream or watching a movie, feeling detached or disconnected from your body, experiencing a sense of floating above the scene, blanking or spacing out, and being unable to remember aspects of the events. Such experiences have been observed in conjunction with traumatic grief,[371] motor vehicle accidents,[402] earthquakes,[403] providing emergency services to disaster victims,[404] terrorist attacks,[405] combat, [377] and criminal assaults, including rape.[406]

Quite worrisome is the finding that peritraumatic symptoms are associated with higher risk for developing PTSD.[407] Yet the link between peritraumatic dissociation and PTSD may reflect just the sheer severity of the traumatic experience:[408] the greater the experience of shock and overwhelming emotion, the more likely you are to dissociate at the time and to develop PTSD subsequently. Clinicians are concerned, however, that peritraumatic alterations of thought processes might interfere with processing the trauma, contributing to disorganized memories and fueling other posttraumatic symptoms. In the midst of traumatic events, many persons have difficulty thinking about what's happening in a meaningful way that is integrated with their sense of identity. For example, the experience may seem like a string of unconnected impressions and may feel as if it were happening to someone else.[409] Such disruption in processing interferes with mentalizing and makes it difficult to talk about the trauma, obtain comfort, and make sense of the experience. Similarly, ongoing dissociation in the months or years after trauma will continue to block mentalizing and processing.

Although researchers have focused on peritraumatic dissociation in adulthood, I believe that attachment researchers somewhat inadvertently discovered peritraumatic dissociation in infancy.[25] As discussed in Chapter 2 ("Attachment"), childhood maltreatment has been linked to disorganized attachment, one form of which is disorientation.[410] Traumatized infants show dazed expressions, freezing, and unresponsiveness when observed with their mothers in a laboratory situation. Notably, disorganized infant attachment is associated not only with active maltreatment but also with a trauma history in the mother. Correspondingly, mothers as well as infants may show altered states of consciousness in the laboratory. For example, the infant may appear disoriented in conjunction with the mother being immobilized and staring into space. Mothers with attachment disturbance conducive to disorganized attachment in their infant are also prone to show dissociative symptoms when discussing their own attachment history.[411] Worryingly, the impact of this intergenerational transmission of dissociation—whether through caregivers' dissociative states or active maltreatment—may continue well beyond infancy. Infants who demonstrated disorganized attachment in the laboratory showed a higher risk for dissociative symptoms in elementary school and high school as well as late adolescence.[412]

Detachment

I think the concept of *detachment* best captures the most common forms of dissociation.[211] Detachment is evident in many peritraumatic experiences:

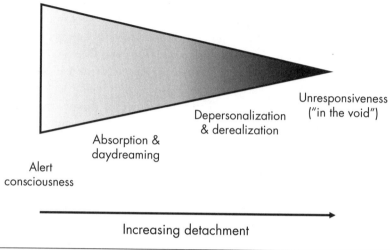

Unresponsiveness
("in the void")

Depersonalization
& derealization

Absorption &
daydreaming

Alert
consciousness

Increasing detachment

FIGURE 10–1. Degrees of dissociative detachment.

feeling dazed, numb, on autopilot, or—at the extreme—outside your body, watching yourself from a distance. I think of dissociative detachment along a spectrum (see Figure 10–1) ranging from alert consciousness (no detachment) to absorption (mild detachment), depersonalization (moderate detachment), and unresponsiveness (severe detachment).

Alert Consciousness

Normal alert consciousness is, above all, flexible. The main function of consciousness is to bring all our knowledge and resources to bear on dealing with novelty, the unexpected, and the unfamiliar.[413] In a state of alert consciousness, you're well grounded in current reality—not just what's going on in the outer world, but also in the inner world, your mind and your body. And you can direct your attention flexibly, as needed, back and forth from the outer world to the inner world. Thus, fully conscious, you're not only aware but also self-aware. To reiterate, consciousness is integrative; dissociation is dis-integrative.

Absorption

What if full awareness of the outer world of events and the inner world of sensations and feelings is painful—even unbearably so? Then you may diminish your awareness, by reflex or by choice. As Kluft put it, you may take mental flight. The first and utterly commonplace step toward detachment is *absorption,* for example, total immersion in a movie, a daydream, or a sporting activity.[414] Within broad limits, absorption is not pathological;[415] on the contrary, absorption is essential to creative activity.[416] In a sense, absorption reflects active *engagement,* the opposite of detachment.

Yet to be engaged in one activity is to be detached from others. It's not the absorption but the detachment that can create difficulty. We all take refuge in fantasy; daydreaming can be a source of pleasure as well as a form of temporary escape. But too much retreating—excessive detachment—becomes problematic, as refuge in fantasy can substitute for coping with reality. And retreating into the inner world can be a slippery slope. Giving up grounding in the outer world can leave you vulnerable to being overtaken by traumatic aspects of the inner world, such as intrusive memories.[417]

Depersonalization and Derealization

Further detachment entails a sense of unreality, evident in depersonalization and derealization. *Depersonalization* involves feelings of unreality associated with your sense of self, your body, or your actions. Feeling as if you're in a dream, acting in a play, disconnected from your body, or merely going along on autopilot are examples. *Derealization* involves a sense that the outer world is not real or is distorted. For example, you might feel as if others are actors in a play or that you're looking at the world through a tunnel. This sense of unreality may include feeling spacey, foggy, or fuzzy, or feeling as if you're floating or drifting. Some persons feel extremely isolated from the world, as if they're in a shell, a bubble, or behind glass. Although depersonalization and derealization can be construed as a form of escape from painful reality, these experiences can be frightening in themselves, as well as leaving you ungrounded and more vulnerable to traumatic memories. Detached, you can feel profoundly alienated:

> A young man sought therapy because he felt that his emotions were out of control. Sometimes he felt tense and irritable. At other times he had inexplicable bouts of crying. He connected some of his feelings with being abandoned by his mother at an early age. He felt unprotected, and he had witnessed a number of violent episodes in his family. Occasional flashbacks contributed to the anxiety that prompted him to seek psychotherapy. But more problematic was his severe depersonalization. He described a continual feeling of being detached from his feelings and behavior. He did not live his life; he watched it. Even when he appeared to others to be animated and involved, he felt distant and hollow. Apart from bouts of anxiety and tearfulness, he felt emotionally bland. He was starved for closeness but felt incapable of intimacy. He went through periods of compulsively seeking sexual liaisons with women, but he could never feel the warmth he longed for. He spent hours in solitude, sitting immobile in the woods, as if in a trance. Yet he could not remember what he thought

or felt during these periods. He found one escape from detachment: he was a talented actor, and he felt fully alive whenever he performed. Ironically, his capacity for dissociation contributed to his acting talent; when he performed in a play, he was totally absorbed, oblivious to his surroundings and the passage of time.

Although feelings of depersonalization are common, depersonalization *disorder* is diagnosed when these symptoms cause intense distress or undermine your functioning.[2] The disorder is frequently but by no means exclusively associated with a history of trauma,[399] and symptoms often begin in adolescence or early adulthood,[418] showing a waxing and waning course, like many other psychiatric symptoms. Derealization is rarely experienced as a distinct problem apart from other dissociative symptoms; hence it's not included in the diagnostic manual as a separate dissociative disorder.

Unresponsiveness

The most extreme form of detachment involves *unresponsiveness*. Patients say they "go away" or are "gone," into the "void" or the "blackness." Or they may just be "blank." In these severely detached states, they may just sit and stare—sometimes for hours. They're beyond reach, as if unconscious. Calling their name may not be enough to alert them. At some point, with or without external prompting, they have a sense of "coming to," although they frequently remain somewhat disoriented or in a daze. It may take hours to become fully alert again; often a period of sleep brings the person back to reality. Having regained full alertness, they feel that they have "lost time."

Memory Impairment

To pick up a point from Chapter 4 ("Memory"), many persons can engage in relatively complex activities during dissociatively detached states. Highway hypnosis is a common—and often disconcerting—example. Many persons hold conversations, write notes, or drive to the store and buy things in detached states. Without anchoring in a sense of self, they're not encoding personal event memories;[419] then they're chagrined when they don't remember having done these things.[211] Such dissociative detachment is an extreme form of *absent-mindedness,* a main contributor to memory impairment.[181] Similarly, peritraumatic detachment contributes to memory impairment, to the extent that the person is not paying attention to what he or she is doing, not thinking about it, and not talking about it—all of which are essential to the process of elaborative encoding of experience that is essential to establishing personal event memories.[179] As described in Chapter 4, without encoding there can be no storage and no retrieval. In addition, to the extent that it's possible to remember events experienced in a state of detachment—including traumatic events—these memories might carry the sense of unreality that went with the original experience.

Compartmentalization

Naturally, you might wish to rid your mind of traumatic memories entirely. But you cannot do so. Next best, you might want to seal away these memories in a compartment. In effect, dissociative defenses do something analogous to this sealing away. A century ago, French psychiatrist Pierre Janet, who pioneered the study of dissociation,[420] described a process of *disaggregation* in which whole realms of experience are excluded from consciousness.[421] As already noted, consciousness is integrative, preserving a coherent sense of self across time. But consciousness can be unbearably painful; you can find it downright intolerable to have traumatic experiences in mind. Then dissociation excludes them by compartmentalizing the mind. Yet dissociative compartmentalization is not a stable solution; these unintegrated experiences are likely to intrude unbidden into consciousness in the form of flashbacks.[200]

Any unbearably painful experience may be compartmentalized, but attachment trauma best illustrates the motivation. Attachment trauma puts the child in an intolerable approach-avoidance conflict: the attachment figure is frightening, and the more frightened the child, the more the need for the safe haven of attachment. Excluding awareness of the frightening aspects of the relationship is one way to preserve the attachment. Psychologist Jennifer Freyd's[31] concept of *betrayal trauma* makes this point plain. Awareness of the betrayal—as in sexual abuse—would endanger the child by threatening the attachment relationship. Thus the abusive aspects of the relationship are kept out of mind—dissociated.

Three forms of dissociative disorder are indicative of dissociative compartmentalization: amnesia, fugue, and dissociative identity disorder.

Amnesia

The psychiatric diagnostic manual[2] describes dissociative amnesia as an "inability to recall important personal information, usually of a traumatic or stressful nature, that is too extensive to be explained by ordinary forgetfulness" (p. 523). Psychiatrist Lenore Terr[422] encountered a dramatic example when she was asked to consult on the case of a woman who was incarcerated for drunk driving and resisting arrest:

Two police officers spotted Patricia parked on the side of the highway and found her to be unresponsive, sitting there like a "zombie." They inferred she was intoxicated and decided to arrest her, at which point she became combative. Patricia awoke in jail the next day and had no idea where she was or who she was. When Terr interviewed her, she had recovered her identity but not her memory. Terr gradually helped her recall the stressful events leading up to the amnesia. Patricia had discovered her boyfriend in bed with another woman and went blank at the time. She did not remember driving anywhere, but she did remember perceiving the arresting officer as a killer. Yet these events were just the tip of the iceberg of her trauma, which dated back to witnessing her intoxicated mother burning to death in a fire, after which she recalled drifting off into never-never land.

Terr's account illustrates a number of features of dissociative amnesia. Although the memories are relatively inaccessible, dissociative amnesia is often reversible,[423] for example, through clinical interviewing. In addition, the example illustrates how detachment is intertwined with amnesia. Because detachment interferes with encoding events, the resulting memories are somewhat patchy. Thus we cannot assume that it's possible to retrieve memories of all trauma, as if they're all in there somewhere. Part of healing is being able to live without knowing.

Fugue

Dissociative fugue[2] goes beyond amnesia to include "sudden, unexpected travel away from home or one's customary place of work, with inability to recall one's past" along with "confusion about personal identity or assumption of a new identity" (p. 526). The travel may range from short trips to wandering over long distances for months. When a new identity is assumed, it often takes the form of an uninhibited and gregarious personality. Like amnesia, fugues are often triggered by stress or trauma.[424]

Although full-fledged fugues are dramatic and uncommon, I find fugue-like states to be relatively common in persons who show extreme dissociative detachment. We might think of a trip to the store in a dissociative state as a micro-fugue. But not uncommon are more extensive and even more disconcerting travels. I interviewed a woman who was very frightened about having driven hundreds of miles from home in a detached state. When she "came to," she was disoriented and had no idea where she was. She found her way to a store, learned where she was, and called her mother, who came to get her. We were able to identify a series of stressors that led to this flight—not just a mental flight but also a physical flight.

Dissociative Identity Disorder

Dissociative identity disorder[2] entails "two or more distinct identities or personality states" that "recurrently take control of the person's behavior"

(p. 529), along with amnesia for behavior in these dissociated states. Dissociative identity disorder was formerly called *multiple personality disorder,* which captures the experience from the inside: sufferers feel as if they are made of different people, often called *alters.* Dissociative identity disorder represents the perspective of the outside observer, who sees a disorder in sense of identity caused by dissociative defenses.

We all show dramatic switches among behavioral states[425] from one time to another and one situation to another—behaving very differently at a football game, a business meeting, in bed with a lover, and in a confrontation with a stranger. Not uncommonly, we do something out of character and may even disown our behavior to some extent: "I wasn't myself." Yet, with consciousness relatively intact, we remember what we've done in these various states and, however apologetically, claim them as our own.

I had a stark introduction to dissociative identity disorder.[426] I had been Joan's psychotherapist for several months during her psychiatric hospitalization, never suspecting that dissociation was among her difficulties:

> The first sign occurred in a psychotherapy session in which Joan—quite out of character—suddenly became angry at me and said, "Goddamn it!" Joan had been extremely reluctant to express anger, and I considered this a breakthrough. Moments later I alluded to what had happened. Joan was totally oblivious to it, denied that it had happened, and accused me of playing a therapeutic game to provoke her anger. As I recounted the events, she began to question her conviction that I was lying, and she became very frightened.
>
> Joan called me the next day to reiterate her confusion and finally accepted that, indeed, she had made this outburst and not remembered it. A few days later she reported that she'd been having periods of amnesia. Minutes before Joan's next session, the receptionist told me that Joan had come in, insisting on seeing me that instant. The patient—now calling herself Mary—entered in an agitated state, handed me a bag containing whiskey and assorted pills, and implored, "Here, take these quickly and hide them! She's going to kill herself with them." I did as she asked, discussing the situation with her, and—for the moment—acceded to Mary's request that I not tell Joan what had taken place. Then the patient switched states, was completely perplexed and disoriented, and identified the experience as being like her other recent blackouts. I accompanied her back to the hospital unit and conveyed to her hospital psychiatrist and staff my astonishment at the emergence of multiple personality disorder.
>
> In working with the patient as Mary, I learned that she came into being when Joan was about 7 years old, apparently in the midst of a traumatic experience. Mary reemerged in college, in a similarly stressful situation. The pattern of dissociation was then reactivated by stresses in the current hospitalization.
>
> A considerable number of the psychotherapy sessions were devoted to work with Mary, who was able to disclose some painful memories. From time to time, she was totally unresponsive, and I had no idea what was going on

in her mind. During one of these states she looked at me and, in a childlike voice, said, "Who are you?" I then realized that a *third* identity had emerged, and I explained who I was. In this state, the patient was transported back in time to age 7. Her whole experience in this state was that of a 7-year-old child, with the associated capacities, memories, and identity. For example, she missed her childhood friends, wanted to return to elementary school, and wondered what she would be when she grew up. It was a challenge to explain to her what was happening—why she was in a grown-up body, where she was, and who I was.

There was a layering of identities: when Joan became anxious, she disso-ciated into Mary; when Mary became anxious, she dissociated into the child state. Each identity employed the same defense. Thus the child bore the most painful early memories that even Mary could not face. At one point, before she had come to trust me, the child emerged in a state of terror. She ran out of my office and could be persuaded to reenter it only if I left the door open. Gradually, she felt more secure and could be reassured quite easily that she was safe.

As her self-awareness increased, the patient gained more control over the switching among identities. Yet one time Mary came into my office in a panic because she could not switch back to Joan. Together, we concluded that she could not switch because she was so angry. As long as Mary was angry, she could not switch back to Joan because Joan could not tolerate anger. Joan had compartmentalized her anger, and our therapeutic work included help-ing her to become less fearful of anger in the present. Ultimately, as her tol-erance of emotions increased, she was able to gain more conscious continuity across these shifts in her state of mind.

Dissociative identity disorder has been documented thoroughly in the clinical literature for more than two centuries,[427] but it was considered ex-tremely rare until recent decades, when clinicians began paying more atten-tion to trauma. Recent estimates of the prevalence of dissociative identity disorder in psychiatric inpatients range from 1%[428] to 5%.[429] Yet controversy among mental health professionals about the legitimacy of this diagnosis and the prevalence of the disorder continues unabated.[430,431] In part, the skepticism about dissociative identity disorder, which often develops in con-junction with severe and prolonged childhood trauma, revolves around con-cerns about false memories. In addition, there's concern that therapists who suspect dissociative identity disorder unwittingly induce their patients to develop the symptoms, for example, by injudicious use of hypnosis. For me, seeing was believing, especially when I was reluctant to see—much less to encourage—the symptoms.

Yet, even if we could agree on the existence of the diagnostic condition, understanding the nature of the dissociative processes involved is another matter. As psychiatrist Frank Putnam,[432] one of the pioneers of contempo-rary understanding of dissociative identity disorder warned, we're seriously mistaken if we think of alters as separate people—even if persons with dissociative identity disorder in fact feel this way. As Putnam pointed out, many other psychiatric disorders, including panic disorder and bipolar disorder, involve dramatic switches in behavioral states, although these disorders do not involve amnesia for different states.

From an attachment perspective, we can think of these switches among dissociated states as involving different working models of relationships. For example, consider a child whose trauma includes terrifying beatings by an intoxicated parent who is dangerously out of control. The child naturally comes to abhor anger. When, as an adult, he becomes angry and flies into a rage, he may be in a dissociative state—a working model of relationships excluded from ordinary consciousness. In his ordinary state of mind, he may be pleasant and compliant. He cannot integrate these two working models of relationships into higher-order consciousness.

I don't believe dissociative identity disorder is carved in stone, as if a bunch of personalities always remain lurking in the background of the mind. Rather, I think of the dissociative fragmentation of consciousness as a defensive process. The traumatized person switches into a different state of mind when she becomes angry or when she has sex, because these experiences are associated with unbearable states of mind in the past. When they are not under high levels of stress, many persons with dissociative identity disorder go for long periods without switching. Like many other disorders—PTSD, depression, and substance abuse, for example—dissociative identity disorder waxes and wanes with stress. It's important that treatment not become an undue source of stress. Treatment approaches that actively pursue alters, encourage switching, and attempt to recover memories of abuse run the risk of abetting dissociation and further undermining the patient's functioning. The goal of treatment should be to gradually promote greater tolerance of a wider range of feelings and memories, all the while promoting greater ability to cope with stress and to develop more secure attachment relationships in the present. Such treatment gradually diminishes the need for dissociative defenses.

What Causes Dissociation?

Unlike PTSD, the diagnosis of a dissociative disorder does not require a history of exposure to traumatic events. Yet trauma is a common cause of dissociative experiences and disorders. This link is most clearly established by research on peritraumatic dissociation, where trauma survivors' experiences during and immediately after the events are carefully studied. Sadly, we can now see this link as early as infancy, in the context of disorganized attachment relationships. Dissociative symptoms also have been observed in children who have been in the custody of child protective services as a result of sexual and physical abuse.[433]

Extensive research also links dissociative disturbance in adulthood to childhood adversity,[434] including sexual, physical, and psychological abuse,[202] as well as loss[435] and neglect.[436] This research uniformly shows that the severity of abuse as well as combining different forms of abuse and neglect—traumatic stress pileup—increases the severity of dissociative symptoms. Not surprisingly, when it occurs in the context of disturbances in attachment relationships, childhood adversity is more likely to result in adulthood dissociative disturbance.[437] As with PTSD, however, trauma is only one contributor to dissociative disturbance. Also important are biological and personality factors.

Biological Factors

It's not unreasonable to suspect that genetic factors contribute to individual differences in vulnerability to dissociative disturbance, like all else psychological and psychiatric. Yet studies of pathological dissociation have yielded contradictory findings, some showing evidence for a genetic contribution,[438] others not.[439] On the other hand, there is strong support for a genetic contribution to the propensity for absorption,[440] as is true of many other personality characteristics.

Although studies of brain functioning associated with PTSD symptoms are well under way, the neurobiological understanding of dissociative states is in its infancy. One research group finds support for a pattern of global *cortical disconnectivity* in dissociative states,[441] a neurobiological parallel to Janet's concept of disaggregation in consciousness. Psychiatrist Douglas Bremner[261] speculates that impaired hippocampal functioning, which has been demonstrated in conjunction with PTSD, may contribute to dissociative symptoms. As described in Chapter 4 ("Memory"), the hippocampus plays an important role in integrating complex facets of situations—the broad context—into coherent memories of events. Dissociative states exclude the broader context of events.

We must also keep in mind that organic brain impairment can contribute to dissociative symptoms.[442] Organic factors include head trauma, migraine, and tumors as well as the use of substances such as alcohol, barbiturates, antianxiety agents (e.g., alprazolam [Xanax]), marijuana, and psychedelics [e.g., LSD]). Dissociative symptoms prominent in temporal lobe seizures may include feeling far away or a sense of observing oneself from outside the body, staring into space, bursting into a rage or fleeing in terror, and even performing routine tasks as if on autopilot.[70] Complicating diagnosis are *pseudoseizures*, that is, seizure-like behavior in the absence of brain changes associated with true seizures. Pseudoseizures may occur in conjunction with dissociative symptoms and a history of trauma, and they are typically precipitated by recent stress, such as current relationships that evoke emotions associated with a history of abuse.[443]

Personality Factors

I've linked dissociative detachment to absorption, and one prominent form of absorption is retreat into fantasy—daydreaming, for example. All of us daydream occasionally, but some persons do so to an inordinate degree, beginning in childhood. As noted in Chapter 4, such *fantasy-prone* children—estimated to be about 4%—live much of their life in fantasy.[210] Their fantasy world can seem more real than reality, as in the example of a girl who felt she was a princess just pretending to be an ordinary child. Given the vividness of their fantasy, fantasy-prone persons are liable to confuse fantasy and reality, leaving them vulnerable to false memories. Underscoring its defensive function, fantasy proneness is associated with a childhood history of loneliness, isolation, punishment, and abuse.

The link between fantasy proneness and creativity is obvious, and those who are fantasy prone can consider themselves in distinguished company. As a child, Mozart endured long journeys through Europe while his father paraded his talent in various courts in search of fame and fortune.[444] In the course of hours spent in uncomfortable coaches, Mozart inhabited an elaborate imaginary kingdom he called "Rücken" ("Back"):

> Rücken had its own geography (conceivably its place names were real ones, spelled backwards), its own laws and its own subjects. It was "Back" possibly too in a Golden Age sense: a return to a world of youthful perfection. Certainly it was a kingdom of, and for, children. Everyone there was good and happy, under their king … there were maps drawn of it—by the servant who travelled with the Mozart family, and perhaps also by Mozart himself, who showed some aptitude for drawing … Rücken was entirely Mozart's own personal kingdom. It offered a respite not only from the reality of slow, cramped, travelling conditions but from all the conditions of reality. Reality included a father who was no royal prince—not even a free agent—but an outwardly humble servant and court-musician attached to the Prince-Archbishop of Salzburg. And reality also meant very early realization that the great people who applauded the boy Mozart often cared little for music as such. (p. 9)

Showing the blurry line between fantasy, absorption, and dissociation, some children learn to cope with trauma by withdrawing into an elaborate world, not just in the aftermath of traumatic events but also in their midst. Illustrating Kluft's idea of mental flight when physical flight is not possible, one woman I treated remembered leaving the room and roaming among the flowers in the garden outside her bedroom while being sexually abused. Here a skill—a capacity for vivid visual imagery—is employed as a defense, for self-protection.

Fantasy proneness, absorption, and the ability to become imaginatively involved in experience are also intertwined with another phenomenon related to dissociation, *hypnotizability*.[414] Hypnosis has a long history in the investigation of multiple personality disorder,[427] and one prominent theory construed this disorder as an abuse of self-hypnosis.[445] Although dissociative states are trance-like,[446] dissociation is not the same as hypnotizability.[447]

A Blessing and a Curse

The ability to take mental flight when physical flight is out of the question seems a blessing—being imaginatively involved in roaming among flowers is highly preferable to being immersed in the experience of sexual abuse. Hence we can think of dissociation as an adaptive response to threat, and we can view the capacity to dissociate as a skill.

From an evolutionary perspective, dissociation has been linked to two forms of defense shown by animals in danger situations, freezing and tonic immobility.[448] Although the immobilized dissociative stare has the appearance of freezing, there's an important difference. The freeze response is a state of high alert, as the animal keeps an eye on the predator and remains immobile to escape detection. The tonic immobility response—a playing-dead reaction—more closely resembles dissociative detachment,[25] which includes numbing associated with stress-induced analgesia.[268] Tonic immobility is observed in animals being subjected to physical restraint, entrapment, harnessing, or confinement; it follows a brief period of struggling and may last from seconds to hours.[449] If animals subjected to these traumas could talk, they might say that they had "gone away."

Although dissociation is self-protective, it's also potentially self-destructive. To a point, detachment might be adaptive in dangerous situation. Going on autopilot and having physical pain blocked by analgesia is far more adaptive than going into a state of helpless terror or freezing. But too much detachment—feeling dazed and disoriented—can block active coping during the time of trauma. Certainly, being "gone" completely undermines your capacity to adapt to any situation.

In addition, many persons with a history of repeated trauma come to dissociate habitually. Even mild stress or anxiety can trigger a dissociatively detached state. Not only does this detachment interfere with coping at any given moment, but it also blocks new learning. Then you're into a vicious circle: because you don't learn to cope, your anxiety continues unabated, and you continue to rely on dissociative defenses. Moreover, dissociating can take you out of the frying pan and put you into the fire; escaping from a mildly stressful situation into a state of dissociative detachment, you can lose your grounding in outer reality, then wind up immersed in traumatic memories. Finally, as discussed earlier in this chapter, dissociation blocks processing of trauma, and potentially becomes intertwined with the development of PTSD—a curse indeed.

Overcoming Dissociation

As with PTSD, overcoming dissociation entails all approaches to healing described in the last section of this book. Some challenges specific to dissociation include accepting responsibility for behavior in dissociative states, using grounding techniques, and achieving a higher level of integration.

Responsibility for Dissociative Behavior

There's a difficult challenge to coping with psychiatric disorders: adopting a sense of *agency*[450] by taking responsibility for your illness without self-destructively blaming yourself for it. This step is hard because, being ill, you feel somewhat out of control—overtaken by your illness. You cannot snap out of any illness by a mere act of will. Nowhere are these problems more challenging than in the dissociative disorders. You might be dismayed by your inability to remember where you've been, what you've said, or what you've done. You might engage in unwanted behaviors in dissociative states. You might be chagrined by your sexual, aggressive, or childlike behavior that you've only heard about from others. Not being fully and flexibly conscious, you might feel wrongly blamed for actions occurring out of your awareness.

Who is responsible for actions in dissociative states? This is a psychological question, an ethical question, and a legal question. The question is not unique to dissociative disorders. Is the intoxicated person responsible for injuring someone in a car wreck? Should a person be incarcerated for a crime committed in a psychotic state? These issues are not new, but they have arisen with particular poignancy in relation to dissociative identity disorder.[451]

Should you be held responsible for actions in dissociated states of mind? Yes. To believe otherwise is to make treatment impossible. Affected individuals often feel that they're punished for their behavior in dissociated states, as if they're being blamed for something someone else did. Certainly, behavior in altered states of mind often results in considerable subsequent suffering. But any person may suffer in one state of mind for actions done in another—regretting the consequences of angry words or feeling remorse for an injury caused by driving while intoxicated.

Accepting responsibility is a major step toward continuity and integration of experience. At first, you may need to accept responsibility *in principle,* even if you have little sense of control in practice. Commitment to treatment entails some acceptance of responsibility, because it attests to an investment in gaining control. You can learn to exercise some control over the switching process, and you can exercise control over destructive behavior in altered states of mind. But it's not easy.

While advocating responsibility, those who treat patients with dissociative disorders must have compassion for their patients' experience of helplessness, and they must have an understanding of the processes that contribute to the felt lack of control.[452] Psychiatrist Seymour Halleck[453] addressed this problem with considerable wisdom:

> In assessing responsibility in the clinical setting, we need not invoke the harsh, "all or none" morality required by the criminal justice system. We can acknowledge that many of our patients, particularly those with severe mental disorders, can make socially acceptable choices only at the expense of a certain amount of pain and suffering. This does not, however, mean that they are without choice. It merely means that their choices are hard ones. (p. 303)

Although the idea of accepting responsibility for dissociated behavior may feel threatening, the prospect of disowning responsibility is even more threatening. Being unable to take responsibility for your behavior—or being told that you're not responsible for your behavior—would promote a profound sense of helplessness and dependency on others.[454] The entire treatment process aims to restore a sense of control and the sense of responsibility that goes with it. Treating the whole person as responsible for all of his or her actions not only enhances this process, it's a prerequisite for it.

Grounding

I discussed grounding—orienting yourself to the present—in conjunction with coping with flashbacks (see Chapter 4, "Memory"). Plainly, as with all other coping strategies, you're in the best position to ground yourself when you're not past the point of no return, for example, "gone" in a state of extreme dissociative detachment. Coping works best as prevention. In a sense, all of the healing discussed in the final section of this book serves as prevention by lowering your general stress level and increasing your capacity to cope with stress.

But we can also think of prevention as early intervention, getting on top of the symptom before it gets to the level of full force where self-control becomes exceedingly difficult. This means that you must learn to become aware of stress as it's piling up and become aware of the first hint of symptoms. I've put dissociative detachment on a continuum ranging from mild to severe, and I've described it as a slippery slope. You're in the best position to stop yourself from sliding all the way down the slope if you can become aware of budding emotional states such as anxiety or irritation that trigger dissociation, as well as becoming aware of the desire to detach or the early stages of absorption, perhaps a budding feeling of spacing out.

The catch-22: dissociative defenses come into play when you do not *want* to be aware of what's happening, because it's stressful and may remind you of past trauma. To cope, you must go against the grain of your desire to retreat, by mentalizing and becoming *more* aware of your feelings and surroundings rather than less so. You cannot simply stop dissociating. Like any symptom, you can only gain imperfect control. But taking responsibility, you can learn to develop better control. The alternative is feeling helplessly out of control, the essence of trauma.

Integration

Imagine a big circle—your self. Imagine a bunch of smaller circles inside—your various states of mind. If you were to label some of these inner states, you'd probably use a lot of emotion words: contented, angry, sad, frightened, cheerful. You might indicate different ages: childlike or adolescent. Capturing both emotion and age, you might label one inner circle "temper tantrums." This isn't a diagram of dissociative identity disorder; it's a diagram of the ordinarily complex self. We all switch from one behavioral state, state of mind, or relationship model to another. We all face conflicts among states—being angry and wanting to hurt someone whom we also love and want to protect. To stay focused on a given task or relationship, we all must compartmentalize, sometimes putting feelings and conflicts out of mind. Imagine feeling frustrated with your boss and going to ask her for a raise. You might do best by compartmentalizing your frustration during that conversation.

But trauma may lead to rigid and extreme compartmentalization of different states, to the degree that your conscious access to the different states—and what you have done in them—may be blocked. The inner circles do not smoothly blend into one another as in a rainbow but rather remain isolated from one another by rigid boundaries, rather like multicolored polka dots. Then you contend with more than the ordinary challenge of integrating various states of mind. Treatment that promotes mentalizing increases flexible access to these dreaded states—memories and ways of feeling in relationships—so as to alleviate discontinuity in daily experience and enhance your potential for conscious control. This process of integration entails expanding awareness and tolerance for emotions, for example, being able to feel angry or sexual without a dissociative switch. It entails an *increase* rather than a decrease in conscious conflict—being able to feel angry and loving toward the same person.

Integration is a matter of degree for all of us; we spend a lifetime at it. There's no simple and fast path to integration for any of us, least of all when dissociative compartmentalization has been wrought by trauma. To reiterate, all the work that goes into healing constitutes the pathway toward better integration: improving your skill at regulating emotions and establishing more secure attachment relationships and broader networks of support, as well as processing the trauma. Dissociative disorders are especially challenging to overcome, because they're generally associated with relatively severe and repeated trauma, and they're typically intertwined with a number of other psychiatric disorders and symptoms. This association is especially true for the severest dissociative disorder, dissociative identity disorder. Not infrequently, patients spend years in treatment working on these problems. Fortunately, the past two decades have seen greatly enhanced awareness and understanding of dissociative disorders and their relation to trauma, leading to improved diagnostic and treatment methods.[455]

Chapter 11

SELF-DESTRUCTIVENESS

When struggling with trauma you're likely to be contending with a high level of negative emotion (anxiety, fear, anger, guilt, shame, and sadness) coupled with a low level of positive emotion (enthusiasm, joy, love, and contentment). Thus you face the challenge of decreasing your negative emotions and increasing your positive emotions. Regulating emotion is a challenge for us all, but trauma makes it far more difficult.[456] Moreover, given that the foundations for regulating our emotional states occur early in life in our attachment relationships, trauma in those relationships can undermine the development of our capacity to regulate our emotions. At worst, stressful events can put you into unbearably painful emotional states, and you may not have effective ways of coping with the events or the emotions. Then you may resort to desperate measures to find relief.

This chapter reviews several desperate measures: substance abuse, eating disorders, deliberate self-harm, and suicidal states. I'll also discuss how these desperate measures can become woven into personality functioning, in which case they're diagnosed as personality disorders. I have called these measures self-*destructive,* because they undermine coping and relationships.

But we should keep in mind that, in one sense, these behaviors are self-*preservative*. Except for suicide, they're not intended to destroy the self but rather to preserve the self by providing relief from overwhelming and unbearable emotional states. We might say they're self-preservative in the short run and self-destructive in the long run. The challenge is to find self-preservative ways of regulating emotion that are not self-destructive, the subject of Chapter 12, "Emotion Regulation."

Substance Abuse

For traumatized persons, the ability to decrease negative emotions and to increase positive emotions is a hard problem. There's one easy solution: intoxication.

Our emotional states and moods, like all else that goes on in the mind, are regulated by the activity of neurotransmitters that facilitate signaling between neurons. By releasing these neurotransmitters, each neuron can stimulate or inhibit the activities of other neurons. Over millennia, we've discovered in nature a wide range of substances that mimic the actions of these neurotransmitters. More recently, we've found ways of manufacturing these substances. These substances either produce stimulation akin to the neurotransmitters or block the actions of these transmitters.[457] The substances that affect our emotions and moods are addictive, because they're rewarding in two senses: they decrease negative emotion and increase positive emotion. If you're anxious and depressed, alcohol and narcotics are highly appealing; they relieve emotional pain and produce pleasure—in the short run. For persons struggling with depression and posttraumatic stress disorder (PTSD), these would be miracle drugs—if they didn't backfire.

It's hardly surprising that a high proportion of persons with PTSD also have problems with substance abuse,[381] and the same is true of persons with depression.[458] Because addictive substances effectively decrease symptoms of these disorders, we often think of substance abuse as a form of self-medication, although it's a poor prescription. Persons with PTSD experience generally high levels of anxiety as well as additional bursts of fear associated with the eruption of intrusive memories. Alcohol, narcotics, and antianxiety agents such as diazepam (Valium) and alprazolam (Xanax) decrease sympathetic nervous system arousal associated with these symptoms.[459] Thus problems with substance abuse commonly arise *after* the eruption of PTSD.[460] Moreover, while we usually focus on its calming effects, alcohol also decreases inhibitions, and some traumatized persons use alcohol to *increase* their experience and expression of emotions. For example, alcohol intoxication makes it easier to express pent-up frustration and anger.[461]

If addictive substances were uniformly effective, I'd be recommending their use. But the long-term costs outweigh the short-term benefits. Although they can decrease negative emotion and increase positive emotion in the short run, addictive substances can have the opposite effects in the long run. For example, intoxication with central nervous system depressants—alcohol and narcotics—decreases negative emotion, but withdrawing from these substances increases negative emotion, for example, producing rebound anxiety. Conversely, intoxication with central nervous system stimulants—amphetamines and cocaine—increases positive emotion, but withdrawal from them decreases positive emotion, inducing depression. Moreover, just like stress, stimulants generate sympathetic nervous system arousal, which may contribute to the process of sensitization that leads to PTSD.[462] Thus stimulants are toxic for traumatized persons, especially when they're already suffering from PTSD. And withdrawal from depressants such as alcohol—which you inevitably do repeatedly when you're abusing them—has similar effects on the sympathetic nervous system. Consistent with this view, patients in treatment for substance abuse generally believe that the substance abuse made their PTSD worse.[463]

The relation between substance abuse and PTSD is a two-way street. Intoxication is a frequent cause of exposure to traumatic events.[459] Drunk driving is a prime example, and motor vehicle accidents account for a substantial proportion of PTSD.[464] Involvement in drug abuse and drug dealing commonly puts people in situations where they witness violence and are exposed to physical assault.[465] And a substantial minority of women who have been raped report using alcohol prior to the rape.[466] Alcohol intoxication increases your vulnerability to sexual assault in a number of ways: it impairs your judgment, blunts your awareness of risk, decreases your capacity to protect yourself, and increases the likelihood of your being perceived as sexually available.[461]

PTSD and substance abuse enter into a vicious circle: PTSD sufferers use substances to decrease their symptoms, but substance abuse makes symptoms worse and also increases the risk of exposure to traumatic events. The same is true of substance abuse and depression.[467] If one of these disorders precedes the other, you might be tempted to think that treatment of the precipitating disorder is sufficient. For example, if depression or PTSD precedes substance abuse, you might think that the substance abuse will take care of itself if you treat the depression or PTSD. Conversely, if the depression or PTSD follows substance abuse, you might think that refraining from substance use will take care of the emotional disturbance. Not so. Once these disorders have developed, each must be treated in their own right—whatever their sequence.

Moreover, each of these disorders complicates the treatment of the other.

Withdrawing from stimulants or using depressants interferes with the treatment of depression. Conversely, depression interferes with substance abuse treatment, for example, by inducing pessimism, undermining motivation, and increasing the desire to self-medicate. Refraining from substance abuse may temporarily increase PTSD symptoms,[468] and processing trauma may increase the desire to abuse substances.[469] Thus trauma and substance abuse are best treated simultaneously.[461]

Eating Disorders

Trauma-related emotions such as anxiety, disgust, and depression all may interfere with appetite and eating.[175] Yet many clinicians and researchers have studied more specific links between trauma, PTSD, and two eating disorders: *anorexia,* that is, weight loss associated with self-starvation, and *bulimia,* that is, binge eating often associated with purging by vomiting or laxative abuse. Clinicians have been particularly concerned about the relation between eating disorders and sexual abuse, given that eating disorders are nine times more common in women than men, and women are at far higher risk than men for sexual abuse and assault.[291]

A wide range of factors contribute to the development of eating disorders, and trauma may or may not be prominent among them.[470] A high proportion of women with eating disorders report a history of childhood sexual abuse, but the relation between eating disorders and sexual abuse is not specific. Sexual abuse contributes to a wide range of psychiatric disorders, and eating disorders are also associated with other forms of abuse and neglect[471] as well as sexual and physical assault in adulthood.[472] Moreover, eating disorders are more likely to develop when women with a history of sexual abuse also have problems with attachment and social support.[473]

Trauma and attachment problems are one potential pathway to eating disorders. We might think of eating disorders as being akin to substance abuse. Eating-disordered behavior often plays a significant role in attempts to regulate trauma-related emotional distress. Also consider that traumatic events, as well as posttraumatic symptoms, involve a feeling of being out of control. It's little wonder that self-starvation may come into play here; self-starvation is a powerful form of self-control, including control over what goes into the body.

Like substance abuse, binge eating can promote an escape from painful self-awareness. Bingeing is a powerful form of distraction; all attention is focused on food.[474] Thus bingeing and purging play an important role in decreasing emotional distress, and these behaviors also provide a way of coping with dissociation by reestablishing a sense of groundedness.[475] Yet, like substance abuse, these distress-relieving effects are short-lived.[476] Bingeing relieves emotional distress by creating a feeling of soothing or by facilitating a state of dissociative detachment. Yet the binge is followed by guilt, shame, disgust, and self-hatred, which then lead to purging. Purging also produces a sense of relief and soothing, as well as a feeling of being back in control. But negative feelings from the whole binge-purge cycle, as well as other sources of stress, only serve to perpetuate the addictive pattern in a downward spiral.

Like substance abuse, eating disorders are highly damaging to the body, adding to the physiological wear and tear wrought by stress.[291] Hence attention to eating disorders is crucial in the treatment of trauma. Just as it is with substance abuse, trauma may complicate the treatment of eating disorders and vice versa:[477] processing trauma evokes distress that eating-disordered behavior temporarily relieves, and refraining from eating-disordered behavior may bring trauma-related problems more into the forefront. As psychiatrist Kathryn Zerbe pointed out,[478] self-destructive as it may be, eating-disordered behavior is intended to preserve the self, and more effective means of self-preservation can be provided in the treatment of eating disorders. When eating disorders and trauma are intertwined, both problems must be addressed in treatment.

Deliberate Self-Harm

A young man with a childhood history of physical abuse and emotional neglect was extremely fearful of close relationships, and he had become a recluse since he left high school. He had a night job that required virtually no contact with anyone. He wasn't content with his isolation; on the contrary, he often felt acutely lonely. His loneliness was intermingled with self-criticism and self-hatred. When the pain became too great to bear, he took a razor blade and made a superficial, several-inch cut down his forearm. As soon as the blood started to ooze, he felt an immediate sense of relief. He did not feel pain; on the contrary, he felt a pleasurable sense of warmth, on his skin and throughout his body. This powerful sensation was his only way of experiencing a sense of warm, soothing touch.

We understand easily how alcohol intoxication or bingeing on food relieves stress; most of us have some direct experience with these ways of coping with distress. But it's hard for most of us to imagine how self-injury could produce tension relief. Thus deliberate self-harm is bewildering and alarming, especially to the loved ones of traumatized persons.

Deliberate self-harm is distinct from attempting suicide. Whereas the intent of suicide is permanent escape from pain through death, deliberate self-harm is intended to provide temporary respite from emotional pain.[479] Self-injury may dramatically relieve emotional distress, and no reward is more powerful than relief from pain. Thus self-injury can become addictive. Moreover, self-harm is often intertwined with other addictive patterns of reducing distress, including substance abuse and eating disorders, as well as other forms of impulsive and aggressive behavior.[480] Virtually any form of self-injurious behavior imaginable can be employed to relieve tension;[481] cutting, banging, burning, and overdosing are among the more common forms. And self-injury is not confined to us humans; it has also been observed in animals who are frustrated, frightened, or socially isolated.[482]

Deliberate self-harm is associated with a wide range of childhood traumas,[483] sexual abuse prominent among them.[484] Self-harm also has been linked to adulthood trauma, including combat[485] and rape.[486] Yet isolation and neglect also play a prominent role in self-harm, both in humans and other animals.[487] Keeping in mind the painfulness of posttraumatic reexperiencing of neglect, we should not be surprised that rejections, separations, and feelings of abandonment often serve as triggers for self-injurious behavior.[488] Psychiatrist and trauma specialist Bessel van der Kolk and colleagues[489] found that, among patients in extended treatment for trauma, those with a history of disrupted parental care had the most difficulty with ongoing self-injurious behavior. These researchers attributed the ongoing self-harm to difficulty maintaining secure attachments.

One of the most puzzling aspects of self-injurious behavior is its capacity to relieve distress. And the behavior relieves distress in many different ways, some of them contradictory. Many persons who engage in self-injurious behavior such as self-cutting do *not* feel pain; rather, they might feel a warm and pleasant sensation. Such pain-insensitivity is a form of analgesia, which is a sign of more severe symptoms as well as a more severe trauma history.[490] Also consistent with diminished sensitivity to pain, self-injury is often associated with dissociation[480] as well as emotional numbing.[491] On the other hand, other persons *do* feel pain at the time of self-injury, but this sensory pain itself can provide relief: it shifts attention from unfathomable and uncontrollable emotional pain to a concrete and controllable physical pain.

Here's another contradiction: self-injury can be employed as a form of escape from emotional pain by putting a person *into* a state of dissociative detachment. Yet states of detachment and numbing may produce a frightening sense of alienation and unreality. Thus self-injury also can provide self-stimulation that brings a person *out of* a painful dissociative state.[492] We can therefore view self-injury as a form of grounding—although not one to be recommended!

Deliberate self-harm is one means of obtaining temporary relief from many different unbearable emotional states.[493] Self-injury provides escape from anxiety, despair, emptiness, and loneliness, as well as a discomfiting absence of feeling.[494] Yet feelings of anger deserve particular attention, because self-injury is self-directed aggression. Hence it's not surprising that frustration, anger, and rage are often expressed in this way.[495] Self-injury also can be an expression of self-hatred and guilt feelings, which fuel a desire for self-punishment.[492] These feelings of self-hatred and anger go hand in hand with feeling neglected and abandoned, which is a common trigger for self-injurious behavior. Many persons with a history of trauma in attachment relationships fear that expressing anger will lead to being hurt worse or to further abandonment; taking their anger out on themselves, they feel relief. Yet sooner or later, the behavior alienates loved ones, adding fuel to the fire. Hence learning to express anger effectively in current attachment relationships is one pathway out of self-harm.

Suicidal States

Whereas self-injury is an attempt to *alter* consciousness by seeking temporary relief from tension and pain, suicide aims to *eliminate* consciousness, escaping pain once and for all. More specifically, psychologist Roy Baumeister[496] believes that suicidal states reflect a wish to *escape from painful self-awareness* when current life problems seem insurmountable. Promising oblivion, suicide is the ultimate weapon in the battle against unbearable emotional states:

> Charlotte entered the hospital in a suicidal depression after extensive prior treatment. She had grown up in an extremely violent household. Her mother was kind but generally unavailable owing to her own depression and alcoholism. As Charlotte recalled it, her mother would often sit for hours staring off into space, apparently in a dissociative state. Largely to get out of the house, Charlotte married young, and she unwittingly married a violent man and then felt trapped all over again. She paid a heavy price for divorcing him when, owing to her own recurrent depression, she lost custody of her beloved children. Although she subsequently developed a relationship with a loving man and remarried, she could not shake her anxiety and depression, and she felt profoundly ashamed that she could not retain custody of her children. Like her mother, she often retreated into a state of dissociative detachment, and she longed for the alcoholic oblivion in which her mother took refuge. She found temporary relief and comfort from self-cutting which gave her the feeling of being in a warm bath. Yet, when she lost her part-time job due to absences from work, she felt utterly humiliated and hopeless. At that point, she made a serious suicide attempt that led to her hospitalization.
>
> Charlotte had little understanding of the reasons for her self-destructive feelings and behavior, and she entered an intensive psychotherapy process in conjunction with her hospitalization. She gradually came to understand the basis of her depression, but her greater awareness of her past only brought

back feelings of fear, rage, guilt, and self-hatred. As she had in childhood, she felt utterly alone, as if no one could possibly care. She sunk into a more severe and protracted depression and developed the unshakable conviction that death was the only solution. She had tried for decades to surmount the unbearable pain, and she now longed for permanent escape. She pleaded with the hospital staff just to let her die.

But neither her husband nor the treatment staff members were prepared to give up. With a tremendous amount of support, Charlotte eventually decided that she would move forward and "try life for a while." After many difficult years, and despite continuing struggles with depression, her life improved to the point that she no longer wished to die. She developed a closer relationship with her children that she'd never imagined possible. Ultimately, two decades after the serious suicide attempt that led to her psychiatric hospitalization, she declared that she was glad to be alive.

As it is for deliberate self-harm, a history of childhood trauma is a common contributing factor to suicidal states.[23] Of course, childhood trauma is only one of many predisposing factors. Others include the full range of psychiatric disorders; biochemical and genetic vulnerability; family history of suicidal behavior; maladaptive personality traits such as perfectionism, impulsivity, and isolation; lack of social supports; and a chaotic family life.[497,498] Many of these predisposing factors are intertwined with trauma and with a history of childhood maltreatment in particular.

I've worked with a number of chronically suicidal patients with a history of severe childhood abuse and neglect. Knowing that it's possible for chronically suicidal persons to come to value their life, I don't side with their wish to give up. Persistence in treatment often plays a key role in their making the shift from wishing to die to valuing their life and more fully appreciating the value of their life to others.

But it's relatively rare for traumatized persons to be in a protracted suicidal state. Far more often, temporary suicidal crises erupt. Typically, the predisposing factors enumerated earlier create a vulnerability to the last straw of a humiliating life experience. Often, the humiliation stems from feeling let down or betrayed in a close relationship. Whatever pathway leads there, the crux of a suicidal state is a feeling of hopelessness,[499] a sense that the only way out is escape through death. The risk of suicide is greatest when several factors conspire—when hopelessness is coupled with a predisposition to impulsive and violent behavior, perhaps fueled by alcohol abuse, and the person has access to lethal means.[500] The first step in prevention is blocking the opportunity for immediate action, for example, by removing guns or pills from the home.

Although I've made a sharp distinction between deliberate self-harm and suicidal states, there's also considerable overlap between them.[501] For example, when self-injury fails to quell the pain, suicide may become the last resort. In addition, some persons take large overdoses in an attempt to knock themselves out, not making a clear distinction between temporary and permanent escape, seemingly indifferent to the prospect of dying.

Psychologist Mark Williams[502] sees a unifying theme in deliberate self-harm and suicidal actions: both signify a *cry of pain*. The cry of pain often expresses the feelings of being overpowered, trapped, and helpless. The cry of pain also expresses the sense of shame and humiliation the person feels about being so helpless, and this feeling of shame prevents the person from reaching out to others for help. Williams describes a typical unfolding sequence: the initial cry of protest is expressed in self-injury, and the ultimate cry of despair and hopelessness is expressed in suicidal behavior. He believes we misunderstand self-injurious and suicidal behavior as a manipulative cry for help. Instead, they're akin to the behavior of an animal caught in a trap and howling in pain. Ideally, these cries *are heard* by others, and help is forthcoming.

The conditions that prompt self-destructive actions—feeling trapped and humiliated in the face of uncontrollable stress—mirror precisely the experience of trauma. The fact that such suicidal crises evolve in the context of rejection, betrayal, and loss fits my belief that the essence of traumatic events is feeling overwhelmed *and alone*. Thus, in the context of trauma, such self-injurious behaviors and suicidal states reflect a 90/10 reaction: when the pain of the past amplifies the pain of the present, you lose sight of your adult resources for coping, including the help of others. In the throes of a 90/10 reaction, mentalizing is especially difficult and especially crucial. You must be aware that the crisis expresses a *mental state* that has joint roots in the present and the past and that other options for coping are now available. Here, other persons can provide needed assistance in mentalizing, countering your feeling of being alone and offering aid in problem solving, pointing a pathway out of hopelessness.

Personality Disorders

As all the preceding material in this book has made plain, trauma—especially in the context of attachment relationships—does not just result in specific psychiatric disorders but also may affect the *whole personality*. Personality problems are diagnosed as personality *disorders* when they're relatively pervasive, leading to significant distress or impairment in functioning. A diagnosis of personality disorder can be especially threatening, to the extent that it may wrongly be translated as having a bad personality—or worse, being a bad person. Judith Herman[58] suggested the alternative diagnosis of complex PTSD to avoid adding insult to injury, in effect, blaming the victim.

It's important to remember, however, that a diagnosis of personality disorder is not a characterization of the whole person; it does not take into account personality strengths but rather singles out specific areas of difficulty. Having a personality disorder does not preclude being kind, compassionate, loyal, and courageous. In addition, it's important to keep in mind that, like those with other psychiatric disorders, patients with personality disorders respond positively to treatment.[503]

Many personality disorders can be viewed as exaggerated personality traits.[504] For example, persons with avoidant personality disorder are afraid to initiate social contact for fear of rejection. Those with paranoid personality disorder remain isolated owing to pervasive distrust. It's little wonder that traumatic experience in attachment relationships might push individuals in the avoidant-paranoid direction. On the other hand, those with dependent personality disorder rely heavily on others for guidance and have great difficulty being separated and alone. Again, little wonder that trauma might result in this dependent pattern of relating. Of course, as described in Chapter 2 ("Attachment"), attachment trauma creates a bind; the need for security is coupled with fear of being hurt and abandoned. Having experienced this bind, you may vacillate from getting close and feeling anxious and resentful to retreating by staying distant and isolated. Thus trauma is often associated with a complex combination of personality problems rather than a single problematic personality trait.[505]

In this section, I focus on two self-destructive personality patterns associated with trauma: masochism and borderline personality disorder (BPD). Both merit careful understanding, because being labeled with either can feel insulting, and the last thing you need is more shame.

Masochism

Masochism is not a psychiatric diagnosis but remains a widely used concept.[506] As commonly understood—or misunderstood—masochism involves feeling pleasure in combination with pain or suffering. It's not uncommon for persons caught in reenactment of abusive relationships, such as those in the throes of traumatic bonding, to be labeled *masochistic*.

I think it's harmful to think of yourself as *wanting* to suffer or *liking* suffering. I think it's better to think of yourself as wanting to suffer *less*—although it may be hard for you to do. From the outside, deliberate self-harm looks masochistic; from the inside, the goal is to *relieve* suffering. Yet I do believe many of us have a *propensity for suffering;* we can be motivated to suffer. Suffering can be a grim compromise. We may suffer if we feel that we deserve punishment, that we don't deserve pleasure or happiness, or that we must pay the price of feeling pain when we've enjoyed a bit of pleasure.

Our propensity for suffering can be cultivated in traumatic relationships. An abused child can learn, for example, that suffering forestalls further attacks.[45] In addition, when it's self-inflicted, suffering can be brought under control.[507] Suffering can be comforting in its sheer familiarity; breaking out of suffering and experiencing positive feelings may provoke anxiety.[508] In my view, if you're caught in masochism, you're not enjoying suffering but rather continually attempting to *regulate and control your level of suffering.* Although this grim compromising may have helped you cope with traumatic relationships, it's likely to backfire in other relationships. Other persons are put off by self-perpetuated suffering, such that masochistic behavior often leads to criticism, rejection, and abandonment. Thus the cycle of self-loathing and suffering escalates.[509]

Masochism, depression, and dissociation share an important common factor: they're passive forms of coping that involve submission and retreat.[25] Anger goes underground; resentment prevails. These passive forms of coping, coupled with self-destructive behavior, exacerbate the feeling of being helpless, and they're conducive to taking on the identity of a victim. Sadly, being helpless and victimized is inherent in trauma. It's the *perpetuation* of this victimized stance beyond the traumatic events—*learned* helplessness[238]—that becomes problematic. True, surrendering rather than expressing anger and aggression is often the safest strategy—or the only possibility—in a traumatic relationship. Yet, when you're out of the traumatic situation, it's crucial to reclaim anger in the service of effective self-protection and self-assertion, rather than continuing to direct it all against yourself. Thus traumatized persons are encouraged to recognize their strengths and to see themselves as *survivors*, a view that reinforces active coping in place of passive surrender.

Borderline Personality Disorder (BPD)

When the term was first introduced, *borderline* referred to the boundary between neurosis and psychosis. Now BPD refers to a complex set of personality problems that include intense anger along with self-damaging impulsivity—such as reckless driving, impulsive spending, and self-endangering sexual relationships—along with recurrent self-injurious or suicidal behavior. These self-destructive patterns are embedded in other personality problems that include frantic efforts to avoid abandonment, unstable and intense relationships, identity disturbance, mood instability, feelings of emptiness, and stress-related paranoid ideas or dissociative symptoms.[2]

This broad array of symptoms illustrates how varied the causes and expression of BPD may be.[510] Childhood trauma is neither a necessary nor sufficient cause of BPD, but diverse forms of childhood adversity are well-established contributing factors.[511] To make sense of this welter of symptoms, it's helpful to focus on problems with abandonment as central to BPD.[512] Especially when BPD arises in conjunction with attachment trauma, the fear of abandonment makes psychological sense. The traumatized person, above all, attempts to avoid the feeling of being afraid and alone, which I've construed as a posttraumatic reexperiencing of neglect. Consistent with this view, Marsha Linehan, who pioneered dialectical behavior therapy for the treatment of BPD,[513] viewed the combination of an invalidating environment and problems with emotional regulation as being central to the development of BPD. Given problems with regulating emotional distress, feeling invalidated triggers self-destructive actions—desperate measures.

To summarize: put problems with attachment at the center. Many—if not all—forms of trauma may profoundly disrupt attachment. Neglect, loss, and a host of other dysfunctional family patterns also can disrupt attachment. Temperamental and environmental factors also conspire. Persons with BPD are exquisitely sensitive to rejection, separation, and loss. Any event that spells abandonment may evoke intense distress, anxiety, and anger. Impulsive self-destructive behavior relieves tension. The distress and dangerous behavior may also evoke the concern of others, *temporarily* alleviating feelings of abandonment. Yet impulsive behavior is also likely to provoke alarm and rejection, ultimately pushing others away. As others withdraw, fears of abandonment escalate. Relationships become increasingly unstable, perpetuating insecure attachment.

Peter Fonagy and his colleagues[514] highlighted the role of mentalizing in the development of BPD. Fonagy and others[515] have found persons with BPD to show severely disturbed patterns of attachment, consistent with their fear of abandonment and instability in their close relationships. Yet those persons who, despite trauma, showed a good capacity to mentalize—to make sense of mental states, including a capacity for awareness of their caregiver's mind—were far less likely to develop BPD than those whose capacity for mentalizing was diminished. These observations are consistent with findings that persons with BPD can benefit from psychological treatment aimed at helping them to develop more stable relationships, better emotional control, and better understanding of their emotional states.[516]

Interpersonal Side Effects

We've examined a wide range of self-destructive actions that may stem partly from trauma and that reflect a desperate effort to regulate emotion: substance abuse, eating disorders, deliberate self-harm, and suicidal states. We've seen how these self-destructive actions can become woven into personality and expressed in attachment relationships. Most conspicuously, feelings of abandonment may evoke the 90/10 reaction of reexperiencing early trauma—feeling neglected and alone in the context of frightening experience.

I'm in full accord with Mark Williams[502] that it's counterproductive to view self-destructive behavior as a manipulative cry for help or an effort merely to get attention. Rather, these behaviors are an effort to put an end to unbearable emotional states. Yet, as Williams observed, the cry of pain also serves a communicative function indirectly. Some persons feel that they cannot possibly express the depth of their emotional pain in words—only actions will do.

Thus the main effect of self-destructive behavior—escape from pain—is paradoxically an effort at self-preservation. But this behavior often has dramatic side effects: it's alarming to others. When we become alarmed, we often become angry as well; think of the mother who yells at her child for running into the street. Thus others' exasperation is expressed in their accusation that self-injurious behavior is a manipulative attempt to get attention. This accusation is experienced not just as a criticism but also as a misunderstanding—another instance of invalidation. There's nothing wrong with wanting and getting attention. For all of us, and particularly for those who have undergone trauma, attention—comfort and a restored feeling of security—is essential. Desiring attention is something to be fostered, not criticized. The problem is finding *effective* ways of getting attention on an enduring basis.

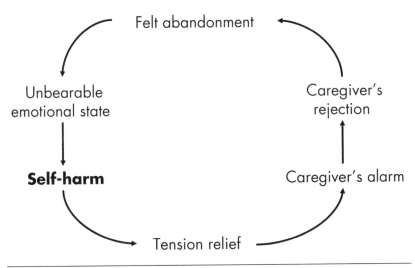

FIGURE 11–1. Vicious circle in self-harm.

Self-destructive behavior is a form of coping that backfires,[25] creating a vicious circle as depicted in Figure 11–1. But self-destructive behavior doesn't just backfire in close relationships. Self-destructive behaviors damage the self, inflicting more trauma on the self, adding to feelings of shame and humiliation. Unfortunately, this sequence often escalates. For example, substance abuse or eating-disordered behavior may escalate into deliberate self-harm as attachments become increasingly unstable; then despair, hopelessness, and suicidal states may ensue as attachments seem irrevocably disrupted, and there seems to be no prospect for things to improve in the future.

Plainly, the pathway out of these vicious circles first involves awareness—mentalizing. Awareness of these feelings and relationship patterns, as well as their origins, can be the first step toward interrupting them. More constructive ways of regulating emotions—ways that don't backfire in relationships—are possible. Then more stable and secure attachment relationships are possible. There's hope. These are the topics of the next section of this book, "Healing."

Part IV

HEALING

EMOTION REGULATION

In the context of coping with trauma, we must give priority to painfully intense and potentially destructive emotions—what I've been calling unbearable emotional states. Yet focusing on these states skews our attitudes toward emotion. To reiterate the main theme of Chapter 3 ("Emotion"), rather than striving stoically to suppress or overcome painful emotions, it's best to *cultivate emotion,* including painful emotions. Instead of pitting reason against passion and viewing emotions as irrational, we can think of emotions as rich evaluative judgments that are essential to our flourishing. We need to know, on a moment-to-moment basis, how we're doing in the world with regard to our countless needs, goals, and projects. No doubt, sometimes we need to reason unemotionally about how we're doing. But emotional reasoning rapidly prioritizes our goals, guiding and motivating our actions. Our feelings provide conscious access to a wealth of knowledge about the success of our strivings. Yet to make use of all the wisdom of our emotions, and to head off their bum steers, we must listen to them. We must mentalize emotionally.

Plainly, with a sensitized nervous system stemming from trauma, emotions can be irrational and destructive—contrary to flourishing. Recall Robert Levenson's[119] helpful distinction between the hardwired core emotional programs, such as our split-second fight-or-flight response, and the surrounding emotional control mechanisms, such as our ability to inhibit our first emotional impulse and to rethink the situation so as to respond in a more effective way. To flourish, we must both cultivate and regulate our emotions—giving them enough rein, but not free rein.

More or less skillfully, we all regulate our emotions. We deliberately monitor, evaluate, and adjust our emotional responses.[517] In any emotional episode—for example, an upsetting phone call—we appraise and reappraise.[133] We appraise the situation's import for our well-being—a dear friend is seriously ill. We appraise our emotional reactions—I'm getting unduly alarmed. We appraise our ability to cope—I wonder if I can give him the support he needs. As we appraise and reappraise, we have feelings about feelings, feelings upon feelings. Potentially, these complex emotional responses lend tremendous wisdom and flexibility to our coping with challenges. Confronted with a threat to the well-being of a loved one, we appreciate the significance of the relationship and we're inspired to provide compassionate support. Unemotional ideas are pale by comparison.

As you know from a lifetime of experience, emotion regulation requires effort. The force of the automatic program may be pitted against the counterforce of control mechanisms—holding back tears or gritting your teeth in anger. I referred to this process in Chapter 3 as *working with emotions*: steering their course. You can't prevent the initial burst of emotion (the flash of anger) or even the bursts of reactive emotions (fear or shame). But you can influence their course, that is, their intensity and duration, as well as the actions you take. And you can cultivate a broader range of emotions, for example, a capacity to feel outrage in addition to timidity. Thus there's a gentler side to emotion regulation as well, what Peter Fonagy and his colleagues[79] call *crafting* emotions. The goal of emotion regulation, from crafting to restraining, is to optimize emotional responses rather than to become stoically emotionless. Tranquility is one desirable emotional state among many, not a model for a whole life.

I have two main agendas for this chapter. First, I'll review several widely employed techniques for self-regulation: sleep, exercise, relaxation, imagery, meditation, and biofeedback. Second, I'll discuss enjoyable emotions and comment on several types: pleasure, excitement, flow, joy, compassion, and love. To set the stage, however, I'll expand on the concept of emotion regulation, first considering the idea of the pause button, then elaborating the concept of mentalizing emotionally.

The Pause Button

In one of our trauma education groups, psychologist Maria Holden was listening to my description of how traumatized persons can resort to self-injurious behavior to find relief from unbearable emotional states. Maria piped up with the clever idea that we need a *pause button,* a metaphor we've used ever since. In an unbearable emotional state, you must push the pause button. Not easy. By emotional design, this requires great effort or counterforce.

Keep in mind that a critical part of the basic emotion package is an action tendency; we're impelled to freeze or to run when afraid, to lash out when angry. Given the intelligence of emotions, these might be the best actions. Yet trauma renders you vulnerable to sensitization and context-inappropriate responding, what we've called the 90/10 reaction. You're not dealing with a charging bear or a raging parent or spouse; you're dealing with a *reminder* of trauma. Then your emotional impulse may be to quell the painful emotion as fast as humanly possible, for example, by getting drunk or some other self-injurious action. In that event, it's essential to put on the brakes—to push the pause button to engage in more constructive coping (see Figure 12–1).

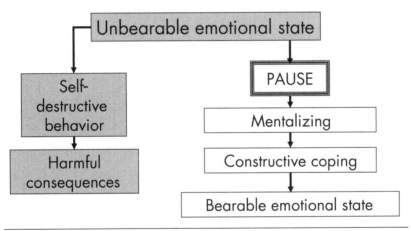

FIGURE 12–1. Pushing the pause button.

There's a technical term for the pause button: *response modulation.*[517] To modulate means to adjust, often in the direction of softening or toning down. Response modulation entails inhibiting a dominant response to permit more adaptive alternative responses to come to the fore. When you feel hurt and angry, your hardwired dominant response is to hurt back. Of course, you may have learned other dominant responses, such as retreating, submitting, or attacking yourself. With the 90/10 reaction, the strong emotions and dominant responses can be triggered in a situation that's not actually dangerous. Response modulation allows you to take full account of the present situational context before you act emotionally. A mild rebuke may be more appropriate than a screaming tirade. Another example of response modulation is using grounding techniques to head off dissociation. You focus your attention on details of your present situation, making an active effort to distinguish the present from the past, focusing on the current 10% as distinguished from the past 90%. This grounding is response modulation insofar as you're suspending your dominant response—dissociation—to allow you to reappraise the situation, better adapting your reaction to the current context.

Obviously, strong emotion makes response modulation difficult. Learning emotion regulation is a major project and requires extensive practice. Many methods have been proposed, from ancient to modern. To employ these methods effectively, however, you must be able to modulate your immediate emotional response, to push the pause button. I call this process *mentalizing emotionally*.

Mentalizing Emotionally

Increasingly appreciating the wisdom of emotion, many psychologists are developing a language to refer to skillful emotion regulation. Although the terminology varies, there's a heartening convergence of spirit. Peter Salovey, John Mayer, and their colleagues are developing the science of *emotional intelligence*.[518–520] In dialectical behavior therapy (see Chapter 13, "Treatment Approaches"), Marcia Linehan emphasizes *wise mind* and *mindfulness* in relation to emotion.[521] Paul Ekman[126] speaks of *attentively considering our emotional feelings—attentiveness* for short. As I will also do, he emphasizes the importance of being attentive and self-aware *during the emotional episode*.

Peter Fonagy and his colleagues[79] proposed the concept of *mentalized affectivity* to refer to our capacity to make meaning out of our emotions. Ideally, we make sense of our emotion when we're in the midst of the emotional state. We mentalize emotionally, for example, feeling and thinking about feeling at the same time. Fonagy and colleagues described three steps: we identify, modulate, and express our emotions. A common example of *identifying* emotions is naming a feeling in your mind, for example, becoming aware, "I'm starting to get angry." But identifying emotions goes far beyond this first step. Typically, in the course of an emotional episode—feeling "upset"—we experience a number of emotions, either in rapid succession or all mixed together. Mentalizing, we can learn to disentangle the various emotions and even to gauge their various proportions in the mix. But we do more than this; we elaborate the deeper meaning of the emotions, their stories and their histories. Just consider the depth of meaning and range of emotions that might go with a feeling of betrayal.

As just discussed, *modulating* emotions refers to changing them, altering their intensity or duration—crafting them, in Fonagy and colleagues' terms. *Expressing* emotions effectively requires that you first identify and modulate them. Of course, sometimes it's prudent to refrain from expressing your feelings to others, in which case Fonagy and colleagues propose expressing them *inwardly*, to yourself. When you are furiously angry, for example, you might imagine yourself pounding your fists while yelling and screaming. Forming the image in your mind might be much preferable to engaging in these actions. All this mentalizing—identifying, modulating, and expressing—transforms and illuminates our emotions, giving us the full benefit of their intelligence.

There's wide agreement that self-awareness—mentalizing emotionally—is necessary for skillful emotion regulation.[522] But self-awareness is a double-edged sword.[517] Self-awareness can be excruciatingly painful, especially when you feel frightened, ashamed, and guilty about your emotional responses—as often happens in conjunction with trauma. Thus self-awareness tends to intensify emotions, and distraction is one of the main ways we decrease their intensity.[323] In desperation, traumatized persons can resort to extreme forms of distraction. Much self-injurious behavior—alcohol and drug abuse, binge eating and purging, self-cutting, and suicidal behavior—is an effort to escape from painful self-awareness.[496] Such desperately avoidant responses also can become dominant. When infuriated, you might feel impelled to get drunk rather than lashing out. This is the time for response modulation, inhibiting the dominant response by pushing the pause button. Mentalizing emotionally is the *way* we push the pause button.

As I noted in Chapter 3 ("Emotion"), you can best mentalize emotionally in a preventive way, regulating your emotions before they reach peak intensity and take you past the point of no return (or difficult return). Mentalizing emotionally is the first step toward three basic pathways to emotion regulation: self-regulation, seeking support, and problem solving.

Self-Regulation

I'll be discussing a number of self-regulation strategies in more detail shortly. They help in two ways. First, used routinely, they can lower your general level of arousal so that you're not so easily propelled beyond the point of no return into unbearable emotional states. Second, when you become proficient in them, you can use self-regulation strategies in the heat of the moment, for example, to calm yourself down. Here's where mentalizing emotionally comes in: when you're attuned to your feelings, you can use your feelings as cues to employ these coping strategies—sooner rather than later.

Seeking Support

Attachment isn't merely the wellspring of emotional learning; as Bowlby[67] emphasized, we rely on attachment relationships throughout life to regulate our emotional distress. Yet you must mentalize emotionally to make use of attachment relationships in this way. Not only must you be aware that you're having emotional trouble and need help, but also you must be able to communicate your needs to another person. That's not to say that you must know exactly what you feel. Sometimes you just feel "upset" or "emotional" and have only the vaguest idea why. You must then elaborate the narrative—the story of the emotions. This is how you learned about emotions in early childhood,[139] and you continue to rely on others to make sense of what you feel throughout life. Here you have a two-way street: mentalizing emotionally enables you to make use of attachment relationships to regulate emotion, and attachment relationships promote mentalizing emotionally. Of course, finding meaning in traumatic emotions sometimes requires professional help, and mentalizing emotionally is largely what psychotherapy for trauma is all about (see Chapter 13, "Treatment Approaches").

Problem Solving

Psychologists find it helpful to distinguish between emotion-focused coping and problem-focused coping,[523] and I think this distinction is crucial to coping with trauma. What I've been discussing so far falls under the category of *emotion-focused coping,* that is, efforts to regulate your emotional state. But we must not give short shrift to *problem-focused coping,* direct efforts to modify the problem at hand. Without problem-focused coping, emotion-focused coping can be futile. If you're being mistreated, intimidated, or exploited in a current attachment relationship, for example, learning how to calm your fear and anger will not suffice. You must deal with the provoking circumstances, for example, by asserting your needs, boundaries, or rights. Symptoms of PTSD are evoked by reminders of trauma, and it's essential to focus on current circumstances that replicate earlier traumas. Patterns of reenactment keep trauma alive (see Chapter 6, "Relationships"). Modifying these relationship patterns and extricating yourself from them is crucial to healing. Dealing with the current circumstances is problem-focused coping, and, without it, emotion-focused coping will be Sisyphus-like.

Mentalizing emotionally is the first step in problem-focused coping. We identify problems emotionally. And emotion-focused coping—working with your emotions rather than avoiding them—can promote problem-focused coping. You can best confront and cope with conflict in relationships when you're aware of your emotions and comfortable with them, know what they mean, and feel confident in regulating and expressing them. Moreover, mentalizing emotionally also entails awareness of others' feelings as well as your own—also when you're in an emotional state. Put simply, interpersonal problem solving goes best when you can empathize with yourself and with the other person, as well as expressing your feelings forthrightly.

Ekman's Guide to Emotional Attentiveness

In his popular book, *Emotions Revealed*,[126] Ekman provided a field guide to basic emotions, including sadness, anger, fear, disgust, and joy. Backed by solid theory and research, it's the most direct approach I've seen to increasing your emotional awareness. There's no substitute for studying the book in depth, but a brief sketch will help concretize what I'm calling mentalizing emotionally.

Ekman proposed a number of exercises to enhance sensitivity to feelings. First, you concentrate on evoking strong feelings. You can use pictures he supplies or your memories. Ekman also guides you in imitating facial expressions of the basic emotions. Voluntarily making the facial expressions induces physiological changes in the brain and body that evoke feelings. You're instructed to pay attention to all the details of these feelings throughout your body. The purpose of these exercises is to enhance your attentiveness, so that you'll become more sensitive to mild degrees of these feelings. Then you'll be in a better position to identify, modulate, and express them.

Ekman's meticulous approach to distinguishing among emotions from facial expressions provides the basis of his manual for learning to identify emotions in others. He provides a self-administered test of your skill in emotion recognition and then guides you through a muscle-by-muscle description of the expression of the basic emotions. Armed with this knowledge, you can develop skill in identifying brief hints of emotions in others. For example, you may identify emotional states that others are trying not to express or states they're not consciously feeling. Ekman makes some suggestions as to how to use such knowledge constructively.

Self-Regulation Strategies

Stress researcher Bruce McEwen[264] rightly pointed out that all the main ways of relieving stress are things our grandmothers could have advised; all that's changed is our having solid scientific evidence for their wisdom. Borrowing from McEwen, in our trauma education groups we now refer to time-honored methods of self-regulation—many of which go back millennia—as *grandmother's list*. Thus it's likely that there's little you don't already know about self-regulation or much you haven't already tried. But I think you can benefit from being aware of some of the obstacles to following grandmother's advice when you're suffering from trauma.

Trauma and stress aren't new. Techniques of self-regulation are ancient. You may not have studied them, but you have used them. Most methods of self-regulation, such as exercise and relaxation, are simple. In relation to meditation, Jon Kabat-Zinn uses the phrase, "simple but not easy."[524] For persons struggling with trauma, I put it more strongly: *simple but difficult.* If it weren't difficult, you'd already be using these strategies successfully rather than reading this chapter. Three sources of this difficulty are worth thinking about: methods of self-regulation require practice; they can be fraught with complications for persons with a history of trauma; and they require caring for yourself.

The first source of difficulty: learning to regulate your emotions is like any other skill—it requires practice and persistence. Levenson[119] regarded developing competence in emotion regulation as a lifetime task. When broaching the subject of self-regulation in trauma education groups, I ask the—somewhat ludicrous—question: which is easier, learning to regulate your emotions or learning to play the piano? Most participants agree with me; learning to play the piano is easier. Then I ask how many hours it takes to learn to play the piano—even without aspiring to be a concert pianist. Many. And, if you don't keep practicing, you get rusty. To become proficient and to maintain your proficiency requires determination and commitment. Such a major effort is no short-term project. If you're dealing with trauma, you're in for the long haul. As Jon Kabat-Zinn[524] said about meditation, "Try it for a few years and see what happens" (p. 104).

The second source of difficulty: trauma-related problems can complicate the use of these techniques. Techniques designed to enhance self-control may instead trigger anxiety, flashbacks, or dissociation. Persons with a trauma history can easily be demoralized when the very things offered as helpful prove instead to be unusable or retraumatizing. Fortunately, because of such a wide range of techniques there's bound to be something for everyone. But finding what works for you may be difficult. It may take time and effort. You may be in for a period of trial and error. Caution is in order. Many self-regulation techniques have been studied extensively in the context of stress management, but they've just begun to be researched in the context of trauma, although they're routinely employed in conjunction with other facets of trauma treatment (see Chapter 13, "Treatment Approaches").

The third and often most serious difficulty: techniques of self-regulation are intended to help you feel better—to even feel *good.* This means taking care of yourself. How can taking care of yourself be a seemingly insurmountable obstacle? Taking care of yourself implies *valuing* yourself. To the degree that the aftermath of trauma entails self-blame or self-hatred, taking care of yourself will go against the grain. "Why should I do anything good for my-self when I don't deserve it?" Your self-concept has a steering function, and this train of thought can lead to a self-perpetuating stalemate. If you hate yourself, you won't take care of yourself, then you'll feel bad, hate yourself, ad infinitum. You might believe that you must feel better about yourself first, then you'll be able to use these techniques to take care of yourself. Logical, but maybe self-defeating. A good way to start feeling better about yourself is to take better care of yourself. Working on self-regulation could come first. It's difficult, but some of the rewards start occurring right away, and they can enhance your motivation to continue.

Many fine books have been devoted to methods of self-regulation. You'd do well to read them, since I can give only a brief overview here. If you've had a traumatic experience, you have a head start. To the extent that you've felt out of control, you have doubtlessly devoted thought and effort to self-regulation. As you read through many of these methods, you may find yourself thinking, "That's what I've been *trying* to do." People have been trying to achieve more self-control for millennia. The professional and academic contribution has been to refine what people have done naturally throughout the ages, and, if you've been traumatized, it's worth your while to become expert with some of these techniques. One bit of expertise relates to goal setting.[525] It's important to set realistic, concrete, short-term goals. But setting goals is not enough; you'll do best if you also specify when, where, and how you'll implement your goal. It's also helpful to reinforce your efforts by keeping a record or diary.

Sleep

The chronic stress associated with posttraumatic symptoms is wearing. I often hear, "I didn't do anything all day. Why am I so exhausted?" Even if you've not run a marathon, your sympathetic nervous system may have been in high gear throughout the day. Anxiety and irritation are tiring. As Darwin[116] asserted, fear is the most depressing of the emotions, and, like anxiety, depression may profoundly interfere with sleep. Yet sleep is the best medicine for stress, and it's arguably the most fundamental practice associated with good health.[526]

Fortunately, by helping regulate anxiety and depression, medications can assist in restoring sleep. Yet sleeping medicine is best used on a short-term basis to help you through a particularly bad patch. Self-regulation comes into play in sleep hygiene, that is, regular practices that promote sleep. Fortunately, sleep researchers have written helpful guides with highly practical advice.[527] For example, in *The Promise of Sleep*,[528] William Dement suggests sticking to a routine sleep schedule, winding down by engaging in relaxing activities prior to going to sleep, refraining from eating large meals within a few hours of going to sleep, avoiding caffeinated beverages for several hours prior to sleeping, avoiding alcohol (which puts you to sleep but interferes with the quality of sleep), ensuring that your sleeping area is comfortable and quiet, and—to introduce what may be a major complication—resolving conflicts with your bedmate. Developing skill in relaxation also can help you get to sleep or get back to sleep in the middle of the night. But relaxation takes practice; it's no time to learn when you're thrashing around in bed, agitated at 3:00 A.M.

Exercise

The benefits of exercise have been widely touted, and they need little reiteration here. Cooper's book *Aerobics*[529] conveys the enthusiasm and provides the prescriptions. Bailey's book *Smart Exercise*[530] is packed with useful information and gives a physiological foundation. Thayer's book *Calm Energy*[338] considers exercise in relating to eating behavior and mood, and McEwen's book on stress physiology, *The End of Stress as We Know It*,[264] makes the convincing case that diet and weight control play a fundamental role in resilience to stress. Moreover, exercise, diet, and sleep are all intertwined, so that working on any one front will help with the others.

Because exercise can decrease anxiety and depression, it's highly pertinent to trauma. And exercise can have other benefits as well; many sexual abuse survivors find exercise to be one of the best ways to regain a sense of control over their bodies.[294] If regulating your mood and mastering your body are not enough incentive, you might be persuaded by recent research suggesting that exercise stimulates the growth of brain cells.[264]

Yet there are potential complications for trauma survivors. Some persons find that exercise *increases* anxiety, probably because of its initially arousing effects. I've worked with persons who have been afraid to exercise because they were catapulted into panic attacks by it. Others have had flashbacks triggered by exercise. Some begin to dissociate and then become confused and disoriented. Arousal is likely to be the culprit. Rapid heartbeat or labored breathing, for example, is often a response to traumatic experience. Anything that increases heart rate or makes a person gasp for breath—even if it has nothing to do with trauma—can evoke traumatic memories and bring back the whole constellation of traumatic experience.

The possibility that exercise can increase anxiety or evoke intrusive memories should be taken as a caution; hard exercise may not work for you. The risk of increased anxiety is also an indication that exercise should be approached gradually—not a bad idea for many reasons. You don't have to run; you can walk. In the process of increasing your level of vigorous exercise, you can desensitize yourself to physiological arousal. A manageable routine for exercise can provide a sense of predictability, control, and accomplishment. Success is just doing it regularly—at whatever level. This regularity is where the need for commitment and determination comes in.

Relaxation

Relaxation is the simplest of the simple techniques, and it's the direct antidote to the fight-or-flight response. You might want to read Herbert Benson's classic *The Relaxation Response.*[531] Benson spells out four components to relaxation: a quiet environment with few distractions; a mental focus on a particular sound, word, phrase, or object; a passive, let-it-happen attitude, free of concern about how well you're doing; and a comfortable position to minimize muscle tension. You may add deep, regular breathing, but you shouldn't force it. Diaphragmatic breathing is best; breathe into your belly, not your chest. Some individuals like to use progressive muscle relaxation: tense and relax the muscles in various parts of your body, just to highlight the difference between tension and relaxation. Begin at your feet or your forehead; work your way up or down.

Relaxation can be simple but difficult. With a house full of children and a ringing telephone, finding a quiet spot and uninterrupted time might be more challenging than mountain climbing. But all is not lost; it takes only minutes to relax. Benson recommends 10 to 20 minutes. As with exercise, a routine for relaxation is essential. Succeeding merely involves doing it regularly. Relaxation is like exercise; as long as you keep doing it, it works. Stop, and the benefits stop—unless you've managed to weave it into your daily routine.

It's hard to imagine anything more innocuous than relaxation. But relaxation can be problematic for persons who have been traumatized. This paradoxical response has been observed frequently enough to acquire a name: *relaxation-induced anxiety.*[532] With this anxiety, you might associate relaxation with letting your guard down; thus, in a relaxed state, you may feel vulnerable to attack. You may feel that you need to be alert at all times. Therefore, before letting yourself relax, you may need to do whatever is necessary to assure yourself that you're in a safe place, protected from any intrusion.

Relaxation entails focusing inward, on your breathing and on your muscles. Your attention is directed away from outer reality onto your body. When you let go of focus on outer reality, you might be prone to dissociate.[533] Rather than feeling relaxed, you might begin to feel spaced out or unreal. Dissociation is the opposite of feeling grounded in outer reality. Relaxation exercises tend to remove this sensory scaffolding.

Fortunately, it's not necessary to do body awareness exercises to relax.

Sitting quietly may be enough. Quiet activities like reading or handicrafts can be relaxing for many persons. Exercise can be relaxing. Routinely setting aside time for quiet activities may be a way to ease into more formal relaxation practice.

Imagery

Picture a field of wildflowers. Hear the sound of a waterfall. You've been using imagery all your life. For most persons, visual imagery is especially vivid and powerful. Interestingly, creating visual images activates the same parts of the brain involved in visual perception.[534] As traumatized persons know best, the power of imagery is a double-edged sword. Imagery is tied to memory and to emotion. Intrusive images of traumatic experience are common symptoms of PTSD. Sights, sounds, smells, tastes, and body sensations all can be associated with reexperiencing trauma.

Think of yourself as having a library of images. Picture a section of the library devoted to traumatic images—but don't open any of the books in that section now! You have a section for imagery associated with positive experiences. This is a section worth browsing in. Spend lots of time there. You may not have checked out some of the volumes for a long time. Put them back in circulation. Check them out regularly in your spare moments.

You can use imagery flexibly and creatively. You can piece together images from memory to imagine something that you've not actually experienced, like floating on a cloud. Much of your anxiety and worry revolves around imagery, anticipating the worst. Your images are also accompanied by changes in your physiological state, so anticipating the worst tends to promote it. But you can create library shelves devoted to imagined scenes that are pleasurable and calming.

Many therapies use *guided* imagery,[224] which simply means that you're provided with suggestions for images that will evoke certain ideas and emotions. You may be told to picture yourself lying on a beach on a beautiful sunny day, watching puffy clouds float by, hearing the sound of waves gently lapping at the shore, feeling the warmth of sand against your skin. Many persons benefit particularly from imagining themselves in a safe place, for example, a secluded and protected place. Although such imagery may initially be suggested by a therapist, ultimately developing your own images is better than using someone else's. For months, I suggested to a patient that she picture herself sinking into relaxation by slowing descending a staircase; eventually, she confessed that she had all the while been picturing herself floating down a river on a raft! To each her own. Given the choice, I suppose I'd opt for the raft, too.

In managing anxiety we use imagery in a virtually instinctive way, and mental escape through imagery is one way of coping with trauma. Some persons in the midst of traumatic experience can dissociate themselves from the trauma by imagining themselves to be elsewhere—outside in the garden among beautiful flowers, wrapped up in a sleeping bag, or traveling through the outer reaches of the galaxy. But comforting imagery developed in situations of desperation may be problematic. Some soothing images will be so closely linked to traumatic experience that bringing them to mind will also tend to reevoke the traumatic memories. These well-worn images may be haunted by trauma. This section of your imagery library may be adjacent to the traumatic images section. You might be better off moving to a new area and creating new volumes of fresh imagery.

Meditation

Of all the techniques described here, meditation probably has the most venerable history,[535] having evolved in the context of early Eastern religions. Meditation and prayer have much in common, and for many, the spiritual dimension forms the foundation of meditation. But meditation can be separated from religion and spirituality. Meditation overlaps with relaxation, and Benson's[531] methods of eliciting the relaxation response combine relaxation instruction and techniques from transcendental meditation.

Meditation is an ancient practice, but a growing body of scientific research now attests to its beneficial effects.[536] Like relaxation, meditation has been shown helpful for stress-reduction in decreasing both anxiety and depression.[537] Kabat-Zinn has described in detail the meditation procedures that he and his colleagues have used in stress-reduction programs.[236] He's done an admirable job of translating Eastern meditation practice into Western concepts and language.[524] In pioneering research on the biological effects of meditation, psychologist Richard Davidson[538] reported that participants in Kabat-Zinn's program showed enhanced immune function as well as changes in brain electrical activity consistent with increased capacity for positive emotion.

What is the essence of meditation? Definitions vary, as do meditative practices.[539] Meditation entails heightened concentration, but concentration can be employed in opposite ways.[540] Most familiar is the technique of stilling your mind by concentrating on a single focus—the breath, a mantra, or a visualization. You can also do the opposite, letting your mind go without trying to control it, just concentrating on the moment-to-moment kaleidoscope of thoughts, feelings, and images—a practice that allows you to steady your mind in a wide variety of situations. Crucial to moment-to-moment concentration is an attitude of *equanimity*—openness, acceptance, and a nonjudgmental stance toward whatever passes through your mind.[539] Also important is the sense of letting go, letting your experience change. This form of insight meditation is a good example of mentalizing, being keenly aware of your mental states. And the process of letting go of thoughts and feelings also counters rumination, which entails getting stuck in one particular train of thought, being unable to shift perspective. Hence meditation has proved to be a useful component of cognitive therapy for depression[350]—in my view, by promoting mentalizing emotionally.[82]

I think *mindfulness* is the single most useful idea in meditation. Buddhist teacher Thich Nhat Hanh[541] defined mindfulness as "keeping one's consciousness alive to the present reality" (p. 11). Not easy. We're the beneficiaries of an evolutionary history that has endowed us with self-awareness and has enabled us to transcend the present by bridging from past to future. This grand evolutionary achievement also can ruin our conscious lives by continually dragging us out of the present into ruminating about the past and the future. Coping with trauma entails separating the past from the present, not being unduly apprehensive about the dangers of the future, and seeing the present for what it is. Alan Watts[535] put it pithily, "There is never anything but the present, and if one cannot live there, one cannot live anywhere" (p. 124). There's no better term for this ideal than *mindfulness*. Simple but difficult. It requires practice and persistence. Buddhist monks devote a lifetime to it, but we Westerners might adopt more modest aspirations. Moderation in all things, as Watts commented, "A certain amount of 'sitting just to sit' might well be the best thing in the world for the jittery minds and agitated bodies of Europeans and Americans" (p. 112).

Mindfulness can be the antithesis of dissociation—the opposite end of the spectrum. Dissociation is associated with a sense of unreality; mindfulness is a state of being highly aware of reality, not spaced out but tuned in. This attunement is why meditation may be helpful in relation to dissociation. Mindfulness could enhance grounding techniques that focus attention on current sensory experience.

Like every other technique of self-regulation, meditation is not without risks.[542] Meditation can be used as an escape from living.[543] Mindfulness is the ideal antidote to dissociation, because it entails heightened awareness of reality, a sense of being fully grounded. Yet sitting motionless for prolonged periods can have a trance-inducing effect. For persons who are prone to dissociation, meditation can lead to a sense of loss of control rather than to enhanced control. Like relaxation and guided imagery, meditation is conducive to opening up the inner world of thoughts and feelings. For this reason, it can evoke anxiety, painful memories, or distressing images and ideas. Although the *intent* may be to foster your ability to concentrate on one thing (your breathing), the actual *effect* may be that you get stuck in painful experience. If you become emotionally overwhelmed, you may not *be able* to gently bring your attention back to the focus of awareness. When coping with trauma, you might best be cautious, starting gradually and seeking the support of a therapist, a teacher, or a meditation group.

Biofeedback

Compared with most of the age-old methods of self-regulation described thus far, biofeedback is a recent innovation—only several decades old. And, unlike the rest, biofeedback requires some technology. The basic idea behind biofeedback isn't complicated. You can change what goes on in your body by your behavior and by what you imagine and think about. Sit down, breathe deeply, imagine being in a pleasant spot, and you'll relax—your heart rate will slow, and your muscles will relax. Start imagining your traumatic experience or anything else frightening, and your level of physiological arousal will zoom back up.

To some degree, you can tell how physiologically aroused you are by paying attention to your body. Of course, partly for neurophysiological reasons, individuals differ in sensitivity to physiology;[544] some are relatively insensitive to internal changes, whereas others are *hyper*sensitive. Yet, to one degree or another, you can feel your heart pound, you can feel your respiration quicken, and you can feel your muscles tense. The more in tune you are with your body, the more you'll be able to regulate your physiological arousal. If your body has been violated, however, you may have difficulty being aware of your physiological state. You may have learned to tune out your body.

But you don't have to rely exclusively on your own inner bodily sensations. Here's where biofeedback comes in: biofeedback is the feedback of biological information to a person.[545] Feedback is essential to learning any skill.[546] In learning to talk, you rely on the sound of your voice to make the needed adjustments in your vocalization. As discussed in Chapter 2 ("Attachment"), in learning about feeling, you rely on social feedback from caregivers' facial expressions. With the aid of biofeedback technology, you can now rely on external feedback such as meters or tones to help you make adjustments in your physiological state. Biofeedback isn't a means of self-regulation; it provides feedback about physiological responses that can facilitate your use of *other* techniques such as relaxation, visualization, or meditation. Thus the proper term is biofeedback-assisted self-regulation.[547] By means of biofeedback, you can gradually learn to broaden your sphere of conscious, voluntary control over any physiological activity you can monitor. In the process, you're not training your body; you're training your brain.

A lot of gear has been developed to measure physiological arousal precisely. You can hook yourself up to a heart-rate monitor and observe exactly how fast your heart is beating from moment to moment. With such equipment, you can detect subtle cardiovascular changes that you might not normally be aware of. You can also become aware of the influence of your own thought processes on your heart rate. With increasing awareness, you can use your thoughts and visual imagery deliberately to exert more exact control over what goes on in your body. This is biofeedback. Instruments provide you with feedback about your "bio" processes. What you do with it is in your hands (or head).

Fortunately, there's a simple and inexpensive window into the physiology of one important aspect of the relaxation response—a little thermometer that measures finger temperature. Finger temperature is a sensitive gauge of autonomic nervous system arousal. With sympathetic nervous system arousal, blood flow is diverted into the large muscles in preparation for vigorous action. With parasympathetic activation, blood flows into the periphery—the tips of your fingers and toes. When you're nervous, your hands get cold; when you can warm your hands, you become calm. You can tape a little thermometer designed for that purpose to a finger and have an excellent barometer of autonomic nervous system activity. If you can get your finger temperature above 95°F and hold it there for several minutes, you can rest assured that you've lowered your sympathetic nervous system arousal, resulting in a pleasant, emotionally relaxed state. Somewhat more elaborate equipment can provide feedback about muscle tension, and more elaborate still are methods that allow you to use feedback about brain electrical activity to regulate your state of mind,[547] approaches that have been applied in the treatment of PTSD.[548]

Once you become aware of how this relaxed state feels, and you've discovered how to get yourself there, you can do it without the little thermometer. You can do it anywhere in the midst of any activity, to remain or restore calm. Although we often think of relaxation in connection with slowing down and resting, it's possible to be relaxed and active.[546]

Like exercise and relaxation, biofeedback is something you could conceivably use on your own. You don't need EEG equipment; you could buy a little thermometer and learn to warm your hands. But it's best to begin by working with a trained biofeedback therapist who can teach you about physiological self-regulation in more depth and who can guide you in the use of the technology. Hand warming will suffice for many persons, but the optimal technique will depend on the specific problematic pattern of physiological arousal.

Like any other technique that enhances relaxation, biofeedback can backfire. It can contribute to a sense of vulnerability as you release tension and let down your guard. And the inward focus may also open up traumatic memories and imagery. This openness to inner experience can be productive and healing in the presence of a competent therapist; otherwise it might lead to overwhelming emotion and retraumatization. When carefully prescribed and monitored, biofeedback has the specific advantages of bolstering awareness of the body and providing a sense of control and mastery. Feedback is ideal for providing tangible evidence of self-regulation and mastery.

Enjoyable Emotions

Fortunately, while legions of psychologists and others have studied the various forms of distress that befall us, a few have worked to understand what Ekman[126] refers to as the enjoyable emotions. We should be devoting at least as much energy to learning about feeling good as we do to learning about feeling bad.[549] Coping with trauma requires not just regulating and expressing painful emotions but also enhancing your capacity for enjoyable emotions—itself one important way of regulating painful emotions.

It's easy to appreciate the biological significance of emotions like fear and anger. Fight and flight can save our skin. But pleasurable emotions are just as biologically necessary. While distressing emotions tell us what to steer clear of, pleasurable feelings tell us what to head for. Pleasurable feelings go with activities that satisfy our basic needs, such as hunger, thirst, and sex. Enjoyable feelings also accompany the healthy forms of relatedness. More generally, pleasurable feelings go with activities that lead to growth, development, mastery, and accomplishment.

Emphasizing their growth-enhancing quality, psychologist Barbara Fredrickson[550] proposed a *broaden and build* theory of positive emotions. Whereas emotions like fear and anger narrow the focus of your attention onto the threat or problem at hand, pleasurable emotions broaden your attention and alter your pattern of thinking such that you become more open to new information, more flexible, and more creative. In a pleasurable emotional state, you're more likely to see problems from multiple perspectives and to come up with novel solutions. Moreover, positive emotional states are conducive to closeness with others and compassionate caring, as well as playfulness. Consequently, pleasurable emotions not only broaden your thinking but also enable you to build resources for coping with challenges, enhancing your resilience to stress.

With her colleague Robert Levenson, Fredrickson[551] also showed more directly that positive emotions can be an antidote to stress, having an *undoing* function. By exposing research participants to a frightening film, they induced a state of physiological stress, evidenced by cardiovascular activation. A subgroup of participants who subsequently viewed an amusing film showed a more rapid return of cardiovascular activity to normal. They also found that participants who spontaneously smiled during a sad film showed a more rapid return to normal activation afterward. Thus positive emotions are an important means of coping with stress—as the frequent use of gallows humor attests.

How might you go about cultivating enjoyable emotions? I suggest three broad strategies: direct mood-induction activities, efforts to find positive meaning, and increased attentiveness to spontaneous pleasurable emotional states. Ekman came up with the most direct pleasure-induction technique: voluntarily positioning your facial muscles into a smiling expression.[126] Remarkably, this technique not only can produce pleasurable feelings but also has been shown to generate patterns of brain activity consistent with positive emotion.[552] Psychologist Peter Lewinsohn and his colleagues[341] developed another direct approach, as I discussed in the context of recovering from depression (Chapter 8, "Depression"): you can take stock of activities that might provide pleasure and make a systematic effort to engage in them. While you can't force pleasure—except by smiling—you can put yourself in situations that might evoke pleasure.

More indirectly, it's possible for persons in stressful situations to enhance their mood by making an active effort to find positive meanings in daily events. Fredrickson,[550] for example, asked college students to find positive meaning in the best, worst, and ordinary daily events on a daily basis. Those who made the effort to do so showed more resilience to stress. In a related vein, psychologist Susan Folkman focused on positive experiences of caregivers of loved ones dying from AIDS.[553] Participants were asked to describe something they did or something meaningful that happened to them that made them feel good and helped them get through the day. Remarkably, in 99.5% of 1,795 interviews conducted, participants reported some meaningful positive event. For example, caregivers found positive meaning in having engaged in loving behavior or preserving the dignity of their ill partner. Caregivers experienced positive emotions when they set realistic goals and focused on small tasks. Successes in problem-focused coping countered their feelings of helplessness. The researchers emphasized how reframing stressful situations to see their positive features played a significant role in coping.

How does this apply to trauma? Certainly, no one would expect to experience positive emotion in the midst of traumatically stressful events. Yet, in the aftermath of trauma, many persons do find positive meaning. While trauma entails lasting negative effects, there is another side to trauma, namely, *posttraumatic growth*.[554] Some traumatized persons report going beyond recovery; feeling strengthened, they develop an enhanced sense of self-efficacy. Some report an increase in empathy, a greater capacity for intimacy, or increased spirituality. Such posttraumatic growth results from successfully wrestling with the various meanings of trauma.

I want to underscore Folkman's hopeful observation that people commonly experience positive emotions while they're coping with stress. Even in the midst of posttraumatic depression—pleasure-robbing as it may be—patients I work with show glimmers of pleasurable feelings and occasional sparks of enjoyment or amusement. I find Ekman's[126] concept of attentiveness to emotions useful here. I encourage depressed patients to *notice* these moments of pleasure. Coping with stress entails not only engaging in potentially pleasurable activities and striving to find positive meanings but also being attentive to whatever pleasurable emotions arise so as to cultivate and enhance them.

Thus I would not restrict the concept of mentalizing emotionally to regulating painful emotions; as I noted earlier, it's just as important to mentalize positive emotions. I'm not advocating replacing painful emotions with pleasurable emotions but rather cultivating the full range of emotion. Developing expertise in emotion is especially crucial for those struggling with trauma, and becoming a connoisseur of pleasurable emotions would be a worthy project. The following sketch of some enjoyable emotions might get you started.

Pleasure

Pleasure is probably the closest we have to a generic term for enjoyable emotional experience. Somewhat fortuitously in the early 1950s, neuroscientists James Olds and Peter Milner[555] discovered what seemed to be a *pleasure center* in the brain. Put a microelectrode in just the right spot on a rat's brain, and the rat will forget about everything else in its life and keep stimulating it. The rat's attitude: forget sex, food, and water, just let me stimulate this brain circuit! One rat in the original study pressed a bar at the rate of 1,920 times an hour to keep the stimulation going; later studies showed response rates as high as 7,000 per hour.[556] Not just rats but all of us vertebrates seem to possess these little pockets of neurons that we like to have stimulated. The idea of a pleasure *center* has fallen out of vogue, but researchers continue to make headway in tracing the complex brain circuits involved in producing the feeling of reward as well as the neurotransmitters and neurohormones involved in activating these circuits.[137]

Pleasure is closely linked to appetites—not just to eating a great meal but also to quenching thirst and having sex. Pleasure is intimately tied to bodily experience. We learn about pleasure through the body, for example, in nursing and being held and stroked. Pleasure comes through the appetites, the body, and the senses. Think of pleasurable sights, sounds, tastes, smells, and touch. Extending sensory pleasure a bit, think of aesthetic pleasure—wrapping your consciousness around something beautiful.

Intimate relationships provide a powerful source of pleasure. Psychoanalyst Joseph Lichtenberg[105] usefully distinguished sensual from sexual pleasure. Sensual pleasure, evident from infancy onward, comes from being touched, held, stroked, and soothed. Sensual pleasure may spark sexual excitement, but not necessarily; it can stand on its own.

For those who have been sexually traumatized, the pleasure that normally goes with sexuality can become linked with painful emotions. Among the most confusing aspects of sexual trauma is the intermingling of sexual pleasure with fear, pain, shame, and guilt feelings. Even in the midst of horrifying experience, the body and brain can respond sexually with excitement and orgasm—the circuits have been established over millions of years of evolution to respond to certain stimuli, and they work.

Sexual trauma can undermine sexual pleasure, because sexual arousal and excitement can become associated with danger, pain, and a host of negative emotions. But sexual trauma also can undermine *sensual* pleasure. Because sensual and sexual pleasure are often linked, sensual pleasure may be avoided. Yet touch is a vital need,[557] and trauma-related aversion to touch can result in severe deprivation. Many persons who have been traumatized find massage to be pleasurable and soothing when they're able to find a massage therapist with whom they feel safe.

Alternatively, if you've been sexually traumatized, you may desire sensual pleasure without sexual involvement. Some individuals put up with sex only for the purpose of obtaining some sensual pleasure in the process. Being held, touched, and stroked is soothing and may rekindle a sense of having a safe haven in attachment. Some persons who've been injured sexually resign themselves to forgoing sexual pleasure entirely, seeking satisfaction in being held and cuddled. Others stay tuned in to the physical contact preceding sex and then detach emotionally as soon as the interaction becomes sexual. Yet, to reiterate a point in Chapter 7 ("Illness"), sexual trauma by no means necessarily undermines the capacity for sexual satisfaction, and professionals now have extensive experience in helping couples find pleasure in sexual relations.

Before continuing with the list of enjoyable emotions, I want to issue an ironic warning: you may need to *go slow with pleasure*. You may need to *take pleasure in small doses*, building up your tolerance gradually. You may have little difficulty understanding your need to accustom yourself slowly to feeling and expressing anger or to gradually confronting situations that evoke fear. You may find it odd to think of pleasure in similar ways. But for many persons who have been through trauma, pleasure has been associated with pain. Pleasurable feelings can become a danger signal. I've talked to patients who've felt suicidal after experiencing intense pleasure, because their positive feelings triggered fear, shame, and guilt feelings. You may need to go slowly with pleasure, gradually desensitizing yourself to it, learning over time to suppress the connection between pleasure and the painful emotions associated with it in the past.

Interest and Excitement

We come wired to experience pleasure in our active engagement with the world. We can array this biologically based pleasure on a spectrum ranging from mild interest to intense excitement. These emotions, evident in infancy, are associated with a gradual and pleasurable rise in arousal.[172] Excitement gives life sparkle and zest. Interest and excitement bolster curiosity and novelty seeking. They fuel enthusiasm and involvement. They spark growth and development, motivating a wide range of activity and learning.

Neuroscientist Jaak Panksepp[137] neatly captured the significance of interest and excitement in what he calls the *seeking* circuit in the brain. He distinguished excitement from pleasure. The seeking circuit propels us, underpinning appetite and wanting. Having gotten what we want, we experience a distinct form of pleasure, consuming and liking. The neurotransmitter dopamine plays a major role in activating the seeking circuitry. Cocaine increases the availability of dopamine and strongly energizes the seeking circuit, providing a feeling of power and propelling the user into a variety of goal-directed activities. Analogously, manic states put the seeking circuit into overdrive.[558] Conversely, anxiety inhibits the seeking circuit, and depression undercuts it.

Relationships provide a main arena for interest and excitement and a foremost source of enjoyable emotions.[132] We come wired with curiosity about other persons—a continual source of novelty. Developmental researcher Robert Emde[559] took the smiling baby as the model of positive emotion. Babies smile at other persons. Smiling is borne of mutual interest and sharing of excitement, the entrée into an attachment relationship.

Excitement and fear have a common denominator—heightened arousal. But the arousal in fear is more abrupt and severe. Novelty can be interesting and exciting or frightening and anxiety provoking. Thus surprise is ambiguous: it can feel good or bad; some people enjoy it, whereas other dislike it.[126] Because of their overlapping arousal, excitement and anxiety have only a fine line between them. Even our language blurs the distinction; we say we're "anxious" to do something when, in actuality, we're eager to do it—excited about it. A sensitized nervous system can erode our sense of excitement, because any arousal can quickly trigger anxiety. And trauma-related emotions—not just anxiety but also depression as well as numbing—run counter to interest and excitement, promoting disengagement rather than engagement.

When you're in the throes of trauma, and especially when you're depressed, experiencing intense positive emotions may be well beyond reach. That's one reason I highlight interest; it's relatively subtle, and closer to hand. When you're depressed, it's important to notice signs of interest in something, however fleeting. Interest heralds the return of pleasure; the seeking circuit is active. Mentalizing emotionally pays dividends here, potentially amplifying glimmers of pleasure.

Flow

Psychologist Mihaly Csikszentmihalyi[560] has devoted his career to the study of optimal experience. His question: what is human experience at its best? This is something we should all know about. Csikszentmihalyi captured it in the word *flow,* a word that epitomizes optimal engagement with the world.

Examples of flow abound. Csikszentmihalyi found them by asking hundreds of individuals about their optimal experiences. He and his colleagues also monitored research participants throughout the day, periodically interrupting them to find out how often they were in flow and, if so, what they were doing at the time. At its most intense, flow involves a high level of challenging activity—mountain climbing, sailing, skiing, or racing are examples. In these instances, flow stands out clearly. It entails a high level of involvement and concentration. When you're in flow, you're completely absorbed in an activity; you're keenly conscious but not self-conscious.

Don't leap to the conclusion that flow is out of the question because you're not climbing Mount Kilimanjaro. You can experience flow in less risky and dramatic activities. Flow is conspicuous in intellectually challenging endeavors—games like chess, writing, lively conversation or repartee, or any sort of problem solving. You can be in flow during quiet activities like reading or meditating. You can experience flow in routine activities of daily living. Many persons experience flow in the course of their work. Contrary to what you may think, you're more likely to be in flow at work than in leisure, especially if you have a challenging occupation. Unsurprisingly, watching TV is usually a low-flow activity.

After studying thousands of flow experiences, Csikszentmihalyi boiled it down to a simple formula: to be in flow, you must balance the *challenge* of the activity with your level of *skill*. You're in flow when you're doing something challenging *and* you have the ability to pull it off. Flow is self-enhancing and growth promoting. As you continue doing the activity, your skills increase; then you need to increase the level of challenge to stay in flow. It doesn't matter whether it's a sport, an intellectual discipline, or a craft.

Being in flow is like walking a tightrope. The balance tips, and you're into something else. If your skills fall below the level of challenge, you're in trouble; you become anxious—or worse, if you're seeking flow in mountain climbing. Anxiety is the antithesis of flow. Anxiety goes with being immobilized, stuck, unable to move forward—behavioral inhibition. But anxiety isn't the only alternative to flow. If the challenge is way below your level of skill, you become bored. If the activity involves neither challenge nor skill, you become apathetic.

The range of potential flow activities is endless. Flow is not in the activity; it's in your consciousness. Flow does not require a high level of skill; it entails finding the right level of challenge. Flow is intrinsic to human consciousness, and it's probably not unique to humans. But it's also partly a personality trait; some individuals are able to find opportunities for flow in the bleakest of situations. Csikszentmihalyi describes individuals in concentration camps who sustained themselves by dreaming up imaginative intellectual challenges. The environment need not be an obstacle to enjoyment, as Csikszentmihalyi[560] wrote, "The Eskimos in their bleak, inhospitable lands learned to sing, dance, joke, carve beautiful objects, and create an elaborate mythology to give order and sense to their experiences" (p. 85). Others can spend megabucks on yachts, electronics, and sporting gear, only to remain bored and apathetic.

Finding your way from anxiety or detachment to flow may not be easy. A history of trauma and preoccupation with emotional survival is hardly conducive to flow. And exciting activities conducive to flow can trigger excessive arousal and anxiety. But flow is captivating and self-perpetuating; it feeds on itself. Once you hit on something, you want to repeat it for its own sake. Here is Csikszentmihalyi's[560] summary of what goes into flow:

> First, the experience usually occurs when we confront tasks we have a chance of completing. Second, we must be able to concentrate on what we're doing. Third and fourth, the concentration is usually possible because the task undertaken has clear goals and provides immediate feedback. Fifth, one acts with a deep but effortless involvement that removes from awareness the worries and frustrations of everyday life. Sixth, enjoyable experiences allow persons to exercise a sense of control over their actions. Seventh, concern for the self disappears, yet paradoxically the sense of self emerges stronger after the flow experience is over. Finally, the sense of the duration of time is altered; hours pass by in minutes, and minutes can stretch out to seem like hours. The combination of all these elements causes a sense of deep enjoyment that is so rewarding people feel that expending a great deal of energy is worthwhile simply to be able to feel it. (p. 49)

Enjoyment and Joy

If interest and excitement are in the anticipation, enjoyment and joy are in the consummation. We might put attachment center stage in joy: Ekman[126] depicts a joyful reunion as the prototype. As I'll discuss shortly, joy is central to love.

Just as interest and excitement are associated with a pleasurable rise in arousal, enjoyment and joy are associated with a pleasurable decrease:[172]

Ahhhh—satisfaction! After great exertion, success! Relief! I put flow between excitement and enjoyment because I think it captures the experience of using your skills to transform challenge to success. But it's hard to be precise here. The term enjoyment has fuzzy boundaries, and Ekman[126] refers to this whole territory of positive experience in terms of the enjoyable emotions. In addition to those mentioned here, he lists amusement, wonderment, ecstasy, *fiero* (the feeling of accomplishment after rising to a challenge), *naches* (the glow of pride a child can give to its parents), elevation, and gratitude. There's much to cultivate in this garden.

Contentment

Nathanson[172] extended the enjoyment-joy curve down to the state of *contentment*, where the arousal of excitement followed by enjoyment has largely subsided. I think it's worth highlighting this end of the curve, whether we call it contentment, tranquility, peace, relaxation, calm, stillness, or quiet. A model of contentment is the calm after orgasm.

If the opposite pole of positive emotion is depression, the opposite pole of distressing emotion is a state of calm,[132] the goal of relaxation exercises. We like best a state of low distress coupled with positive emotion, what Thayer called *calm energy*,[338] the antidote to tense tiredness.

Pride

I discussed this greatest of deadly sins in conjunction with shame (Chapter 3, "Emotion") and wish to emphasize it further here. To reiterate, we must distinguish between healthy pride and the destructive arrogance that has given pride a bad name. Many traumatized persons, crippled with shame, are inhibiting pride; yet pride is crucial to cementing memories that build self-esteem. Emde's[559] studies of smiling babies led him to appreciate the pleasure in *getting it right*. This marvelous phrase captures the pleasure in learning, understanding, and reaching a goal—even babies feel *fiero*! Getting it right promotes feelings of competence, control, and efficacy. The pleasure in getting it right is the flip side of helplessness—the essence of trauma.

Nathanson[172] construed pride and shame as being polar opposites. Shame involves a plummeting of pleasure associated with deflation. Pride follows the enjoyment of success after striving during challenging goal-directed activity. Thus we can think of pride as the afterglow of flow.

Pride, like shame, is a social emotion. When you feel proud, you want to be noticed and admired. You want to share your accomplishments. Shame is the opposite. When you feel ashamed, you're inclined to withdraw, to hide your face. Traumatic experience can interfere with pride the same way it interferes with all other emotions. Just as pleasure can become connected to shame, the pleasure in pride also can be connected to shame. Self-doubt, self-criticism, and self-hatred are incompatible with pride. With a history of trauma, pride may be extremely hard to come by. It's well worth cultivating this source of pleasure as an antidote to shame.

Compassion

First and foremost, the traumatized person needs compassion. For the sake of understanding compassion, it will help to make a few distinctions.[140] We can start with *sympathy,* a feeling of concern for someone in distress. *Empathy* is more complex, stemming from the comprehension and sharing of another person's emotional state, a key form of mentalizing. Empathy and sympathy often blend together and motivate helping. Yet it's not uncommon for us to respond with *personal distress* to others' distress; then we're more concerned about alleviating our distress than theirs.

Philosopher Martha Nussbaum[561] construed *compassion* as an emotion directed at the suffering of another person, but she emphasizes the complexity of the judgments that go into this feeling. We feel compassion when we judge that the other person is in a seriously bad way, prototypically, having suffered a tragedy or having suffered evil (see Chapter 14, "Hope"). We also experience compassion to the extent that we believe that the suffering is not deserved. Our compassion is facilitated by a sense that we, too, might suffer a similar fate. Finally, our compassion depends on encompassing the sufferer within our sphere of concern; we feel compassion to the extent that the sufferer's well-being is important to our own well-being.

I've been recommending self-compassion throughout this book. When you're suffering, self-compassion is a fitting companion. Self-compassion requires mentalizing emotionally—comprehending what you feel—and self-concern. In advocating compassion, for others or for oneself, we must distinguish it from pity. *Pity* connotes a feeling of superiority or even contempt, as in *pitiful.* By contrast, compassion implies respect.[562]

I think trauma sufferers unnecessarily resist self-compassion, confusing it with self-pity. Like confusing pride with arrogance, this blurring runs the risk of self-deprivation. When you're suffering, you deserve compassion and caring, from yourself as well as others. Compassion—not self-pity—can motivate caring for yourself, just as it motivates caring for others. As noted in Chapter 5 ("Self"), it's important to take your relationship with yourself most seriously and to improve it as best you can; you're continually immersed in it.

Love

Love is not a single emotion but rather a term we use to capture a highly emotional attachment relationship. Certainly, a loving relationship can be the source of the most profoundly rewarding and enjoyable feelings—affection, lust, awe, reverence, bliss, and ecstasy to note a few. Yet, as Freud[15] and other sages[16] have warned, given the inevitability of loss, to love is to risk profoundly painful feelings. Moreover, as we've seen throughout this book, loss is just one source of risk; love can be tangled up with all manner of attachment traumas. Thus love cannot be construed as unalloyed pleasure, but it's potentially the deepest and most enduring source of pleasurable emotion.

In his marvelous book *A Small Treatise on the Great Virtues*,[562] French philosopher André Comte-Sponville eloquently captured the essence of loving relationships. Unsurprisingly, the ancient Greeks had it well sorted out, distinguishing among three forms of love: eros, philia, and agape. Driving *eros* is an all-consuming desire, a passion for possessing, ultimately a quest for oneness. Eros is the strongest, most violent form of love: "The greatest source of suffering, failure, illusion, and disillusionment ... want is its essence, and passionate love is its culmination" (p. 238).

Philia encompasses friendship in its broadest sense; Aristotle's model was the delight mothers take in loving.[170] In the sense of philia, love means to derive joy from something—from seeing, touching, feeling, hearing, or imagining. In short, as Comte-Sponville put it, *love brings joy to the soul.* Accordingly, here's a fitting declaration of love: "I rejoice in the thought that you exist" (p. 251). Philia and eros are not mutually exclusive; we can love both passionately (eros) and joyously (philia).

Agape represents love in its broadest sense: universal love, as would bind all humanity together. Agape overlaps with charity and with compassion. Given our all-too-narrow sphere of concern,[561] we're bound to fall most short with respect to agape. Yet Comte-Sponville argues that love in general is most conspicuous by its absence; that's what makes loving virtuous.

We're liable to reject the concept of self-love as pathological narcissistic; yet we should no more reject self-love than pride. Brilliantly, New Zealand philosopher Christine Swanton[563] construed self-love as *bonding with oneself.* Thus self-love could be construed as an attachment relationship with oneself. Just as secure attachments do, self-love promotes strength, vitality, and energy. Thus self-love enables you to invest fully in your projects and goals. Moreover, as an inner secure base, self-love will promote mentalizing, your capacity to explore your own mind with a feeling of safety—freedom from fear of self-attack.

Self-love is not a vice. On the contrary, Swanton considers it essential to all other virtues, including love for others. Imagine being able to express self-love in Comte-Sponville's sense: I rejoice in the thought that I exist. Why not? As biologist Richard Dawkins[564] pointed out, the likelihood of your existing is infinitesimally small: "It's overwhelmingly probable that you are dead....In spite of these odds, you'll notice that you are, as a matter of fact, alive" (p. 3). Should you not rejoice?

Needing Help

You began learning and practicing emotion regulation in early infancy;[565] yet, achieving emotional competence is a lifelong task. Keep in mind that these venerable ways of regulating emotion are not easy for anyone. The Stoics and Buddhist monks devoted a lifetime to it. And I'm setting the bar high by advocating mentalizing emotionally: making sense of your own emotions and those of others while you're in the midst of an emotionally aroused state. As ample informal observations will attest, skillfully mentalizing emotionally is no small feat. Trauma poses additional challenges by evoking strong emotional reactions and creating a pattern of sensitization that renders you vulnerable to sudden eruptions of intense feelings and impulses that are especially hard to control. Moreover, trauma in early attachment relationships may interfere with the development of mentalizing and emotion-regulation skills.

I'm impressed by the persistent effort many trauma patients have made over the course of their lifetime to do many of the things I've been recommending in this chapter, often with considerable success. My fondest hope would be that this chapter would bolster your determination to stick with these efforts. I know, however, that stress can pile up to the extent that self-care falls by the wayside; then you can feel utterly overwhelmed and out of control. You may hit a patch when you need help to do what ordinarily comes naturally, if not easily. Then you may need professional treatment to help you employ these strategies so that you can return to the path of self-regulation, self-compassion, and self-care—always with the aid of attachment relationships.

Chapter 13

TREATMENT APPROACHES

Given the broad array of problems, symptoms, and disorders associated with traumatic experience, virtually all forms of psychological treatment have been applied to trauma.[566] Because of the complexity of trauma-related disturbances, the many forms of trauma, and inherent differences among individuals, treatment must be tailored to each patient's needs. Individual psychotherapy is the mainstay of treatment for trauma-related problems. But persons who have been severely traumatized may need a combination of diverse treatment approaches over an extended period of time.

The core of trauma treatment comes down to talking about traumatic experience in a trusting relationship—mentalizing in the context of secure attachment. Here we face a dilemma: reminders of trauma trigger symptoms of posttraumatic stress disorder (PTSD), and talking about traumatic experience is a direct reminder. Thus trauma-focused therapy can worsen symptoms, particularly for persons with a history of attachment trauma that has led to problems managing emotional distress.[567] There may be some wisdom in the view that you must get worse before you get better, but I wouldn't push that idea very far. It's better to *minimize* the likelihood that talking about trauma will make your symptoms worse. The goal of treatment is to improve your functioning and enhance your quality of life. For this reason,

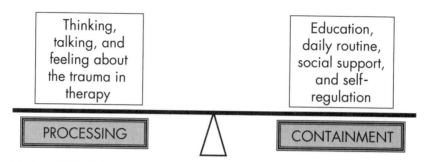

FIGURE 13–1. Balancing processing and containment in trauma treatment.

as depicted in Figure 13–1, *trauma treatment must balance processing with containment.*[25] Processing entails thinking, feeling, and talking about trauma. Containment entails regulating emotional responses, for example, by means of methods just discussed in Chapter 12, "Emotion Regulation." Thus containment renders processing emotionally bearable and productive, such that you move forward rather than backward.

This chapter spells out how treatment fosters containment and then discusses different facets of the therapeutic relationship, which provides the foundation for trauma treatment. I'll review several treatment approaches: cognitive-behavioral techniques for processing trauma, group psychotherapy, family interventions, medication, and hospitalization. Consider this chapter a sampling to acquaint you with a range of possibilities rather than a definitive guide to trauma treatment. We're on shifting sands as treatments continually are being refined and new interventions are being developed. I believe you'll be in the best position to find optimal treatment if you understand the general principles, especially the need to balance processing with containment and the overriding goal of enhancing the quality of life rather than immersing yourself further in trauma.

Containment

Containment has two related meanings: 1) holding or enclosing and 2) holding *back*, controlling, and restraining. The first meaning, the gentler one, is appealing. We could think of a mother containing her child's sadness by holding and comforting him while he cries. Processing trauma goes best in the context of such holding—emotional and physical—in a secure attachment relationship. But the second meaning of containment is also apt. Think of the mother's containing the child in the middle of a tantrum, holding him in the sense of restraining, so that he doesn't hurt himself. No doubt, self-containment also can be a struggle, sometimes requiring heroic self-restraint. And, when self-containment fails, we need external containment.

Sometimes containment entails holding back the full expression of emotions. Yet containment also *enables* fuller expression of emotion, as when a grieving widow holds back tears until she's in the loving embrace of a friend. Processing trauma, and feeling the associated emotions, requires both internal and external containment. The internal containment stems from a compassionate relationship with yourself and the capacity to mentalize, both of which facilitate various forms of self-regulation. External containment stems from supportive relationships, ideally, secure attachments.

I emphasize the importance of containment in trauma treatment because processing traumatic experiences will evoke strong emotions. But there's an equally important reason for emphasizing containment. Persons with a history of early attachment trauma are liable to have particular difficulty coping with painful emotions. Thus I consider developing the capacity for internal and external containment—self-holding and being held by others—to be the *primary goal* of trauma treatment. And, for persons with complex PTSD who are emotionally overwhelmed, trauma treatment might need to focus *exclusively* on containment rather than processing.[567] With better containment, trauma can be processed gradually, in small doses.

The natural recovery process from exposure to potentially traumatic events includes processing in close relationships—with loved ones and friends—in conjunction with employing naturally developed self-regulation skills. When the natural recovery process doesn't suffice, you need professional help. The first step in any treatment process is understanding the problem, and this understanding alone provides some degree of containment. Knowledge can make a big difference. Knowing you're having a panic attack and not a heart attack, or knowing that you're dissociating and not losing your mind, can be reassuring and somewhat calming.

Yet treatment generally must go beyond helping you understand your symptoms, and developing the capacity for containment may be a long process. To reiterate, processing without containment can backfire—particularly if you have not developed the capacity naturally to regulate your emotions and to make use of others' help in doing so. At worst, you may find yourself back in a state reminiscent of the original trauma: feeling afraid and alone. To highlight the dangers, I'll focus on a problematic—if intuitively appealing—treatment approach: abreaction.

Problems With Abreaction

Why talk about trauma? The simple answer: to get rid of the bottled-up feelings. In technical terms, *abreaction* describes this process of reexperiencing the trauma and expressing the strong emotions. In nontechnical terms, this idea of purging blocked emotion can be construed as *catharsis*. Treating symptoms by liberating blocked emotion goes back a century to Freud's early work.[220]

As I stated in discussing anger (Chapter 3, "Emotion"), I think it's misleading to think of yourself as being *filled up* with emotion. Maybe you feel strong emotions much of the time. Maybe you can easily become intensely emotional very quickly. You have a *capacity* to experience intense emotion. You may wish you didn't have this capacity. But just having another episode of extremely intense emotion will not diminish your capacity. You may protest, "I *feel* much better after an emotional outburst!" Releasing tension can lead to temporary relaxation. Like vigorous exercise, it can lower arousal. You may feel calmer after wearing yourself out. But emotional catharsis in itself does not lead to lasting change, and it often poses serious risks, especially for patients with PTSD.[568]

We have ample reason for caution: abreaction may be retraumatizing rather than helpful. Repeated exposure to traumatic levels of emotion may further sensitize you to the slightest reminder of traumatic memories. Your capacity to function may be increasingly undermined. Especially when dealing with repeated and prolonged trauma, you may find the goal of remembering and abreacting every traumatic experience not only overwhelming but also impossible. At worst, as discussed in Chapter 4 ("Memory"), you might add insult to injury by constructing inaccurate memories and burdening yourself with additional trauma.

The following scenario commonly precedes extended hospitalization: in the service of "getting it all out," exploring trauma leads to worsening symptoms and self-destructive behavior; the patient becomes increasingly desperate and dependent on the therapist; the therapist makes increasingly heroic efforts to keep the patient going; therapeutic boundaries are eroded by extended sessions, late-night phone calls, and sometimes efforts to provide physical comforting; the therapist becomes overwhelmed, worn out, and starts to withdraw; the patient feels abandoned and becomes distraught; and the patient is finally hospitalized in a suicidal crisis. At the point of hospitalization, everyone belatedly realizes that the emphasis must shift away from uncovering, exploration, and abreaction to containment.

The goal of talking about traumatic experience isn't to *release* pent-up emotion; instead, it's to gain better *control* over emotion. But the benefits of talking about trauma go beyond emotional control. Previously fragmented and unintelligible experience becomes more meaningful. In the process of talking about the trauma, you come to better understand yourself and your problems. Dissociated experience becomes integrated. Most important, talking about the trauma in an emotional way provides the opportunity to be *heard by someone*.

When—and if—the time is right to talk about trauma, you need to do so in an emotionally meaningful way. Yet, you should not assume that you must experience extremely intense emotions to benefit from talking about trauma. Some clinicians propose that talking about trauma in a calm state of mind can be therapeutic, and that the *authenticity* of the experience is more crucial than the emotional *intensity*.[569] As discussed earlier, two safeguards provide some assurance that you can talk about the trauma without adding to it: adequate preparation and pacing the work. Keep in mind Kluft's[452] maxim: "The slower you go, the faster you get there" (p. 42).

Safety First

Judith Herman[58] rightly declared that establishing safety is the first priority in treatment and that no other therapeutic work can be done without this first step. Albeit paramount in the beginning of treatment, safety remains crucial throughout. Above all, progress in treatment depends on putting an end to ongoing trauma, for example, battering or any other form of abuse. Your safety cannot be predicated on others' declarations that they will no longer inflict harm; rather, it must be based on your capacity for self-protection.

Safety includes not only protection from others but also protection from yourself. Many persons who have been severely traumatized continue to feel endangered by their own self-destructive impulses. This vulnerability reaches the extreme in dissociative identity disorder when the individual feels terrorized by dissociated suicidal states. Herman emphasized caring for basic needs, and doing so without exposing oneself to endangerment from abuse at the hands of others or oneself. Caring for basic needs includes finding safe living quarters, eating and sleeping properly, obtaining needed medical care, and providing for financial security. Another crucial component of safety is a social support network—the wider the better. This network may include friends, a partner, trusted family members, self-help groups, and mental health professionals. The process of establishing safety as a foundation for treatment isn't easy; Herman likens it to preparing to run a marathon.

Establishing safety can carry a high price. Many individuals face the dilemma of being economically dependent on persons who continue to inflict trauma. Herman poignantly described the potential costs of security:

> Creating a safe environment required the patient to make major changes in her life. It entailed difficult choices and sacrifices. This patient discovered, as many others have done, that she could not recover until she took charge of the material circumstances of her life. Without freedom, there can be no

safety and no recovery, but freedom is often achieved at great cost. In order
to gain their freedom, survivors may have to give up almost everything else.
Battered women may lose their homes, their friends, and their livelihood.
Survivors of childhood abuse may lose their families. Political refugees may
lose their homes and their homeland. Rarely are the dimensions of this sac-
rifice fully recognized. (p. 172)

Dialectical Behavior Therapy (DBT)

Psychologist Marcia Linehan's[513] approach to treating borderline personality
disorder (BPD), dialectical behavior therapy (DBT), is highly pertinent to
coping with trauma. As described in Chapter 11 ("Self-Destructiveness"), the
effects of trauma and the symptoms of BPD overlap considerably. For many
individuals, BPD could be construed as a complex posttraumatic stress syndrome.[567] Problems regulating intense emotion are the focus of DBT, and
Linehan recognizes their common origins in childhood trauma. That is, Linehan construes BPD as arising from a combination of difficulty regulating
emotional arousal and an invalidating environment. The child's intense emotional distress isn't contained by emotional attunement but rather exacer-
bated when natural emotional reactions are dismissed or punished. Plainly, a
childhood history of attachment trauma involving abuse and neglect would
typify the combination of emotional dysregulation and an invalidating environment. This combination undermines the development of mentalizing.
With these developmental problems in view, DBT interventions are carefully
designed to build skills in emotion regulation, taking into account trauma-
related problems and emotions, including dissociative symptoms that interfere with coping.[570]

Linehan cautions that pat answers and simple solutions will not do; the
problems are complex, and the work of treatment is arduous. She emphasizes that problematic behavior is an understandable effort to cope with often overwhelming feelings, and her intent is to help individuals find more
effective and less self-injurious ways of coping. Crucially, DBT requires that
skills for coping with painful emotional states that lead to self-destructive
behavior be learned before delving into traumatic experience in therapy[521]
—containment before processing.

Consistent with the principle of safety first, DBT's first priority is decreasing self-destructiveness, including deliberate self-harm and suicidal behavior. Systematic research has demonstrated considerable success for DBT
in this regard.[571] The second priority is to interrupt behavior that interferes
with therapy, such as failing to attend treatment sessions, not cooperating in
the work required, or not adhering to the therapist's limits. These problematic behaviors, like any others, become the focus of active problem solving.

The third priority is to decrease behavior that interferes with the quality of life, such as substance abuse, high-risk or criminal behavior, or financial problems. The next priority is increasing behavioral skills—not only enhancing interpersonal skills but also building tolerance for distress and learning techniques for emotional control. Patients are encouraged to adopt a perspective of *radical acceptance*—accepting as part of life the realities that one cannot control along with painful emotions.

As a behavioral approach to treatment, DBT is noteworthy for its emphasis on *actively teaching and reinforcing adaptive behavior.* As with other forms of treatment, the therapist works hard, but the patient must work even harder. The patient is encouraged to be highly active in concrete problem solving: carefully analyzing in step-by-step fashion the chain of events leading to problematic feelings and self-destructive behaviors and then identifying new ways of thinking and acting to avert such difficulties in the future. Patients use role-playing to practice different ways of handling troublesome situations.

DBT combines individual psychotherapy with educational group meetings that teach coping skills including mindfulness, emotion regulation, and distress tolerance. Patients are also encouraged to make use of telephone contact between sessions for on-the-spot consultation regarding hitches in problem solving. Especially pertinent to containment is DBT's emphasis on emotional regulation training,[572] which involves learning to identify and label emotions, analyzing the functions of emotions, preventing negative emotional states, increasing emotional hardiness, increasing positive emotions, letting go of negative emotions by paying attention to them and accepting them, and changing painful emotions by acting in a manner opposite to the feeling. Because DBT skills are so practical and helpful in day-to-day coping with emotional distress, DBT skills groups are a mainstay of trauma treatment at The Menninger Clinic.

The Therapeutic Relationship

The universal prescription for trauma: *talk about it.* To whom? To any trusted person who will listen—the sooner the better. This universal prescription works best in conjunction with single-blow traumas, such as a natural disaster, an assault, or a rape. Even then, it's not always easy to do. Talking about it may bring back the feelings of terror or rage engendered by the trauma. Shame may get in the way. As you begin to think or speak about it, self-protective defenses may block the memory.

It's not always easy for others to listen, even when they're caring and eager to help. Trauma can be abhorrent. Listening to another person's horrific stories of trauma can itself be traumatizing. It can threaten the listener's sense of safety and security. Friends may urge you to "just get your mind off it" so that *they* do not have to think about it. You may need to impress on them the importance of your need for someone to listen. But listeners' feelings of fear and outrage also can interfere with their capacity to listen. A woman who has been raped may find that every time she tries to discuss it with her husband, he becomes so embroiled in his wish to kill the rapist that he can hardly pay attention to her feelings. In such cases, trying to talk about the trauma can make it worse, not better.

When talking through the trauma with others isn't possible, you may need to turn to a psychotherapist who can help with the process. Like others who will listen, the psychotherapist's role is to bear witness. Not that it's easy for the psychotherapist. Psychotherapists also can feel horrified and outraged. But their training, experience, and professional role afford a degree of objectivity that provides a safeguard against their becoming so distressed that they, too, cannot listen.

Psychotherapists are continually challenged to find the right balance between professional detachment and emotional involvement. Empathy for another's feelings requires a delicate blend of intellectual understanding and emotional sympathy. If your psychotherapist goes too far in either direction, you may not feel safe talking about the full extent of your traumatic experience. If your psychotherapist is too detached, you may not feel supported. If your psychotherapist is too emotionally involved, you may feel a need to protect her or him from your feelings. In doing their best to bear witness, psychotherapists inevitably lose the middle ground of empathy to a degree: sometimes they withdraw into detachment, and at other times they're pulled into distressing emotional involvement. But as long as your psychotherapist spends a good deal of time in the middle range of empathy, you'll sense that the therapist has your mind in mind. Then you'll be able to talk in a way that proves beneficial.

The Therapeutic Alliance

Talking about trauma will go best when you have a solid alliance with your psychotherapist. The two essential ingredients of the therapeutic alliance are a positive relationship and a sense of working together with the therapist.[573]

Trust and a feeling of acceptance form the foundation of a positive relationship with a psychotherapist. The feeling of trust should be based on your perception that your psychotherapist is trustworthy, reliable, and striving to be helpful. For a good alliance, your psychotherapist must indeed be trustworthy and capable of providing help. Obtaining a referral from a reliable source and checking out your psychotherapist's reputation can help with trust. But ultimately you must make a judgment on the basis of your own experience with the psychotherapist. It's important to find a good match; a psychotherapist whom someone else finds helpful may not necessarily work well with you.

A therapeutic alliance also includes active collaboration. In psychotherapy research at The Menninger Clinic,[574] we've defined the patient's collaborative role as one of *making active use of the psychotherapy as a resource for constructive change.*[575] You should feel that you and your psychotherapist are working together toward common goals. You should be an active participant in the process. Probably every patient in psychotherapy wishes she or he could just be cured by the psychotherapist. Who wouldn't? But you're the major contributor to the success of your therapy. Your psychotherapist's job is to provide the guidance and support you need to do your hard work. Talking about trauma is hard work. Coping with trauma is hard work. Like any other hard work, you can't do it continuously. You need breaks, you need rest, and you need respite. Continuously avoiding traumatic memories blocks needed processing, but processing must be done in tolerable doses. Much of the time, distraction and avoidance are in order. It's the balance that's crucial. Regardless, the ultimate outcome of treatment depends on your persistence over the long haul.

Obstacles to the Therapeutic Alliance

Establishing a positive, collaborative relationship with trustworthy persons is easy if you have a history of good relationships. But if you've been traumatized in relationships—especially attachment relationships—then forming a positive alliance can be a huge challenge. You cannot ignore all prior experience and just plunge into psychotherapy with a good therapeutic alliance. You'll bring with you all the problems with attachment and relationships discussed earlier. Three of these problems deserve special emphasis: distrust, dependency problems, and boundary difficulties.

Working productively with your psychotherapist requires *trust*. If you've been traumatized in intimate relationships or by persons in a caregiving role, trust will not come easily. If you go on the basis of your previous experience—and no one is equipped to do otherwise—distrust is inevitable. You're likely to feel vulnerable to being injured or abandoned—or both, in that order. Here's a catch-22: if you can't trust, you can't do the work of therapy; if you can't do the work, you can't learn to trust. Once in this bind, you'll find that developing trust is a gradual process that takes a lot of courage. You may go back and forth. Trust will build slowly; as trust builds, you'll be able to do more work; and trust will continue to evolve. And your trust will be challenged from time to time by disappointments and frustrations in response to your therapist's inevitable failings and limitations—what I call the "H-factor," the therapist's being human.

As I noted in Chapter 6 ("Relationships"), it's common for individuals who have been traumatized by other persons to swing from one extreme to another—from distrust to excessive *dependency*. This alternation should not be surprising. When you finally develop a relationship that meets your needs, you're loath to let go and may rely exclusively on it.

Psychotherapy *requires* dependency. And psychotherapy can substitute belatedly for the safe haven of attachment that was not available at the time of the trauma. In a sense, the psychotherapist takes on the role of the attachment figure—mother, father, or friend. It's tempting to think of psychotherapy as a kind of reparenting. But taken much beyond a metaphor, the hope for reparenting is sure to lead to disillusionment.[576] Psychotherapists' time, the extent of their caring, and their availability are all limited. Their livelihood depends on payment for their services. Their capacity to be helpful as psychotherapists requires the professional role, without which it wouldn't be possible to provide the essential blend of emotional involvement and professional detachment. Because of the inherent limits on how much you can depend on your therapist, therapy also requires a considerable degree of self-dependence—the capacity to bridge the gap between separation and reunion—from the outset. And it's not easy to be self-dependent when you're struggling with trauma. Ideally, therapy will help you depend on others more easily.

Boundaries in the therapeutic relationship are especially crucial to trauma treatment. Boundaries maintain the integrity of the self. Your boundaries regulate closeness and distance in your relationships. By establishing boundaries, you maintain your privacy and your space. You set limits. Your boundaries shift from one relationship to another—you maintain less distance in intimate relationships. Boundaries need to be flexible, neither too rigid nor too fluid. A cell membrane is a good example of a flexible but durable boundary; it allows connection and interchange with the outside but also regulates what comes in and what goes out.

Trauma always entails intrusion and boundary violation—whether the trauma results from a tornado, from an assault, or from childhood abuse. Those who've been traumatized repeatedly by other persons, however, are likely to have difficulty with interpersonal boundaries. A boy whose mother routinely walked in on him whenever he was in the bathroom has had his boundaries violated. A girl whose father continually went through her private belongings has had her boundaries violated. A woman whose jealous husband spies on her is having her boundaries violated. A more extreme boundary violation is that of the body—physical or sexual assault. The most extreme boundary violation is that of the mind—brainwashing and totalitarian control such as occurs in psychological abuse, whether it be in a prison camp or in a home.[58]

Many persons whose boundaries have been violated are exquisitely sensitive to the boundaries of others. They may feel extremely reluctant to intrude on others or to make any demands of them. They keep their distance. They may not call, visit, or ask for help. Still other persons may have experienced such pervasive and severe boundary violations that they've never learned to become aware of interpersonal boundaries. They may lack any sense of privacy. They may intrude on others—using belongings without asking, calling at all hours, making unreasonable demands—and then be surprised or dismayed when rebuffed. Or they may allow themselves to be intruded upon or exploited in this way by others.

Maintaining therapeutic boundaries is essential in the treatment of persons who have been traumatized in childhood attachment relationships. The relationship must remain thoroughly professional. Psychotherapy is incompatible with business dealings or social contacts. With rare exceptions, such as emergencies, psychotherapy should take place at scheduled times in a professional setting.

The desire to be reparented goes awry when boundaries are not maintained. Many persons who have been traumatized understandably long for the physical comforting that they should have had. They feel extremely deprived and may have a hunger for soothing touch. This desire can be extremely powerful; it's natural and healthy, well worth fulfilling. But within psychotherapy, touch is problematic.[577] Psychotherapy is a *verbal* process. The comfort must come from being heard and understood, the sense that your therapist has your mind in mind. Many individuals who have been severely hurt and neglected feel that comforting words are a poor substitute for much-needed touch, and the therapy relationship can be frustrating in that respect. Physical comforting is highly desirable, but it should come from *other* relationships. The therapy process can help build the needed trust to make that possible.

Just as we've learned about the alarming prevalence of sexual abuse, we've also become aware of the troubling occurrence of sexual exploitation of patients by psychotherapists.[578] Moreover, patients with a history of sexual abuse are at highest risk for such exploitation.[579] As much as you might crave touch, you're likely to perceive it as a signal that further boundary violations are in the offing. Then your sense of safety is jeopardized, and you lose the fundamental prerequisite for therapy. Thus the therapist's insistence on maintaining boundaries—which at times may be frustrating to the patient—is an effort to preserve the therapeutic relationship. The same is true of any relationship. If boundaries are seriously violated, the relationship is likely to self-destruct, sooner or later.[577]

Confidence in Resolving Conflicts

Maintaining a solid therapeutic alliance continually challenges both patient and therapist. Even with patients for whom trauma isn't a main focus, the therapeutic alliance is likely to fluctuate considerably over the course of treatment.[574] You might find yourself starting with a relatively positive working relationship, only to find your trust and collaboration plummeting when you get further into the painful work and your relationship with your therapist deepens. Then you'll be challenged to grapple with your feelings and conflicts so as to reestablish the positive relationship. You may find that there are times when your therapy is on the brink of falling apart. Perhaps you're infuriated at your therapist or extremely disappointed, and you have some good reason to be. Talk it through. Developing the ability to work through such difficult periods can be the most significant part of the healing process. Conflicts are inevitable in *all* close relationships. Psychotherapy provides a relatively unique opportunity to talk freely about conflicts in a relationship with someone whose task it is to help you address interpersonal conflicts. Thus addressing and resolving conflicts in psychotherapy can be of paramount importance in building your confidence in resolving conflicts in other relationships.

The Benefits of a Therapeutic Relationship

Psychotherapy isn't a cure by love. Rather than belatedly attempting to provide the level of attachment security that was missing at the time of trauma, your psychotherapist can help you mourn that lack of mothering, comforting, and affection. No amount of psychotherapy can entirely redress that loss.

Although not a cure by love, the relationship established in psychotherapy can be healing and growth promoting. All too often, traumatic events are endured alone. Belatedly, these experiences can be revisited in the context of a trusting relationship. Secure attachment provides the needed context for processing and mentalizing—being able to have the traumatic memories in mind and to make some sense of the experience.

You may extend the capacity to trust and the feeling of security that you establish with your psychotherapist into your relationships with others. You may translate the acceptance provided by your psychotherapist into *self-acceptance*. Your therapist can serve as a model by helping you to think about yourself in a more tolerant and compassionate way. As you become more accepting of yourself, you can better confront your problems, conflicts, and limitations. At first, you need your therapist's help; later, you can do these things more on your own and with the help of others.

You might think of psychotherapy as a *bridge* to other relationships in which your natural and healthy needs for intimacy and physical comforting can be met.[25] As Bowlby stated, the need for comforting attachment—including touch—is lifelong.[71] Optimally, psychotherapy is but a way station that fosters a capacity to depend on others even more deeply and intimately. Yet patients in our trauma education groups are quick to point out that, while it's hard to have the trust to get on the psychotherapy bridge, it's even harder to get off the bridge once trust has evolved. Developing other attachments enables patients to leave the security of the bridge—ideally with the knowledge that the bridge will still be there if they need it in the future.

Cognitive-Behavioral Techniques

A century ago, Freud pioneered psychoanalytic treatment of trauma-related problems. Although he shifted focus from external trauma to internal conflict, the insight-oriented approach to psychotherapy that he developed continues to be a mainstay in the field of trauma. Ideally, as just discussed, psychotherapy provides a context in which you can talk about traumatic experience and make sense of it in the context of a trusting relationship.

In recent years, clinicians have developed cognitive-behavioral therapies focused specifically on treating symptoms of trauma, and most research on the effectiveness of therapy for PTSD has focused on these approaches. Like insight-oriented psychotherapy, these approaches offer a balance of containment and processing in the context of a safe and trusting relationship. Their unique techniques, however, have been developed to structure the processing of traumatic memories more systematically. Whereas individual psychotherapy for trauma is widely used but rarely researched,[580,581] cognitive-behavioral techniques have the advantage of considerable research support.

Exposure Therapy

Many techniques have been developed to help patients cope with frightening experiences and situations, and all these techniques require *exposure* to the feared stimulus. You must become *desensitized* to whatever frightens you. If you want to conquer a fear of public speaking, you might do so by speaking in front of groups, perhaps starting with small informal gatherings and gradually working your way up to more challenging groups. That's how most of us desensitize ourselves to fear—it's called *in vivo* (in life) exposure. With repeated exposure, your anxiety gradually decreases, and you respond less strongly to the feared situation.

As PTSD attests, it's not necessary to be in a frightening situation to feel afraid; imagining frightening situations also brings fear. Thankfully, owing to the emotional richness of imagination, you don't need to expose yourself to traumatic situations to become desensitized. *Imaginal exposure* is also effective in reducing fear and anxiety. By talking about traumatic events and integrating them into your self-understanding, you can become desensitized to them. Keep in mind, however, that processing must be balanced by containment: if you try to go too fast and are unable to regulate the level of your emotional distress, you can become *sensitized* rather than desensitized. You may then respond *more intensely*—rather than less so—to the images and memories.

Focusing on women with a history of assault, psychologist Edna Foa and her colleagues developed a method of exposure therapy based on solid theory and careful research.[17] Foa[582] highlighted three components essential to successful processing of traumatic experiences, each of which plays a role in a positive treatment outcome: 1) engaging emotionally with the traumatic memories, 2) organizing a coherent narrative of the trauma, and 3) modifying core negative beliefs associated with the trauma, namely that the world is dangerous and the self is incompetent.

Although focusing on processing, Foa's treatment approach attends to the need for containment, for example, by providing educational material about trauma and its treatment as well as relaxation exercises for the purpose of stress management. Both in vivo and imaginal exposure are employed. As an example of in vivo exposure, the rape survivor is instructed to return to the scene of the assault—under safe conditions—and to remain there for 30–45 minutes until her anxiety subsides. The imaginal exposure entails a series of therapy sessions during which the patient repeatedly recounts the details of the traumatic event as if it were happening in the present. The sessions of imaginal exposure are audiotape recorded, and the patient continues the exposure at home, listening to the tape recordings of sessions.

When exposure therapy proceeds according to plan, the patient's anxiety gradually subsides over the course of the therapy, and the narrative—the story—becomes increasingly organized. The patient's perspective on the dangerousness of the world becomes more realistic, and she feels less incompetent and blameworthy. But the effectiveness of this process hinges on emotional engagement—feeling the distressing feelings. Demonstrating this point, Foa and her colleagues videotaped sessions to study the relation between patients' facial expressions of fear and the outcome of the treatment. They found that patients who experienced fear in conjunction with talking about the traumatic events had a good treatment outcome—their posttraumatic symptoms decreased. Surprisingly, those who showed more anger were less likely to improve, not because there's anything wrong with feeling and expressing anger but rather because the anger was blocking the processing of fear.

It's not welcome news that effective treatment entails emotional pain, but it makes some sense: you must feel the emotions in order to learn how to regulate them and to become less frightened and intimidated by them. To say that you must feel the fear, however, does not mean that you must feel panic or terror; that would be counterproductive. The emotion is best kept at a manageable level. For persons who have great difficulty regulating their emotions, exposure therapy may not be the best approach.[567] An alternative is systematic desensitization, where there's a greater focus on maintaining a state of relaxation while imagining the traumatic situation.[583] Although not as extensively researched as exposure therapy, there's some evidence that systematic desensitization can be helpful in the treatment of trauma,[584] such that it might be considered as an alternative for those who cannot tolerate standard exposure therapy.

Cognitive Restructuring

Researchers have found that persons with negative beliefs (cognitions) about themselves and the world are more vulnerable to developing PTSD in the aftermath of trauma, and that these negative beliefs also perpetuate PTSD.[585] Negative views about the self promote feelings of helplessness and guilt, and unrealistic beliefs about the dangerousness of the world contribute to a feeling of ongoing threat, fueling worry, anxiety, and dread. Any therapy for trauma will address these beliefs, but cognitive restructuring makes them a primary focus.

There are many cognitive approaches to trauma treatment,[566] but psychologist Patricia Resick and colleagues' cognitive processing therapy[586] is noteworthy in having a very clear rationale, blending a range of therapeutic elements, and having solid research evidence for its effectiveness. Like exposure therapy, the process begins with the patient writing a detailed description of the traumatic event and her reactions to it, then reading it aloud to herself and to the therapist. The cognitive component involves educating the patient about the role of maladaptive thinking in PTSD and then systematically exploring and challenging the negative thoughts so as to help the patient rethink the meaning of the experience in a more balanced way.

Eye Movement Desensitization and Reprocessing (EMDR)

Psychologist Francine Shapiro developed eye movement desensitization and reprocessing (EMDR) somewhat fortuitously.[587] When walking in a park, she noticed that her rapid eye movements reduced her emotional distress at a point when she was thinking disturbing thoughts. Then she developed a systematic way of incorporating eye movements into trauma treatment.

EMDR is similar to exposure therapy in that patients are instructed to think about the details of a traumatic event and their reactions, and then they bring images of the event to mind. EMDR incorporates aspects of cognitive restructuring in identifying negative beliefs connected with the trauma, such as self-blaming thoughts, and formulating alternative beliefs that are more positive. The desensitization process involves bringing the traumatic memory to mind while simultaneously moving the eyes from side to side, following the therapist's fingers moving back and forth in front of the face.

After a series of eye movements, the patient is instructed to let go of the traumatic images and to say whatever comes to mind. Quite often, memories and ideas not previously connected with the traumatic events come to mind and provide new perspectives on the meaning of the trauma. Over the course of successful treatment, the emotional distress associated with the traumatic memories abates, the traumatic images become less intrusive, and beliefs about oneself become more positive.

A number of research studies have shown EMDR to be an effective treatment for trauma,[588,589] and a large number of clinicians have been trained in the method. Yet many professionals remain skeptical of EMDR, in part because of continuing controversy as to whether the eye movements contribute to the effectiveness of the treatment.[590,591] Like other effective treatments for trauma, the full EMDR procedure includes aspects of containment, such as education and help with stress management, as well as therapeutic exposure and processing. EMDR can be a relatively brief treatment for some traumas,[592] and the relatively brief exposure to traumatic memories in EMDR may make it a relatively tolerable procedure for many patients.[593] Nonetheless, some patients find EMDR to be highly stimulating and difficult to tolerate. Like any other treatment method, EMDR will be helpful for some patients and not others.

Challenges in Choosing an Intervention

Considering the large number of treatment techniques employed in treating trauma, patients and therapists alike are keen to know which ones are most effective. Cognitive-behavioral therapists have been most assiduous in researching their treatment outcomes and comparing techniques. Exposure therapy, cognitive restructuring, and EMDR are all effective. However, are they all *equally* effective?

We have more research on the effectiveness of various interventions than we have horse race–like comparisons between methods. The results of well-controlled studies[594,595] show more similarities than differences between exposure and cognitive restructuring approaches in effectiveness. The clinical difference between these two treatments is essentially a matter of emphasis;

exposure therapies make use of cognitive restructuring and vice versa, so their similarity in effectiveness is not surprising. Although research isn't consistent on this point, there may be some advantage in systematically combining exposure and cognitive techniques.[596]

EMDR also includes a modified exposure component as well as cognitive restructuring, and its effectiveness is well demonstrated. Researchers are beginning to compare outcomes of EMDR directly to other techniques, which will put patients and therapists in a stronger position to make informed choices. One study noteworthy for its careful research methods compared EMDR, exposure therapy, and relaxation training.[597] All three interventions were effective, with exposure therapy showing some advantage over EMDR and relaxation training. Notably, although relaxation training may be a helpful adjunct to trauma treatment, it's not generally effective as a stand-alone treatment insofar as it does not include the processing of trauma.[580]

Research to date provides the strongest evidence for exposure as the crucial element in treating PTSD.[580] To reiterate, exposure entails bringing traumatic memories to mind and talking about them in the context of safety, which entails mentalizing in the context of attachment. This process occurs in the full range of cognitive-behavioral techniques as well as in psychotherapy more generally. As emphasized throughout this book, trauma-related problems may go far beyond PTSD, such that there's far more to therapy than exposure techniques. Moreover, some persons find any form of exposure to be too anxiety provoking, such that the emphasis must be placed on containment, at least in the short run if not also in the long run. Thus, for complex trauma-related problems, the treatment must be individualized in a way that calls for sophisticated clinical judgment.[581]

Group Psychotherapy

We develop our first attachments in the context of dyadic relationships—twosomes, such as mother and infant. But attachment gradually extends beyond caregivers and family members to encompass affiliation with groups. Cohesive and stable groups can provide a powerful sense of belonging as well as a sense of safety. Like a secure attachment relationship, they can provide a safe haven and a secure base. Although systematic research on the effectiveness of group therapy for trauma survivors lags behind research on individual therapy, the studies that have been reported are encouraging.[580]

There's tremendous diversity in the kinds of groups that are beneficial to trauma survivors. Many groups are established according to the type of trauma experienced—groups for victims of specific natural disasters, for Vietnam veterans, and for incest survivors. Groups also can be beneficial for persons with dissociative disorders who may feel that their seemingly unusual symptoms are particularly alien.[598] Herman[58] emphasized that the type of group should be matched to the stage of recovery. In the first stage, group therapy should focus on safety; in the second, on remembering and talking about traumatic experience; and in the third, on developing sustaining relationships. Moreover, persons who have been traumatized should not begin group therapy until they've achieved initial stability with individual psychotherapy and other social supports. Prematurely entering a group in which traumatic experience is discussed can be overwhelming and retraumatizing—sensitizing rather than desensitizing. Just talking about the topic of trauma in groups can stir traumatic memories, and listening to other group members talk about traumatic experiences can be extremely distressing. Thus having developed some capacity to process trauma and contain the associated emotions is a crucial prerequisite for doing additional work in a group.

Yet when ready, traumatized individuals can benefit enormously from group psychotherapy. Telling the story and having others bear witness takes on a new dimension within the context of a group. Anyone who has been traumatized has felt helpless, alone, and isolated. But many who have been traumatized have been isolated by virtue of their own feelings of shame and guilt. Being able to talk in a group helps overcome this sense of isolation, as does learning that others have gone through similar experiences.

Overcoming the sense of isolation and establishing a base of emotional support are probably the most important benefits of group therapy for trauma. Group therapist Irwin Yalom[599] referred to the appreciation that others have struggled with the same problems as *universality*. But he also found that the most common benefit offered by a therapy group is interpersonal learning. Withdrawing from others is a nearly universal response to trauma. Moreover, those who have experienced prolonged childhood trauma often have been systematically isolated from their peers. Therapy groups provide a forum for learning to trust, to manage interpersonal conflicts, and to interact in satisfying ways. Thus a cohesive group can provide a secure base for exploring problems and conflicts in relationships as well as providing a great deal of support. Like individual psychotherapy, a group can be a stepping stone to a wider array of relationships and community groups.

Family Interventions

Family work in relation to trauma is extremely complex, owing to the diversity of trauma, the multiplicity of family members and their roles, and the many purposes of intervention. Here, as elsewhere, safety is the overriding issue. If family members—spouse, siblings, parents—are involved in ongoing violence or abuse, any treatment effort will be stalemated. Enlisting the support of any family members who *can* be supportive is essential, whether they're in the contemporary family or the family of origin. Yet it's essential, first, to consider the impact of trauma on those who are in the role of caregivers.

Strain on Caregivers

Those to whom we are closest usually bear the brunt of our problems. Of course, any serious psychiatric disorder may place a significant burden and strain on family members, and this effect is true for trauma-related disorders as well.[600] Many trauma-related problems such as dissociative experiences are bewildering. Deliberate self-harm is frightening, and suicide attempts can be downright terrifying. Partners who are willing to bear witness to the trauma may find themselves traumatized vicariously. They may experience painful emotions, have nightmares, or be aware of intrusive thoughts about the trauma. Short of vicarious trauma, they may feel taxed by emotional turbulence in the relationship. Most poignantly, couples struggle with the barriers trauma poses to healthy intimacy:

> A woman who had been raped became panicky and rageful when her husband lay on top of her with his face close to hers during sexual intercourse. His weight on her chest interfered with her breathing and triggered memories of feeling suffocated. This fearful reaction was explained to her husband as being analogous to a Vietnam veteran's flashback on hearing a car backfire. Recognizing this connection enabled the couple to find ways of being sexually intimate without triggering symptoms of PTSD.

Vulnerability to emotional contagion and reenactment of traumatic relationship patterns are common problems in intimate relationships.[601] Emotional contagion is a problem for us all, especially in close relationships. Traumatic stress is contagious, and trauma-related symptoms are all the more distressing to caregivers because they're hard to understand and don't seem justified by the situation. The 90/10 reaction is seen as an unjustified overreaction. In addition, as discussed in Chapter 6 ("Relationships"), reenactments are common in close relationships. Not only is it distressing to the traumatized person to feel as if the abuse and neglect is occurring yet again, it's also distressing to the caregiver to be experienced as abusive and neglecting—or worse, to be drawn into *behaving* in abusive and neglectful ways. These problems of contagion and reenactment are particularly intense when both members are struggling with a history of trauma. Then 90/10 reactions on both sides can magnify each other.

Quite naturally, caregivers struggling with contagion and reenactment will feel stressed out and helpless, and they're likely also to become irritable and frustrated. Their entreaties—"Just do something to get your mind off it!" or "Stop acting crazy!"—will fall on deaf ears. Extensive research on the role of the family in psychiatric disorders has focused on the harmful effects of criticism and hostility directed toward the person with the disorder, and these findings apply to trauma as well. Not uncommonly, persons with PTSD become engaged in hostile and critical interactions with family members,[602] and these interactions have an adverse effect on treatment as well as family relationships. Frustration and argumentativeness burden everyone.

The obvious strain on caregivers places an additional burden on traumatized persons, who are already likely to feel unrealistically guilty as well as to fear that they will be abandoned yet again. It's easy to lose sight of the fact that many caregivers are steadfast, and their emotional reactions stem partly from the level of their concern and caring as well as their sense of helplessness.

As described in Chapter 8 ("Depression"), caregivers walk a tightrope, potentially alternating between being overly critical and withdrawing. To remain steadfastly supportive, caregivers also need help.[603] Just as the traumatized individual needs to be educated, so, too, does the family.[604] Just clarifying the basis of the traumatized member's difficulties can often prove helpful. Better understanding brings more acceptance and a prospect of calmer interactions. When the family's anxiety abates, the traumatized individual's anxiety also decreases.

How Partners Can Be Supportive

No special characteristics are needed to support a traumatized person—just tolerance, patience, understanding, dependability, empathy, compassion, and affection! These characteristics are likely to be needed in considerable measure. I have greatly admired a number of supportive partners, but I have yet to meet a saint. Many persons have these admirable characteristics in large measure, but no one has them in limitless amounts. And support is inevitably intermingled with periods of apprehension, frustration, and discouragement. Patience and tolerance wear thin.

Partners must maintain their own boundaries; they must know their limits and set them. Partners who overextend themselves will not be able to sustain their support and are likely to withdraw or break off the relationship. Partners can be helpful in fostering other supportive relationships and in encouraging involvement in whatever form of treatment may be needed.

To be supportive, partners need to be supported. They must take care of themselves to be able to be caregivers. They also need supportive relationships. When we conducted family workshops for traumatized patients,[25] partners told us that the single most important thing for their well-being was ensuring that their life did not become dominated by the trauma. Maintaining outside interests and other supportive relationships were crucial. Many also find it helpful to participate in treatment with the trauma survivor or to find their own individual or group treatment.

Disclosure and Confrontation

Seeking support requires you to let others know something about the trauma you've undergone. This openness may not be so difficult if the trauma was an accident or a criminal assault. But much traumatic experience—rape or child abuse—is associated with a great deal of shame. In such cases, disclosure is no easy matter. Children who disclose sexual abuse often experience adverse consequences: they're not believed, not supported, or blamed for ensuing family problems. When these reactions occur, the whole experience becomes even more traumatic.[605]

If the traumatic experience involved maltreatment within your family of origin, then disclosing the trauma within the family will prove particularly challenging. Experienced clinicians recommend that you make a list of family members, then begin telling persons who are most likely to be receptive or who may be able to provide validation by offering additional information.[606] Such planning makes disclosure a thoughtful, step-by-step process. Moreover, at various points, disclosure shades into confrontation. For example, when a history of abuse is revealed to unknowing family members, such as the mother, resentment or outrage at their failure to protect or their complicity also might come to the fore. Some individuals might even decide to confront those who abused them as the final step in bringing the traumatic experience to light.

Disclosure and confrontation are likely to have a powerful impact, for better or for worse. To ensure a better chance of their being therapeutic instead of destructive, careful preparation is essential. *If done at all,* disclosure and confrontation be should be done in the later stages of treatment rather than at the beginning. It's particularly important to resist being pressured into premature confrontation by an outraged friend, family member, or survivors' group.

Progress in therapy can be a gauge for your readiness to disclose the trauma outside of therapy. Readiness for disclosure is marked by being able to talk about the trauma without becoming emotionally overwhelmed or dissociating. Disclosure and confrontation require that you be comfortable with expressing anger and experiencing the sense of power that goes with it. The motto, safety first, applies to this situation as it does elsewhere. You should have built up a reliable support network and trustworthy allies—in the family or outside it. The process of disclosure can be extremely stressful and will necessitate additional support. Also, you should be at a point where you feel in control of any self-destructive inclinations and can ensure your own safety. Finally, some individuals may use the help of a therapist in the disclosure process.

Setting realistic goals helps pave the way for disclosure and confrontation. Disclosure can be empowering to the degree that unburdening yourself facilitates giving up secrecy, shame, guilt, and a feeling of responsibility for the trauma. Disclosure may also bring forth validating information, bolstering your sense of reality. Ideally, disclosure and confrontation can open up communication within the family and provide an opportunity to establish more healthy adult relationships.

Some goals are understandable but counterproductive. Revenge is a likely motive for confrontation. The desire for revenge may be more or less conscious, but it's probably always present to some degree. If vengeance is in the forefront, an explosive situation may be in the offing, which heightens the potential for retraumatization. A related goal may be to have an emotional catharsis—in effect, "If I could just let him have it, I'd feel better." But the idea of a cure by catharsis is just as dubious in the context of family work as it is in any other type of therapy.

No matter how extensive your preparation, you cannot be assured that disclosure and confrontation will lead to any particular outcome—or even a good outcome. At best, the result is likely to involve a mixture of satisfaction and disappointment. Keep in mind that you cannot control others; you can only control what *you* do. If your well-being depends on a certain outcome, such as being believed or hearing expressions of remorse, you could be risking additional disillusionment. If you can settle for being satisfied with having spoken out and told the truth, regardless of the consequences, then you'll have more control over the whole process.

Emancipation and Connection in Adulthood

Extricating yourself from traumatic relationships isn't easy. At worst, traumatic bonding may be like emotional superglue. Many adult children who felt mistreated by their parents remain highly dependent on them yet angry and resentful toward them—the adult counterpart of resistant attachment. They encounter extreme frustration and disillusionment as they continue to hope—despite ongoing evidence to the contrary—that family relationships will be more fulfilling. It's not easy to gauge how much change is possible and how much energy to devote to it. Persistence is admirable, but it can be carried too far. When faced with the impossible, giving up is not an unreasonable strategy.

Often, adults struggling with ambivalent attachments to their parents go from one extreme to another. Feeling frustrated and hurt, they're tempted to break their ties completely and cut themselves off from the family. In some cases, a period of distance may be needed to maintain safety and to prevent retraumatization. In some instances, minimizing close contact over the long term may be the only solution. Yet family cutoffs are incompatible with life-long needs for attachment, and most persons prefer not to sever family ties. Becoming more self-dependent does not mean becoming completely independent. In some instances, family therapy may help adult children strike a better balance, becoming more separate and autonomous so as to remain emotionally connected in a more stable and satisfying way.

Medication

We have antianxiety medications, antidepressants, antipsychotics, and anticonvulsants. There are no anti-PTSDs or antidissociatives. But, in conjunction with psychological interventions, many medications initially developed for other psychiatric disorders and general medical conditions also provide some benefit for trauma-related symptoms. Our drug classifications should not be taken too seriously. The brain has a mind of its own and shows little respect for our labels. Regardless of the name we assign a medication, the brain determines what to do with it. *Antidepressants*, for example, have turned out to be effective in preventing panic attacks and treating anxiety more generally; thus it's been suggested that selective serotonin reuptake inhibitors—SSRIs such as fluoxetine (Prozac)—could well be considered "antinervousness" agents.[607]

Psychopharmacology, the treatment of psychological symptoms with medication, is evolving at a fast pace. New medications are continually coming onto the market, and older medications are being tried in new ways. Although psychiatrists have accumulated a great deal of clinical experience in using medications for treating PTSD in the treatment of trauma, relatively little controlled research on the effectiveness of various medications for treating PTSD has been conducted.[608] And there are two glaring limitations of studies conducted to date. First they tend to focus on one disorder—PTSD—whereas many traumatized patients have multiple disorders. Second, they study one medication in isolation from others, whereas many patients are prescribed combinations of medications. Moreover, psychiatrists recognize the need to target medications to the specific biology or to the specific symptoms of PTSD rather than continuing only to rely on medications for other disorders.[608]

This section describes the extensions of the major classes of psychiatric medications to the treatment of trauma. I present this material not to imply that you should be taking any specific type of medication; that decision is between you and your psychiatrist. I'm primarily interested in getting across a few general points. First, an awareness of medication treatment underscores the significance of biological factors in trauma-related problems. Second, there are lots of possible avenues of help with medication. Third, you should appreciate the complexity of treating trauma-related symptoms with medication. As with the rest of treatment, you may need substantial doses of patience and persistence. But the effort is worthwhile, because medication can be one pillar of containment; taking medication is a cornerstone of self-regulation.

Antidepressants

As described in Chapter 8, depression is a common result of trauma, so it's not surprising that many traumatized patients are prescribed antidepressants. Yet, failing to stay within the bounds of our labels, antidepressants are the closest we have to an anti-PTSD medication, and their effectiveness in treating PTSD is far better supported by research than any other type of medication.[608] Other types of medication are used to target problematic symptoms that may accompany PTSD, but antidepressants have become the standard pharmacological treatment.

Earlier antidepressants employed in the treatment of PTSD include tricyclics such as imipramine (Tofranil) and amitriptyline (Elavil), as well as monoamine oxidase inhibitors such as phenelzine (Nardil). The newer antidepressants, the SSRIs, have now become the first-line treatment for PTSD.[580] The SSRIs include sertraline (Zoloft) and paroxetine (Paxil), which, at the time of this writing, are the only two medications to receive indication for treatment of PTSD from the U.S. Food and Drug Administration.[609] Serotonin plays a major role in the overall regulation of brain activity,[610] and SSRIs increase its availability by inhibiting the reuptake mechanism that terminates its action. In addition to serving as antidepressants, these serotonergic medications can help with the full spectrum of PTSD symptoms, including not just hyperarousal and intrusive symptoms but also avoidance and numbing.[611] Because they also appear to help with control of impulsive behavior, the SSRIs play a useful role in treating symptoms such as self-directed aggression, explosiveness, and behavioral reenactment of trauma.[612]

Other Classes of Medication

PTSD is an anxiety disorder, and antianxiety medications (e.g., benzodiazepines such as diazepam [Valium], alprazolam [Xanax], lorazepam [Ativan], and clonazepam [Klonopin]) are widely employed to reduce anxiety and promote sleep. Although the antianxiety agents would seem to be the logical choice in treating PTSD, research on their effectiveness has yielded mixed results,[392] and these medications can create additional problems.[612] The benzodiazepines resemble alcohol in their neurophysiological effects, and, like alcohol, they can be addictive. You can develop a tolerance to them so that you need increasingly high doses to get the same effect. In addition, abrupt withdrawal can be dangerous, for example, leading to seizures. Withdrawal also can stimulate rebound anxiety, worsening PTSD symptoms. Other potentially adverse side effects for persons coping with trauma include depression, decreased ability to exert control over aggressive impulses, and memory problems. Benzodiazepines also can react dangerously with alcohol and can lead to falls, suppression of breathing, and loss of consciousness.

As noted repeatedly throughout this book, the basic response to traumatic stress is fight or flight, which entails sympathetic nervous system arousal. Medications used primarily to treat hypertension (high blood pressure) have been enlisted in the treatment of PTSD because of their effects on sympathetic arousal.[613] Beta blockers, for example, dampen physiological arousal, thereby alleviating subjective distress and attenuating the physiological triggers for panic attacks. Like many other psychiatric medications, these antihypertensives may have serious side effects and must be carefully prescribed and monitored.

Some agents employed as antiseizure medications (anticonvulsants) as well as lithium, an antimanic agent used to treat bipolar (manic-depressive) disorder, also appear to be of benefit in stabilizing mood. PTSD is neither a seizure disorder nor a mood disorder but, given the potential role of some anticonvulsants and lithium in stabilizing mood-related symptoms, these medications may also be employed to treat such symptoms in patients with PTSD.[611]

Psychotic symptoms reflect a loss of contact with reality. Hallucinations (e.g., hearing voices) and delusions (extremely unrealistic beliefs, such as believing one's food to be poisoned) are not included in the diagnosis of PTSD, but a number of persons also experience these symptoms in association with PTSD.[614] Although antipsychotics are not indicated for routine treatment of PTSD,[580] low doses of these medications may be helpful in the treatment of associated psychotic symptoms.[615] New-generation antipsychotics with fewer side effects are gaining more widespread use and thus may find increasing clinical application in the treatment of trauma.[608]

Individual Differences

There are already lots of potentially helpful medications, and lots more will undoubtedly come on the market. Not only are there many individual medications to choose from, but also these medications are frequently used in combination. The huge number of possible medications, combinations, dosages, and lengths of treatment makes choosing the optimal treatment extremely complex.

The particular treatment must be matched to the individual's symptoms. In addition to having different symptom patterns, individuals differ widely in how they respond to specific medications. What works for someone else may not work for you, even if your symptoms are similar. These individual differences are undoubtedly related to constitutional factors such as genetic makeup and metabolism. Because of the genetic contribution, a family history of medication response may be a useful guide. If a parent or sibling benefited from a particular medication, you may also respond well to it. Note that pharmacotherapy invariably involves some trial and error to find the optimal medications, as well as some tinkering to find the best combinations and dosages. In addition, various medications should receive an adequate trial; for some, several weeks or even months may be needed to achieve the optimal benefit.[616] Moreover, you may need to continue taking medication for a considerable time after recovery to guard against recurrence of symptoms. Finally, your medication needs may change over time, depending on your condition and your response to treatment.

Integrated Treatment

It's utterly natural to wish for a cure by medication—or by anything else, for that matter. Anyone would. For trauma, however, the current medications are only moderately effective, at best. And medication is only part of more comprehensive treatment. Medication isn't an alternative to psychotherapy and other forms of psychological treatment; instead, psychological and pharmacological treatments potentially enhance each other. If your symptoms are severe and you feel completely out of control, working productively in psychotherapy may be out of the question. Medication may be essential to provide the stability for psychotherapy to be feasible. Moreover, psychotherapy may entail exploring traumatic memories, and this exploration can temporarily heighten anxiety and arousal. Medication may provide containment by helping to keep arousal within bounds. And it works both ways: psychotherapy, by fostering self-understanding and self-control, may help control arousal so that the medication will be most effective. At best, from a psychosomatic perspective, psychotherapy and pharmacotherapy work synergistically: mind stabilizes brain, and brain stabilizes mind.

One final point about medication: it won't work if you don't take it. This obvious point is worth addressing, because patient compliance with any kind of medical treatment is notoriously poor. Yet it's crucial not only to take the medication as prescribed but also to keep track of its benefits and side effects and report them to your psychiatrist. Making optimal use of medication therefore requires a high level of collaboration between patient and physician. Your psychiatrist will have no way to judge the potential effectiveness of the medication without your collaboration and feedback. Without such active collaboration, the often complicated process of finding the optimal medications and dosages will be unduly prolonged.

Yet severe trauma-related problems can interfere with needed collaboration. For example, if dissociation leads to gaps in memory, you may not remember what medication you have taken, and you may have more difficulty evaluating its benefits. When such problems significantly interfere with medication compliance, treatment in a structured setting, such as an inpatient unit or day hospital, may be needed so that regular observation is possible. Otherwise, it's another catch-22 situation: you need to be taking the medication for the symptoms that interfere with your taking the medication.

Hospital Treatment

Occasionally, some persons with a history of attachment trauma and severe symptoms need hospitalization during periods of crisis. Hospitalization provides added external containment when self-regulation and social support are not sufficient.

A number of different precipitants may create trauma-related crises that merit hospitalization. Under the weight of stress pileup, you may feel overwhelmed and, at worst, resort to self-injurious behavior as a way of coping. Hospitalization may be needed for self-protection, and, for some persons, hospitalization is required to prevent destructive behavior toward others. Ideally, the person in crisis can be hospitalized during periods of high risk *before* acting on destructive impulses.

Remembering long-forgotten traumatic experience is another potentially disruptive stressor[197] that sometimes precipitates a crisis eventuating in hospitalization. An individual who has gone for years or even decades with no thought of childhood trauma may have this past experience brought to awareness by some stressor in adulthood such as an accident, an assault, a loss, or a divorce. The mind may be flooded by traumatic images and feelings of confusion and panic. And, for those predisposed, any emotional crisis—including being flooded by memories of trauma—may lead to episodes of dissociation. Recurrent flashbacks, uncontrolled switching among dissociative states, and continual interruption of ongoing experience by amnesia can make it virtually impossible to cope with the demands of daily life. Then hospitalization may be needed to get you back on track.[617]

The principle, safety first, applies as much to hospitalization as it does to any other form of treatment. Initially, however, the individual will be confronted with an unfamiliar environment, many strangers, and a number of restrictions. It's not uncommon for patients to want to leave the hospital soon after they've been admitted. But during a crisis, the inpatient setting can become a much needed safe haven. The main function of hospital treatment is to provide protection and to enhance self-control. But hospitalization also serves a variety of other functions by providing protection from intruders, a structured day with constructive activities, an opportunity for 24-hour observation to monitor dissociation and switching, a healthy daily cycle of sleep and wakefulness, medication management, and medical care. Perhaps most important, individuals in crisis typically are isolated—back in the fundamental traumatic situation of feeling afraid and alone. Hospital treatment counters isolation by encouraging the individual to reach out and make contact with others, promoting social engagement rather than isolation. The hospital environment ensures involvement in relationships, which ultimately hold the key to healing.

Not uncommonly, patients enter the hospital with the anticipation of delving into memories of trauma in a safe environment. There's no question that a hospital can be a safe place to do painful therapeutic work. Yet hospitalization for that purpose alone is questionable.[618] The goal of a curative catharsis is an illusion. If hospitalization is needed because of the likelihood that further processing of trauma would lead you to become emotionally overwhelmed or put you at risk for further destructive behavior, then the balance in treatment has tipped too far away from containment. The function of hospitalization should be to bolster your capacity for containment.

Most trauma treatment will be carried out on an outpatient basis, and, in general, hospitalizations for crises will be brief. Some individuals, however, may need longer hospitalizations. Factors that may necessitate longer hospital stays in the treatment of trauma-related disorders are similar to those that make for extended hospitalization in the treatment of other psychiatric disorders.[619] These factors include protracted destructive or self-destructive behavior, complex dissociative symptoms that do not allow for a rapid restoration of continuity, other severe symptoms that do not respond to outpatient treatment (such as severe depression or eating disorders), family problems that preclude discharge to a supportive environment, or complications in establishing appropriate outpatient treatment.

As the role of trauma in psychiatric disorders has become more apparent over recent decades, specialized inpatient treatment programs for trauma have been developed.[257] These programs have the advantages of providing clinical expertise in conjunction with a milieu in which patients with similar experiences can support and learn from each other. The effectiveness of these programs has been somewhat hard to gauge, as relatively little research has been conducted and we always have difficulty knowing which aspects of these multifaceted programs are helpful. Moreover, because the programs are geared to the treatment of patients with more severe and chronic trauma, their effects are understandably modest.

Most research on specialized inpatient programs has been conducted on combat trauma in Department of Veterans Affairs hospitals, and this research attests to the challenges in treating chronic trauma.[620] Studies of specialized treatment for traumatized women have yielded encouraging results, although these findings must be considered preliminary.[621] We found that patients benefited substantially from hospitalization but continued to struggle with symptoms 1 year after discharge.[257] Given the inherently waxing and waning course of complex trauma-related disorders, however, we don't expect any treatment to be curative; the goal of hospitalization of any duration is to foster sufficient containment so that treatment can proceed on an outpatient basis.

Just as we can think of the need for containment as ranging along a wide spectrum, mental health services also can provide a broad continuum of care, including inpatient treatment, day-hospital programs, residential treatment, halfway and quarterway houses, activity and vocational programs, medication clinics, and social work services, as well as individual and group psychotherapy. In principle, you could have whatever level of support you might need during a given period of treatment. In practice, the availability of services varies widely from one region to another, and costs typically impose significant constraints.

Quality of Life

Here's one way to think about trauma treatment: your capacity for containment must be developed so that you can get on with the real work of therapy, processing the trauma, for example, by exposure therapy. However, I've come to think of this formulation as backwards. The main goal of therapy is to develop the capacity for containment, through building supportive attachment relationships and self-regulation skills that promote emotion regulation. Processing isn't something to be done for its own sake; the value of processing is to build greater capacity for containment—through secure attachments and self-regulation.

This thought brings me to a key conclusion: some individuals get so caught up in trying to uncover everything in the service of "getting it all out" that they completely lose sight of the goal of treatment—improved quality of life.[580] This point is so obvious that you can breeze right over it without even thinking about it. So let me emphasize again: *the goal of treatment isn't to uncover memories or to purge emotion but rather to improve the quality of your life.* At worst, catharsis can become a *way of life* or a substitute for living. As such, it's not much of a life, and it could be endless.

Treatment is likely to play a significant role in working toward the goal of enhancing your quality of life. But treatment isn't sufficient. As discussed in Chapter 7 ("Illness"), your health-related behavior also plays a major role in your well-being. To reiterate stress researcher Bruce McEwen's[264] point, the advice our grandmothers could have given us now has a solid scientific foundation: eating well, sleeping well, moderating use of alcohol, refraining from smoking, exercising routinely, and maintaining supportive relationships all contribute significantly to our physical and mental health. Few of us can live being completely free of illness, and many traumatized persons live with a considerable amount of illness. But we'd best aspire to live well—with illness if need be. This approach brings us to the topic of hope.

```
┌─────────────────────────────────────────────┐
│  ┌───────────────────────────────────────┐  │
│  │   •    C h a p t e r    1 4    •       │  │
│  ├───────────────────────────────────────┤  │
│  │                                       │  │
│  │             HOPE                      │  │
│  │                                       │  │
│  └───────────────────────────────────────┘  │
└─────────────────────────────────────────────┘
```

HOPE

This chapter brings hope from the background into the foreground. I've intended each chapter to provide some grounds for hope by promoting understanding and suggesting coping and treatment strategies. But I've adopted a low-key approach, based on years of working with traumatized persons. I've found that a cheerfully upbeat and naively optimistic attitude fails to inspire hope by not respecting the gravity of traumatic experience. Excess optimism can be demoralizing, teetering on the "just-put-the-past-behind-you" injunction that so alienates traumatized persons by neglecting the sheer difficulty of recovering from trauma. You know from experience what I've endeavored to reinforce throughout this book: recovering and remaining well can require hard work over a long period of time on many fronts—trying to make sense of the trauma, striving to take care of yourself, and cultivating close relationships.

I trust you've gathered that there are grounds for hope, not least that trauma can be understood and that there are many potential avenues of healing. And I find reason for hope in the prodigious amounts of energy and intelligence that legions of clinicians and researchers are devoting to expanding our understanding of trauma and to developing increasingly effective treatments. At the time of this writing, the American Psychiatric Association is finalizing guidelines for treatment of posttraumatic stress disorder (PTSD) that pull together current knowledge and chart the course for future research.

Psychotherapeutic approaches will continue to be refined, and we can count on significant progress on the biological front. The Decade of the Brain has come to a close, but researchers are forging ahead on the neurobiology of trauma, an endeavor that will enhance understanding and treatment in ways we can hardly foresee. Sadly, it has taken neuroscience to demonstrate what every trauma sufferer knows beyond a doubt: trauma is a real illness. And Columbia University psychologist Susan Coates[622] proposed that the events of September 11, 2001, yielded an overdue benefit to trauma survivors: "The long-standing stigma on traumatized individuals has come to an end" (p. 11).

The topic of hope is too important to leave implicit in what I've written thus far, because healing from trauma depends on it. As with all else, we must understand hope as best we can. I recognize that I'm rushing in where angels fear to tread; writing about hope is a bit like writing about love (and I wasn't deterred from that either). There's a limit to how much analysis some emotional experiences can withstand, and we always run the risk of trivializing. Undaunted, I'm applying the approach I've taken to all the other emotions, convinced that thinking about hope more clearly might help you cultivate it.

This chapter proceeds in four steps. First, I'll give some definition to hope by contrasting psychological and existential perspectives. Second, I'll make a bold suggestion as to what traumatized persons might *hope for*: flourishing. Third, I'll discuss two aspects of trauma that most threaten hope: depression and evildoing. Finally, I'll discuss three foundations of hope: meaning, benevolence, and self-worth.

Understanding Hope

I'll begin sharpening the concept of hope by distinguishing it from wishing and optimism. Then I'll discuss the psychology of hope, emphasizing how feeling and thinking must be conjoined in hope. Yet, believing that psychology cannot take us far enough, I'll construe hope as an existential stance adopted in tragic circumstances.

Wishing and Optimism

My mentor, psychologist Paul Pruyser, drew a sharp contrast between hoping and wishing. Wishing focuses on specific objects or desirable things—we wish for everything from a winning lottery ticket to a new home or a suitable mate. When we think or say, "I hope that ...," we're often just wishing. Certainly, nothing is wrong with wishing; on the contrary, desires that prompt wishing fuel our worthy goals and projects. Yet to wish is not to hope.

Hope and optimism are not so easily distinguished; they overlap in three ways. First, both entail positive expectations about the future. Second, both can be more or less realistic, and, if they are too unrealistic, both can be counterproductive, undermining prudence, planning, and constructive action. Third, both can be traits or states. That is, like optimism, hopefulness can be a relatively enduring trait; some persons are characteristically more hopeful than others. Too, like optimism, hopefulness is a potentially changeable state of mind; in the aftermath of a major loss or setback, you can sink into hopelessness, and then you can rebound into hopefulness. Ideally mentalizing, you might recognize that such feelings of hopelessness are a state of mind that is biasing your appraisal of reality.

In the face of all these similarities, here's the main difference: optimism pertains to less serious matters, and hope applies to more grave concerns. To take extreme examples, you might be optimistic that you'll have a sunny day for your picnic, whereas you might maintain hope that humanity will find a way to avert its self-annihilation with weapons of mass destruction.

To take the lighter side for a moment, much can be said in favor of optimism. Extensive research shows that optimism is associated with good mood, good health, popularity, perseverance, and success in a wide range of endeavors.[623] Conversely, pessimism is associated with alienation, passivity, failure, and ill health. Although a mildly unrealistic positive bias is healthy and beneficial,[235] optimism works best when it's tempered by pessimism, as reality dictates.

As I contended at the outset, optimism seems too lighthearted a word to capture what's needed in the oftentimes grueling process of healing from trauma. Just like healing from any other serious illness or psychological wound, healing from trauma requires hope.

Psychological Perspectives: Agency and Pathways

Your heart and head must work together here. Hope requires a synthesis of emotion and reason, feeling and thought. Emotion and reason come together in Karl Menninger's[624] definition: hope provides a motive force (emotion) for a plan of action (reason) that has prospects of succeeding. As Menninger saw it, hope sustains a confident search based on sound expectations. The research of psychologist Rick Snyder and his colleagues[625] on hope parallels Menninger's view. Snyder and his colleagues propose two ingredients: *agency* (the emotional motive force) and *pathways* (the reasoned plan of action). Borrowing from the proverb "Where there's a will there's a way," Snyder defined hope colloquially[626] as "the sum of mental willpower and waypower that you have for your goals" (p. 5). *Willpower* (agency) refers to determination and commitment, a feeling of having what it takes to achieve your goals. *Waypower* (pathways) requires effective means for reaching your goals. Thus hope must not be blind; to act hopefully, you need more than the motivation; you also must have some sense of direction—a pathway.

Oncologist-hematologist Jerome Groopman's work with gravely ill patients led him to an elegant formulation in his brilliantly wise book, *The Anatomy of Hope*.[627] His definition also combines feeling and thinking, both grounded in reality:

> Many of us confuse hope with optimism, a prevailing attitude that "things turn out for the best." But hope differs from optimism. Hope does not arise from being told to "think positively," or from hearing an overly rosy forecast. Hope, unlike optimism, is rooted in unalloyed reality. Although there is no uniform definition of hope, I found one that seemed to capture what my patients had taught me. *Hope is the elevating feeling we experience when we see— in the mind's eye—a path to a better future.* Hope acknowledges the significant obstacles and deep pitfalls along that path. True hope has no room for delusion. (p. xiv; emphasis added)

Most germane to our concerns, Groopman's observations attest to the cardinal role of hope in recovering from serious illness. Also directly pertinent, Snyder[626] described how supportive attachment relationships foster hopefulness and, conversely, how trauma in childhood and adulthood tends to erode hope. But Snyder's research also documents a broader range of benefits. Hope is associated with positive emotion, high self-esteem, a sense of control, and greater problem-solving ability as well as more success in attaining goals. Little wonder that hope fosters coping and recovery. Unsurprisingly, Snyder found that hopefulness is diminished by painful emotions like depression, hostility, anxiety, and guilt feelings.

Existential Hope

Drawing on his substantial contributions to the psychology of religion, Paul Pruyser[628] considered hope to be an existential condition. Here's the link between trauma and hope: hoping presupposes a tragic situation and serious suffering. When all is well, you might do a lot of wishing, but you have no need for hope. *Hope is a response to felt tragedy.* For example, one might have hope that life can be worth living despite the handicaps and troubles imposed by illness, hope that life-threatening disease can be faced with courage, or hope that bitterness can be overcome.

When you consider that hope is a response to felt tragedy, you can appreciate how hope and fear are close companions. We most need hope when we're threatened and endangered; thus hope is always infused with fear to a greater or lesser degree. When we focus on the danger, we feel more afraid; when we can envision averting the danger, we feel more hopeful. Thus we tend to alternate between fear and hope in varying proportions. Ironically, as Stoic philosopher Seneca claimed, "You will cease to fear if you cease to hope" (quoted by Nussbaum,[117] p. 28). But giving up hope, and thereby giving in to despair, is too great a price to pay for ridding oneself of fear.

Hope requires restraint. Pruyser contrasted the demanding impatience of wishing with the modest and more peaceful waiting that hoping sustains. Based on a tragic sense of life and an undistorted view of reality, hoping entails an attitude of modesty and humility, coupled with recognition that reality—and the future—is open ended, not fully knowable. Accepting our inherently limited grasp of reality allows for the possibility of novelty, leaving some space for hope. An absolute conviction that things will turn out badly immodestly fails to take into account our limited grasp of reality.

Hope also requires imagination. As rational agents, we're able to "imagine realistically alternative possible futures," to borrow contemporary philosopher Alasdair MacIntyre's[244] apt phrase (p. 83). Depression and fear undermine hope by constraining your imagination: to the extent you *can* imagine, you envision only the worst.

To summarize: to hope is to adopt an existential *stance*. The grounds for hoping do not lie in the *facts* of reality but rather in the *meaning* we ascribe to reality. Hence hoping is an active process of making meaning. As an active process, hoping is not static; hoping may alternate with fearing when the threat looms large and with despairing when meaning collapses. In the face of tragedy and suffering, hoping is difficult and precious; it's a virtue, hard won and challenging to sustain.

Aspiring to Flourish

We encourage traumatized persons to think of themselves as survivors, not victims. When we were discussing this distinction in a trauma education group some years ago, one patient protested, "It's not enough to survive: I want to *thrive*." She had it just right. Thriving is a high aspiration for someone who has been traumatized. Yet, in the long run, nothing less will do.

Plainly, surviving is not sufficient—and even recovery may not be. Recovering from illness doesn't automatically restore purpose in life, and, often enough, it's essential to find meaning in a life that includes illness. The aspiration of thriving confronts us with the age-old quest for the good life, a perennial preoccupation of philosophy and a dawning concern in psychology.

Philosophical Perspectives

In the fourth century B.C.E., Aristotle[170] launched his discourse on ethics with the question, "Are we not more likely to achieve our aim if we have a target?" (p. 64). I can't tell you how to flourish or become hopeful or how to lead the good life. But having a clearer idea of what you're aiming for will help, assuming that—like the protesting patient in my group—you're not content with being a survivor but rather aim to thrive. Fortunately, we're in a position to take fairly careful aim because, evolving from Aristotle's magnificent legacy, we're blessed with a rich history of thought on what thriving entails.

In his treatise on ethics, Aristotle[170] took aim on *eudaemonia*, a term that lends itself to various translations, "happiness" being the most common. But, unlike us, Aristotle didn't consider happiness to be an emotional state like enjoyment or contentment. Such feelings are a potential *by-product* of eudaemonia, which entails living well. As we all know—or should know— we can't aim straight for happiness; rather, happiness is an accompaniment to engaging in valuable projects and developing meaningful connections with others. Because we tend to confuse happiness with enjoyment, eudaemonia is better translated as *flourishing*. More specifically, Aristotle construed eudaemonia as acting in accordance with virtue, where virtues are defined as excellences of character (e.g., courage, persistence, and truthfulness).

Psychological Perspectives

After more than a half-century of focusing on illness, psychologists have begun to embrace the project Aristotle so masterfully launched, conducting research that identifies the basis of flourishing. We can start with the idea that flourishing stems from *vital engagement* in activities, most often in conjunction with active exploration of the world.[629] Vital engagement in activity has value beyond reaching specific goals; such activity contributes to flourishing in being *expressive* of your individuality. Self-expression has innumerable avenues—not just through creative products like artworks but also through whatever individual style you give to your various words and deeds.

Helpfully, psychologists are reaching consensus on three domains of activity that contribute to flourishing: intimacy, generativity, and spirituality.[630] All three domains entail a sense of connection with other persons and the world.

- *Intimacy* first. Central to intimate relatedness is the capacity to confide and to express emotions, coupled with a sense of being understood, validated, appreciated, and valued.[241] This is precisely what we construe as mentalizing in secure attachment relationships: creating a feeling of connection, with each person having the other person's mind in mind.

- Going beyond intimacy is *generativity*, one of psychoanalyst Erik Erikson's[72] later stages of life development. Generativity entails an investment in future generations, for example, as expressed in teaching, mentoring, counseling, leadership, or creating products that will be of lasting benefit.

- *Spirituality* can be defined in many ways and in both religious and secular contexts. Broadly, spirituality entails relatedness with something transcendent, often with a feeling of reverence or awe. If we put self-centeredness at one end of a spectrum, spirituality would belong at the other end. Spirituality involves a sense of connection with something beyond the self—something vast or grand—as in the sense of connection with nature or the divine. Loving another person can be spiritual in this sense. Philosopher Robert Solomon[143] emphasized the process of reaching beyond the self and offered this view: "Spirituality means to me the grand and thoughtful passions of life and a life lived in accordance with these grand thoughts and passions. Spirituality embraces love, trust, reverence, and wisdom, as well as the most terrifying aspects of life, tragedy, and death" (p. 6).

Vital engagement in intimacy, generativity, and spirituality promotes flourishing. Ironically, investing in the stereotypical American dream—pursuing goals related to physical attractiveness, financial success, social recognition, and power—tends to undermine flourishing and to contribute to dissatisfaction, anxiety, and depression.[630] And we should not overlook the role of positive physical health—functional abilities, aerobic capacities, and healthy behavior in relation to sleep, exercise, and diet.[258] We Americans are not doing well on that score either, considering our sedentary lifestyle and epidemic obesity.

How common is flourishing? Not very. Psychologist Corey Keyes[631] estimated that roughly 20% of the population in the United States is flourishing, that is, showing emotional vitality along with positive psychological and social functioning. On the opposite end of the spectrum, roughly 20% are *languishing*, that is, devoid of positive emotion, having a sense that life is empty and hollow, and living a life of quiet despair. Importantly, these languishing individuals are *not* reporting any symptoms of depression. They're not ill; yet, lacking in positive mental health, they're certainly not doing well.

Unfortunately, it's possible to be languishing (not flourishing) and depressed (ill), whereas it's rare for a person to be ill with severe depression and still flourishing. Plainly, posttraumatic depression and the host of trauma-related disorders reviewed in this book pose significant impediments to flourishing. But it's important to keep in mind that mental illness and positive mental health are somewhat independent of one another. Flourishing in the midst of a major depressive episode is highly uncommon. But all is not lost. Trauma-related illnesses tend to have an episodic quality—you do better in some periods and worse in others, often in tandem with levels of stress. Like illness, flourishing may be episodic. For all of us, flourishing is a matter of degree and will vary from one time to another.

Yet, short of a patch of profound depression, illness isn't necessarily a barrier to flourishing, at least in some domains. Even in the face of terminal illness, some persons are able to find meaning and purpose that sustains hope. Groopman's book[627] is full of examples in the general medical setting. As I've noted earlier in this book, psychologists consistently observe that many persons find positive meaning even in the midst of stress, challenges, struggling, and suffering. It's not uncommon for survivors to report significant growth experiences following trauma.[554] Examples include increased self-reliance, awareness of mortality, closer ties to others, greater empathy and compassion for others, developing a clearer philosophy of life, renewed appreciation of life, and a deeper sense of meaning and spirituality.

Paradoxically, traumatic stress can be one contributor to flourishing, perhaps most prominently by enhancing your appreciation for being alive, an appreciation that all too easily slips out of mind in the fray of day-to-day living. Remarking on the perennial complaint that life is too short, Stoic philosopher Seneca[632] countered that human life is plenty long, but "slight is the portion of life we live" (p. 49). His Stoic successor, Roman Emperor Marcus Aurelius[633] challenged, "Think of yourself as dead. You have lived your life. Now take what's left and live it properly" (p. 94). Flourish.

Threats to Hope

I've been commenting throughout on ways in which trauma undermines hope, and I want to elaborate on two major challenges here, one psychological (depression) and the other existential (evil).

The Challenge of Depression

As should be amply evident by now, depression is a powerful enemy of hope. Hope depends on positive emotion, including the anticipation of rewarding feelings that support your striving to attain goals. Yet, as we've seen, the core of depressed mood is a diminished capacity for positive emotion—the catch-22. Thus depression undercuts expectation of reward and the feeling of agency, the motive power for hope. Moreover, depression undercuts imagination, eroding your capacity for flexible and creative thinking. You're liable to focus all your attention on the negatives, at worst, spinning your wheels in rumination. Thus, to use Snyder's terms, depression is capable of undermining both your willpower (agency) and your waypower (seeing pathways out of your plight).

Working with cancer patients, Groopman[627] came to appreciate how hopelessness and hope are grounded in the body. Metastasizing cancer affects many tissues and organs, potentially compromising the vital functions of respiration, circulation, and digestion. He speculated that the brain registers this compromised body state in the feeling of hopelessness. When tissue and organ function begin to recover in response to treatment, the feeling of hope returns. I'm inclined to extrapolate Groopman's view to posttraumatic depression. As described in Chapter 7 ("Illness"), chronic stress can have a pervasive impact on the body, affecting many organ systems, leading to a state of generalized ill health. Perhaps the brain registers also this state of ill health in feelings of hopelessness. Note the hopeful side to this speculation: all the things you can do to improve your physical health may contribute powerfully to hope.

My clinical experience also mirrors Groopman's. As patients' depression begins to lift, they become more hopeful in both feeling and thought. They have more energy for coping—a greater feeling of agency and more motive force. Their vision broadens. They begin to see pathways—ways of handling difficult situations and challenges—that never occurred to them in the midst of the hopeless state. This healing process is remarkable. The external reality has not changed, but their *experience* of reality is transformed.

I've pointed to physical health as one route to rekindling hope, and another also bears mention: setting reasonable goals. Menninger, Snyder, and Groopman are in accord in linking hope to goal striving. I want to reiterate the importance of setting and achieving small goals as ways of recovering from depression and rekindling hope. One depressed patient emphasized how heartened he was one day when he was able to walk out to the mailbox and back. This accomplishment seems small to persons who are not depressed; it was big from his perspective, and he was able to build on it. Success breeds success—and hope.

The Challenge of Evil

Up to this point, I've focused on psychological trauma. But we must also consider the significance of *existential trauma*, the damage to meaning. Psychologist Ronnie Janoff-Bulman's book, *Shattered Assumptions*,[221] goes to the heart of this matter. She proposed that psychological well-being rests on three fundamental assumptions: the world is meaningful, the world is benevolent, and the self is worthy. At worst, trauma can shatter all these assumptions. And nothing is more shattering than trauma wrought by evil.

Contemporary philosopher Susan Neiman[634] contended that the challenges of living with evil have been the driving force in modern philosophy over the past few centuries. This philosophical preoccupation endures because of the fact that *we are most traumatized by evil.* If Karl Menninger[624] was right in proposing that hope is the enemy of evil, we must find some basis for hope in this context.

The problem of evil has been an enduring concern of theology and religion as well as philosophy.[635] Neiman formulated the theological problem of evil thus: "How could a good God create a world of innocent suffering?" (p. 3). How many trauma survivors have anguished over this question? Neiman argued pointedly, "The problem of evil occurs when you try to maintain three propositions that don't fit together. 1. Evil exists. 2. God is benevolent. 3. God is omnipotent" (p. 119). *Theodicy* is the branch of theology devoted to reconciling the seeming contradiction between the existence of evil and the benevolence and omnipotence of God. In religious or secular terms, every traumatized person needs a theodicy, some way to make sense of the fact that *what ought not to happen nevertheless did happen.* Trauma strikes arbitrarily, undeservedly.

Not surprisingly, many persons who suffer trauma stemming from evil struggle mightily with their religious faith, and it's not uncommon for trauma to shake the foundations of religious beliefs. Yet we can't make generalizations about the impact of trauma on religious beliefs and spirituality.[166,636] Trauma diminishes religious convictions for some persons and strengthens those of others. Religion and spirituality may protect the individual from illness by promoting resilience; alternatively, when they fail to serve this protective function, religious convictions may be employed to cope with illness. In light of these challenges and complexities, I find that many trauma survivors benefit enormously from sensitive religious and spiritual counseling.

Whether from within religion or from without, the alternative to making sense of evil is despair. Recognizing that traumatized persons will approach the problem from a wide variety of religious beliefs and unbelief, I find it best to approach evil from a secular perspective. Others have thoughtfully approached the problem of trauma and evil from a religious (Christian) perspective.[637]

Philosopher Claudia Card[162] usefully defines *evils* as "foreseeable intolerable harms produced by culpable wrongdoing" (p. 3). No doubt, trauma as described throughout this book counts as intolerable harm. Card clarifies that intolerable harms, as distinct from ordinary wrongs, deprive persons of basics needed to make life tolerable. Such basics include uncontaminated food and water, sleep, freedom from prolonged pain and fear, emotional ties with other persons, freedom to make choices, and a sense of worth. Sadly, it would take an encyclopedic work to enumerate all the large-scale evils encompassed by Card's concept of *atrocities*. Some of her examples: the Holocaust; bombings in World War II (e.g., Hiroshima and Dresden); the My Lai massacre; the genocide in Rwanda; and the global destruction of the environment. She also discussed at length the atrocities of rape in war and of terror in the home; that is, childhood maltreatment and domestic violence.

Card highlighted a subcategory of *diabolical evil:* knowingly and deliberately corrupting the character of victims, for example, with the intent of being able to look down on victims—or to *bring* them down so as to avoid having to look up to them. The practice of putting Jewish prisoners in Hitler's death camps in positions of authority over other prisoners exemplifies diabolical evil at its worst. Such diabolical evil puts persons into situations in which, to survive, they must make choices that risk their own moral degradation. This process also occurs in psychological abuse, where children and adults are coerced into participating in acts that they find morally abhorrent. The most perniciously traumatic result is profound shame and guilt, a sense of *oneself* as evil.

To understand evil fully, we must understand *evildoers,* such as rapists, sexual abusers, torturers, and terrorists. Many survivors are not just outraged by their experiences; they're utterly bewildered: "Who could do something like that?" We're prone to demonizing, tempted to see all evildoers as *evil persons.*

However, the likelihood of an evildoer being an evil person is an exception rather than the rule. Whereas Card focused her study on persons traumatized by evil, psychologist Roy Baumeister[638] carefully studied evildoers. The sadist, who derives pleasure and a sense of power from tormenting others, typifies the evildoer who is an evil person. Baumeister estimates that only about 5% of evildoers are sadists. Of course, this small proportion comprises a large enough absolute number to inflict horrific trauma, and it's little solace to their victims that sadists are a small minority of evildoers.

Far more common than sadism is evildoing that stems from gross negligence or indifference—a lack of emotional attunement to the victims, the grossest failure of mentalizing. Nonsadistic motives for evildoing include greed, lust, ambition, egotism, and revenge. Even idealism can motivate evildoing, as evidenced by terrorists who are convinced of the rightness of their cause. Baumeister discovered a gap between the perpetrators and victims in their perception of evil: the perpetrator—oblivious to the victim's mental state—is likely to minimize the degree of harm; whereas the victim is likely to overestimate the sheer malevolence of the perpetrator, for example, seeing the perpetrator as an evil person.

Baumeister's convincing argument that the majority of evildoers are not evil persons is profoundly disquieting. It implies that the capacity for evildoing is not an aberration but rather part of the human condition. Under the right circumstances, most of us are capable of evil. Diabolical evil capitalizes on that fact; evildoers can draw others into evildoing, and evil thus can perpetuate evil. We must make sense of evil to counter it, and facing the ordinariness of evil and our own vulnerability to evildoing is a necessary step.

The Foundations of Hope

To reiterate, as Janoff-Bulman has proposed, trauma may shatter the assumptions that the world is meaningful and benevolent, and that the self is worthy. In parallel, I propose that meaning, benevolence, and self-worth are foundations of hope. By shattering these assumptions, trauma undermines the existential foundations of hope. Finding meaning and benevolence in the world and establishing a sense of self-worth will rekindle hope.

In this conclusion, I'm elaborating the central theme of this book: healing from trauma evolves from attachment relationships in which you have the experience that another caring person has your mind in mind—what we've been calling mentalizing. Such relationships enable you to make sense of your experience, a process through which you develop and maintain a sense of self and, ideally, develop loving feelings for yourself as well as others. Put simply, meaning and self-worth stem from benevolent attachments; hope is founded on all three.

Meaning

Part of the horror of trauma—particularly trauma stemming from evildoing— is its seeming senselessness. *Innocent suffering,* one facet of evil, is hardest to understand. Innocent suffering shatters our assumption—dating back to Aristotle—that virtue should lead to flourishing. As the existence of trauma and evil lay bare, striving to live a good-enough life may be *conducive* to flourishing, but it's no *guarantee.* Innocent suffering abounds. How are we to understand the Washington, D.C., snipers' random gunning down of so many people? How are we to understand the plight of the teenager crippled by a drive-by shooting? How are we to understand the situation of the battered infant? How are we to understand the fate of the children in daycare who were killed in the Oklahoma City bombing? How are we to understand the thousands of men, women, and children maimed and killed in terrorist attacks? How are we to understand thousands upon thousands dying in genocides? And how are we to understand the traumatic grief of all their loved ones?

We find it nearly impossible to sit with meaninglessness and senseless-ness. We're all too prone to ascribing guilt. We blame the victim. And victims blame themselves in an effort to find meaning: "I'm bad"; "I deserved it"; "It's my punishment." Children do this quite naturally, and they don't necessarily stop doing it when they reach adulthood. Religious persons may be confronted with the choice between abandoning their convictions and concluding that God is punishing them—or worse, doesn't care.

Natural as it may be, self-blame cannot effectively resolve the meaninglessness and senselessness of trauma or evil. We must go deeper. Neiman[634] invoked the *principle of sufficient reason:* the conviction that we can find a reason for everything the world presents. She maintained that *hope lies in our refusal to accept a world that makes no sense*. We are driven to make sense of the world in the face of the fact that things go intolerably wrong. It was the cardinal assumption of the Enlightenment that hope is based on the intelligibility of the world and that intelligibility promotes controllability. Understanding evildoing does not justify it. On the contrary, evildoing promotes outrage, which can provide fuel for our efforts to use understanding to prevent or contain it. Psychology has a key role to play here. The events of September 11 so painfully made clear to everyone what trauma sufferers have long known: the domain of nature we most need to understand and control is human nature.

Of course, trauma poses not only problems of intelligibility but also profound emotional problems—guilt feelings, shame, resentment, hatred, and vengeance, along with the challenges of forgiveness and reconciliation. These problems, too, go beyond psychology and psychiatry, beyond the realm of psychopathology. These, too, are existential problems that will not yield to glib prescriptions but require painful individual resolution. All this painful work must be sustained by hope. While hope is founded on our capacity to make sense of suffering, we need more than the power of our reasoning to sustain it. To reiterate, we need more than the head; we need the heart.

Benevolence

Psychoanalyst Erik Erikson[72] believed *basic trust* to be the first stage of development—the foundation. And he construed hope as the virtue that stems from basic trust. In this same vein, Paul Pruyser[628] concluded that "hoping is based on the belief that there is *some benevolent disposition toward oneself somewhere in the universe, conveyed by a caring person*" (p. 467). In Erikson's and Pruyser's formulations, we can see the foundation of hope in attachment.

Thus hope rests squarely on the capacity to depend on others. I've worked with many persons who view the need to depend on others as a weakness. In his book *Dependent Rational Animals*,[244] MacIntyre argues just the opposite: the capacity to depend on others is a virtue. He succinctly articulated the full extent of our dependency, which we're all too prone to deny:

> We human beings are vulnerable to many kinds of affliction and most of us are at some time afflicted by serious ills. How we cope is only in small part up to us. It is most often to others that we owe our survival, let alone our flourishing, as we encounter bodily illness and injury, inadequate nutrition, mental defect and disturbance, and human aggression and neglect. (p. 1)

Sometimes trauma sufferers must depend directly on others for hope; feeling hopeless, they must rely on *borrowed hope*—hope that others hold out for them. In the midst of profound depression, traumatized persons might not be able to envision anything beyond unending suffering. They depend on other persons to imagine realistically alternative possible futures, to reiterate MacIntyre's phrase. I'm able to lend hope, because I've seen so many patients who felt hopeless become hopeful again. I've worked with a number of traumatized patients who were suicidally depressed, wishing to die and resenting efforts to keep them alive, sometimes for weeks and even months on end. I've seen them recover to enjoy lives that included flourishing, although not without the ups and downs of illness. I'm not about to give up hope when I've seen so many patients feel glad to be alive after wanting so fervently to die. Rarely do I know what the pathway will be in the midst of the crisis, but I can count on some pathway being found.

Pruyser[628] left this quest for hope entirely open-ended, predicating it on a benevolent disposition *somewhere in the universe*. Some traumatized persons find hope in their faith in God. Others may find hope in the benevolence of nature. But I'm convinced that Pruyser was right. Our prototype will always be a *caring person*—an attachment relationship. I've reiterated throughout this book the dilemma that recovery requires depending on others despite a history of having been hurt and let down. I find hope in the fact that, despite this dilemma, so many survivors of trauma persist in seeking attachments.[101] And I find hope in the sheer flexibility of attachment that accommodates such wide variety of relationships.[259]

Focusing on trauma—and evil in particular—skews our perspective on human nature. We can easily lose sight of all the evidence that we humans and closely related primate species demonstrate ample benevolence and goodness.[639] Altruism evolved alongside competitiveness and aggression.[640] If Pruyser and Erickson were right, this evolutionary legacy has made loving relationships the wellspring of hope. Sadly, when these relationships have been traumatizing, establishing and maintaining secure attachments that will sustain hope will be especially difficult. Yet, difficult as it may be, most survivors are able to do so, sooner or later.

Even the most devastatingly traumatic events do not obliterate benevolence. In Chapter 3 ("Emotion"), I mentioned Haidt's[641] concept of *elevation*—the expansive, warm feeling we experience in observing moral goodness. I find it noteworthy that Groopman included an "elevating feeling" in his definition of hope. I'll never forget my visit to Oklahoma City after the bombing of the Alfred P. Murrah Federal Building, when I went to talk about trauma with the employees of the adjacent federal courthouse. While horrified by the devastating effect of the evil deed perpetrated by two men, I was emotionally overwhelmed by the outpouring of compassion by thousands of persons who came to help. On a tragically larger scale, the horrific attacks of September 11 showed how the evil done by a small band of individuals evoked heroic rescue efforts and compassionate caring from countless numbers. Haidt is certainly right; hope springs from elevation. We must keep the benevolence of others in view, and we must also cultivate it in ourselves, as providing compassionate care to others is one way we all flourish.[642]

Self-Worth

Finally, you shouldn't lose sight of the fact that Pruyser's reference to benevolence "somewhere in the universe" might be construed to include inside yourself. I've advocated self-compassion and self-love as crucial in healing from trauma. Both promote self-worth. To reiterate philosopher Christine Swanton's[563] contention, we can construe self-love as *bonding* with oneself, thereby giving oneself strength and vitality—and, I would add, hope. I don't think self-love can substitute for attachment relationships, although it might help to get you through a fairly long bad patch. To sustain a feeling of self-worth, we need fuel from without as well as fuel from within. But I think a benevolent disposition toward yourself *from within yourself* is profoundly important in sustaining hope. Without it, you're liable to languish. With it, you're in a better position to flourish.

GLOSSARY

90/10 reaction   Colloquial for CONTEXT-INAPPROPRIATE RESPONDING, wherein 90% of the emotion comes from the past and 10% comes from the present

abreaction   Emotional catharsis; expression of intense emotion often followed by a feeling of relief

amygdala   A structure deep in the temporal lobe of the brain that rapidly registers threatening stimuli and mediates conditioned fear responses

anxiety sensitivity   Fear of being anxious, which further increases anxiety; opposite of ANXIETY TOLERANCE

anxiety tolerance   The capacity to experience anxiety without being unduly distressed; facilitates constructive emotion regulation

appraisal   Judgment of the emotional significance of a situation

attachment trauma   Trauma in ATTACHMENT relationships; often interferes with establishing and maintaining secure attachments

attachment   The emotional bond that develops in close relationships, the prototype being the mother-infant bond

---

SMALL CAPS type indicates terms defined elsewhere in this glossary.

biofeedback Using biological information to enhance emotion regulation (e.g., using readings of finger temperature or muscle tension to enhance relaxation)

catch-22s of depression The idea that all the things one must do to recover from depression (e.g., feel hopeful, engage in pleasurable activities, eat properly, and sleep well) are made difficult by the symptoms of depression (e.g., feelings of hopelessness, diminished capacity for pleasure, decreased appetite, and insomnia)

complex PTSD A broad cluster of trauma-related symptoms that goes beyond narrowly defined PTSD (e.g., also including depression, DISSOCIATION, self-destructive behavior, identity disturbance, and problematic patterns of interpersonal relations)

containment Support needed for effectively PROCESSING trauma; provided by secure ATTACHMENT relationships, self-regulation strategies, education, daily structure or routine, and a solid THERAPEUTIC ALLIANCE

context-inappropriate responding Responding with intense emotion to one facet of a current situation that bears similarity to a past situation in which trauma occurred; colloquially, a 90/10 REACTION

deliberate self-harm Self-injury (e.g., cutting or overdosing) for the primary purpose of escaping from unbearable emotional states; not based on suicidal intent

desensitization Decreasing fear by means of gradual exposure to a frightening situation or stimulus

diabolical evil Evildoing that entails knowingly and deliberately corrupting the character of victims

dissociation Alteration of consciousness (e.g., feelings of unreality) in response to extreme stress; a self-protective defense that ultimately interferes with adaptation and coping

dual liability Adverse effects of ATTACHMENT TRAUMA in childhood, which evokes marked distress and simultaneously undermines the development of the capacity to regulate that distress (e.g., undermines the development of MENTALIZING capacity)

elevation The warm feeling one gets when observing acts of virtue or moral beauty

EMDR   Eye movement desensitization and reprocessing, a cognitive-behavioral technique designed to facilitate PROCESSING of traumatic memories

eudaemonia   Aristotelian concept of flourishing, for example, in conjunction with intimacy, generativity, and spirituality

evil   Culpable wrongdoing that results in intolerable harm

exposure therapy   Procedures designed to help patients engage with a frightening stimulus and tolerate the anxiety this provokes with the goal of DESENSITIZATION (e.g., visiting the vicinity of a trauma when the situation is safe or talking about traumatic events with a trusted therapist and feeling less frightened as a result)

flow   Intensely enjoyable experience based on absorption in activity that optimally balances challenge and skill

grounding   Focusing attention on the present situation so as to interrupt traumatic memories or dissociative symptoms (e.g., by naming the objects in a room, splashing cold water on the face, or holding a conversation)

hippocampus   A structure deep in the temporal lobe of the brain that plays a central role in encoding coherent memories of complex events and facilitating conversion into long-term autobiographical memories

ill health   A wide array of physical symptoms (e.g., pain, dizziness) that are stress related and not associated with a specific diagnosable disease process

illness   A state from which one cannot recover by a mere act of will and a social role that provides a legitimate excuse from many social and occupational obligations while obligating the ill person to seek and cooperate with treatment

infantile amnesia   The common inability to remember much from one's past before age 5 years

internal working models   Mental representations of relationships, based on images of the self and others, that provide patterns for perceiving and interacting with other persons, for example, based on early ATTACHMENT experience

interpersonal trauma   Trauma inflicted deliberately or recklessly by another person (e.g., a sexual assault or accident stemming from drunk driving)

intrusive memories   Disturbing memories of trauma that come into aware-ness unbidden, often in response to a reminder of a traumatic situation (e.g., flashbacks)

involuntary subordination strategy   In the face of being overpowered or op-pressed, submitting involuntarily for the adaptive purpose of avoiding a dangerous confrontation, resulting in a state of depression

learned helplessness   A response to repeated uncontrollable stress; learn-ing to be helpless, evident in a failure to learn to escape the stress once it be-comes avoidable

masochism   Unwitting self-perpetuation of suffering (e.g., based on guilt feelings)

mentalizing   Apprehending mental states in oneself and others, for exam-ple, thinking about feelings; in relationships, the experience that each per-son has the other person's mind in mind

mentalizing emotionally   MENTALIZING in the midst of an emotional state (e.g., feeling and thinking about feeling at the same time)

pause button   Colloquial for RESPONSE MODULATION; blocking immediate ex-pression of an emotional impulse, for example, by MENTALIZING

peritraumatic symptoms   Symptoms that occur during or immediately after exposure to traumatic events

potentially traumatic event   An extremely threatening event in which one feels helpless or horrified—often emotionally alone as well—that may or may not result in TRAUMA

processing   Thinking, talking, and feeling about traumatic events for the purpose of making sense of TRAUMA; MENTALIZING

psychological unavailability   Lack of emotional attunement or responsive-ness in the ATTACHMENT figure

PTSD   Posttraumatic stress disorder; a psychiatric disorder that may devel-op after exposure to potentially traumatic events, symptoms of which in-clude reexperiencing the traumatic event (e.g., in the form of flashbacks or nightmares), hyperarousal, avoidance, and numbing of emotional respon-siveness

reenactment Unconsciously repeating past traumatic patterns in current interpersonal relationships; plays an important role in perpetuating post-traumatic symptoms

resilience Capacity to cope effectively with adversity; enhanced by secure ATTACHMENT and the capacity to MENTALIZE

response modulation Inhibiting an emotional impulse or diminishing the intensity of emotion to allow for reappraisal of the situation and more adaptive coping

safe haven Feeling of security provided by contact with an ATTACHMENT figure

secure base Foundation for autonomy and exploration—including exploring the mind of oneself and others—provided by a secure ATTACHMENT relationship

self-dependence The capacity to bridge the gap between separation and reunion (e.g., by self-soothing or by holding in mind a comforting memory of being with a caring person)

self-efficacy A feeling of being able to influence the external environment (e.g., other persons) or internal experience (e.g., emotions)

self-love The virtue of emotional bonding with oneself that fosters strength, vitality, and hope

sensitization Increased emotional responsiveness to a stressful stimulus resulting from repeated exposure to extreme, repeated, and uncontrollable stress; opposite of DESENSITIZATION

SSRIs Selective serotonin reuptake inhibitors, widely used antidepressants (e.g., sertraline [Zoloft] and paroxetine [Paxil]) that current research indicates to be the most effective type of medication for treating PTSD

stoicism Ancient Greek and Roman philosophical movement advocating eliminating emotional reactions to uncontrollable events

stress pileup An accumulation of stress that erodes the capacity for coping, often manifested in episodes of depression

stress-induced analgesia Diminished sensitivity to pain associated with a high-stress state, in part mediated by endogenous opioids (narcotic-like substances in the brain)

temperament   Biologically based personality characteristics evident early in life that place constraints on development (e.g., proneness to anxiety)

terrorism   Inflicting psychological trauma for political ends

therapeutic alliance   Optimal patient-therapist relationship based on feelings of trust and acceptance coupled with active collaboration on shared goals

trauma   Lasting adverse effects of exposure to POTENTIALLY TRAUMATIC EVENTS

traumatic bonding   Clinging to a traumatizing relationship as a result of feeling frightened and having no other source of ATTACHMENT security

universality   A benefit of group therapy and related experiences, namely, learning that other persons share one's experience, resulting in a feeling of belonging that counters feelings of alienation

vicious circle   Two factors interacting such that each one makes the other worse (e.g., depression promotes alcohol abuse, which, in turn, deepens depression; DELIBERATE SELF-HARM stemming from feelings of abandonment leads to criticism and rejection, which, in turn, increases feelings of abandonment and impulses to engage in self-harm)

REFERENCES

1. *Webster's New Twentieth Century Dictionary of the English Language Unabridged.* New York, Simon & Schuster, 1979.

2. American Psychiatric Association: *Diagnostic and Statistical Manual of Mental Disorders*, 4th Edition, Text Revision. Washington, DC, American Psychiatric Association, 2000.

3. Lear J: *Happiness, Death, and the Remainder of Life.* Cambridge, MA, Harvard University Press, 2000.

4. Terr LC: "Childhood Traumas: An Outline and Overview." *American Journal of Psychiatry* 148:10–20, 1991.

5. Bolin R: "Natural and Technological Disasters: Evidence of Psychopathology," in *Environment and Psychopathology.* Edited by Ghadirian AA, Lehmann HE. New York, Springer, 1993, pp. 121–140.

6. Kilpatrick DG, Resnick HS: "Posttraumatic Stress Disorder Associated With Exposure to Criminal Victimization in Clinical and Community Populations," in *Posttraumatic Stress Disorder: DSM-IV and Beyond.* Edited by Davidson JRT, Foa EB. Washington, DC, American Psychiatric Press, 1993, pp. 113–143.

7. Worden JW: *Grief Counseling and Grief Therapy: A Handbook for the Mental Health Practitioner.* New York, Springer, 1991.

8. Jacobs S: *Pathologic Grief: Maladaptation to Loss.* Washington, DC, American Psychiatric Press, 1993.

9. Amick-McMullan A, Kilpatrick DG, Resnick HS: "Homicide as a Risk Factor for PTSD Among Surviving Family Members." *Behavior Modification* 15:545–559, 1991.

10. Adam KS, Sheldon Keller AE, West M: "Attachment Organization and Vulnerability to Loss, Separation, and Abuse in Disturbed Adolescents," in *Attachment Theory: Social, Developmental, and Clinical Perspectives.* Edited by Goldberg S, Muir R, Kerr J. Hillsdale, NJ, Analytic Press, 1995, pp 309–341.

11. American Psychiatric Association: *Diagnostic and Statistical Manual of Mental Disorders,* 3rd Edition. Washington, DC, American Psychiatric Association, 1980.

12. Brende J: "A Psychodynamic View of Character Pathology in Vietnam Combat Veterans." *Bulletin of the Menninger Clinic* 47:193–216, 1983.

13. Basoglu M, Paker M, Paker O, et al.: "Psychological Effects of Torture: A Comparison of Tortured With Nontortured Political Activists in Turkey." *American Journal of Psychiatry* 151:76-81, 1994.

14. Townshend C: *Terrorism: A Very Short Introduction.* Oxford, UK, Oxford University Press, 2002.

15. Freud S: *Civilization and Its Discontents* (1929). Translated and edited by Strachey J. New York, WW Norton, 1961.

16. Grayling AC: *The Reason of Things: Living With Philosophy.* London, Weidenfeld & Nicolson, 2002.

17. Foa EB, Rothbaum BO: *Treating the Trauma of Rape: Cognitive-Behavioral Therapy for PTSD.* New York, Guilford, 1998.

18. Russell DEH: *The Secret Trauma: Incest in the Lives of Girls and Women.* New York, Basic Books, 1986.

19. Avina C, O'Donohue W: "Sexual Harassment and PTSD: Is Sexual Harassment Diagnosable Trauma?" *Journal of Traumatic Stress* 15:69–75, 2002.

20. Fitzgerald LF: "Sexual Harassment: Violence Against Women in the Workplace." *American Psychologist* 48:1070–1076, 1993.

21. Gutek B: "Responses to Sexual Harassment," in *Gender Issues in Contemporary Society* (*Claremont Symposium on Applied Social Psychology,* Vol. 6). Edited by Oskamp S, Costanzo M. Newbury Park, CA, Sage, 1993, pp. 197–216.

22. Menninger KA: "The Suicidal Intention of Nuclear Armament." *Bulletin of the Menninger Clinic* 47:325–353, 1983.

23. Bifulco A, Moran P: *Wednesday's Child: Research Into Women's Experience of Neglect and Abuse in Childhood, and Adult Depression.* London, Routledge, 1998.

24. Kempe CH, Silverman FN, Steele BF, et al.: "The Battered-Child Syndrome." *Journal of the American Medical Association* 181:17–24, 1962.

25. Allen JG: *Traumatic Relationships and Serious Mental Disorders.* Chichester, UK, Wiley, 2001.

26. Kaplan SJ, Pelcovitz D, Salzinger S, et al.: "Adolescent Physical Abuse: Risk for Adolescent Psychiatric Disorders." *American Journal of Psychiatry* 155:954–959, 1998.

27. Malinosky-Rummell R, Hansen DJ: "Long-Term Consequences of Childhood Physical Abuse." *Psychological Bulletin* 114:68–79, 1993.

28. Eth S, Pynoos R: "Children Who Witness the Homicide of a Parent." *Psychiatry* 57:287–306, 1994.

29. Herman JL: *Father-Daughter Incest.* Cambridge, MA, Harvard University Press, 1981.

30. Gorey KM, Leslie DR: "The Prevalence of Child Sexual Abuse: Integrative Review Adjustment for Potential Response and Measurement Biases." *Child Abuse and Neglect* 21:391–398, 1997.

31. Freyd JJ: *Betrayal Trauma: The Logic of Forgetting Childhood Abuse.* Cambridge, MA, Harvard University Press, 1996.

32. Finkelhor D, Hotaling G, Lewis IA, et al.: "Sexual Abuse in a National Survey of Adult Men and Women: Prevalence, Characteristics, and Risk Factors." *Child Abuse and Neglect* 14:19–28, 1990.

33. Kinsey AC, Pomeroy WB, Martin CE, et al.: *Sexual Behavior in the Human Female.* Philadelphia, PA, WB Saunders, 1953.

34. Feldman W, Feldman E, Goodman JT, et al.: "Is Childhood Sexual Abuse Really Increasing in Prevalence? An Analysis of the Evidence." *Pediatrics* 88:29–33, 1991.

35. Nash MR, Hulsey TL, Sexton MC, et al.: "Long-Term Sequelae of Childhood Sexual Abuse: Perceived Family Environment, Psychopathology, and Dissociation." *Journal of Consulting and Clinical Psychology* 61:276–283, 1993.

36. Noll JG, Trickett PK, Putnam FW: "A Prospective Investigation of the Impact of Childhood Sexual Abuse on the Development of Sexuality." *Journal of Consulting and Clinical Psychology* 71:575–586, 2003.

37. Widom CS: "Posttraumatic Stress Disorder in Abused and Neglected Children Grown Up." *American Journal of Psychiatry* 156:1223–1229, 1999.

38. Dinwiddie S, Heath AC, Dunne MP, et al.: "Early Sexual Abuse and Lifetime Psychopathology: A Co-twin-Control Study." *Psychological Medicine* 30:41–52, 2000.

39. Rind B, Tromovitch P, Bauserman R: "A Meta-Analytic Examination of Assumed Properties of Childhood Sexual Abuse Using College Samples." *Psychological Bulletin* 124:22–53, 1998.

40. Kendall-Tackett KA, Williams LM, Finkelhor D: "Impact of Sexual Abuse on Children: A Review and Synthesis of Recent Empirical Studies." *Psychological Bulletin* 113:164–180, 1993.

41. Browne A, Finkelhor D: "Impact of Child Sexual Abuse: A Review of the Research." *Psychological Bulletin* 99:66–77, 1986.

42. Moran PM, Bifulco A, Ball C, et al.: "Exploring Psychological Abuse in Childhood, I: Developing a New Interview Scale." *Bulletin of the Menninger Clinic* 66:213–240, 2002.

43. Goodwin JM: "Sadistic Abuse: Definition, Recognition, and Treatment." *Dissociation* 6:181–187, 1993.

44. Fromm E: *The Anatomy of Human Destructiveness.* New York, Holt, Rinehart & Winston, 1973.

45. Millon T: *Disorders of Personality: DSM-IV and Beyond.* New York, Wiley, 1996.

46. Bifulco A, Moran PM, Baines R, et al.: "Exploring Psychological Abuse in Childhood, II: Association With Other Abuse and Adult Clinical Depression." *Bulletin of the Menninger Clinic* 66:241–258, 2002.

47. Wolock I, Horowitz B: "Child Maltreatment as a Social Problem: The Neglect of Neglect." *American Journal of Orthopsychiatry* 54:530–543, 1984.

48. Egeland B: "Mediators of the Effects of Child Maltreatment on Developmental Adaptation in Adolescence," in *Developmental Perspectives on Trauma: Theory, Research, and Intervention,* Vol. 8. Edited by Cicchetti D, Toth SL. Rochester, NY, University of Rochester Press, 1997, pp. 403–434.

49. Barnett D, Manly JT, Cicchetti D: "Defining Child Maltreatment: The Interface Between Policy and Research," in *Child Abuse, Child Development, and Social Policy* (*Advances in Applied Developmental Psychology,* Vol. 8). Edited by Cicchetti D, Toth SL. Norwood, NJ, Ablex, 1993, pp. 7–73.

50. Stein HB, Allen D, Allen JG, et al.: *Supplementary Manual for Scoring Bifulco's Childhood Experiences of Care and Abuse Interview (M-CECA): Version 2.0* (Technical Report No. 00-0024). Topeka, KS, The Menninger Clinic, Research Department, 2000.

51. Erickson MF, Egeland B: "Child Neglect," in *The APSAC Handbook on Child Maltreatment.* Edited by Briere J, Berliner L, Bulkley JA, et al. Thousand Oaks, CA, Sage, 1996, pp. 4–20.

52. Rose DS: "Sexual Assault, Domestic Violence, and Incest," in *Psychological Aspects of Women's Health Care.* Edited by Stewart DE, Stotland NL. Washington, DC, American Psychiatric Press, 1993, pp. 447–483.

53. Browne A: "Violence Against Women by Male Partners: Prevalence, Outcomes, and Policy Implications." *American Psychologist* 48:1077–1087, 1993.

54. Walker LE: *The Battered Woman.* New York, Harper & Row, 1979.

55. Walker LE: "Psychology and Domestic Violence Around the World." *American Psychologist* 54:21–29, 1999.

56. Holtzworth-Munroe A, Smutzler N, Bates L, et al.: "Husband Violence: Basic Facts and Clinical Implications," in *Clinical Handbook of Marriage and Couple Interventions.* Edited by Halford WK, Markman HJ. Chichester, UK, Wiley, 1997, pp. 129–156.

57. Mahoney P, Williams LM: "Sexual Assault in Marriage: Prevalence, Consequences, and Treatment of Wife Rape," in *Partner Violence: A Comprehensive Review of 20 Years of Research.* Edited by Jasinski JL, Williams LM. Thousand Oaks, CA, Sage, 1998, pp. 113–161.

58. Herman JL: *Trauma and Recovery.* New York, Basic Books, 1992.

59. Olson DH, Lavee Y, McCubbin HI: "Types of Families and Family Response to Stress Across the Family Life Cycle," in *Social Stress and Family Development.* Edited by Klein DM, Aldous J. New York, Guilford, 1988, pp. 16–43.

60. March JS: "What Constitutes a Stressor? The 'Criterion A' Issue," in *Posttraumatic Stress Disorder: DSM-IV and Beyond.* Edited by Davidson JRT, Foa EB. Washington, DC, American Psychiatric Press, 1993, pp 37–54.

61. Goldberg J, True WR, Eisen SA, et al.: "A Twin Study of the Effects of the Vietnam War on Posttraumatic Stress Disorder." *Journal of the American Medical Association* 263:1227–1232, 1990.

62. van der Kolk BA: "The Compulsion to Repeat the Trauma: Re-enactment, Revictimization, and Masochism." *Psychiatric Clinics of North America* 12:389–411, 1989.

63. Glodich A, Allen JG: "Adolescents Exposed to Violence and Abuse: A Review of the Group Therapy Literature With an Emphasis on Preventing Trauma Reenactment." *Journal of Child and Adolescent Group Therapy* 8(3):135–154, 1998.

64. Perry S, Difede J, Musngi G, et al.: "Predictors of Posttraumatic Stress Disorder After Burn Injury." *American Journal of Psychiatry* 149:931–935, 1992.

65. McNally RJ: "Stressors That Produce Posttraumatic Stress Disorder in Children," in *Posttraumatic Stress Disorder: DSM-IV and Beyond.* Edited by Davidson JRT, Foa EB. Washington, DC, American Psychiatric Press, 1993, pp. 207–212.

66. Coates SW, Rosenthal JL, Schechter DS (eds.): *September 11: Trauma and Human Bonds.* Hillsdale, NJ, Analytic Press, 2003.

67. Bowlby J: *Attachment and Loss, Vol. 1: Attachment,* 2nd Edition. New York, Basic Books, 1982.

68. Cassidy J, Shaver PR (eds.): *Handbook of Attachment: Theory, Research, and Clinical Applications.* New York, Guilford, 1999.

69. George C, Solomon J: "Attachment and Caregiving: the Caregiving Behavioral System," in *Handbook of Attachment: Theory, Research, and Clinical Applications.* New York, Guilford, 1999, pp. 649–670.

70. MacLean PD: *The Triune Brain in Evolution: Role in Paleocerebral Functions.* New York, Plenum, 1990.

71. Bowlby J: *A Secure Base: Parent-Child Attachment and Healthy Human Development.* New York, Basic Books, 1988.

72. Erikson EH: *Childhood and Society.* New York, WW Norton, 1963.

73. Grossmann KE, Grossmann K, Zimmermann P: "A Wider View of Attachment and Exploration: Stability and Change During the Years of Immaturity," in *Handbook of Attachment: Theory, Research, and Clinical Applications.* New York, Guilford, 1999, pp. 760–786.

74. Field T, Reite M: "The Psychobiology of Attachment and Separation: A Summary," in *The Psychobiology of Attachment and Separation.* Edited by Reite M, Field T. New York, Academic Press, 1985, pp. 455–479.

75. Hofer MA: "The Emerging Neurobiology of Attachment and Separation: How Parents Shape Their Infant's Brain and Behavior," in *September 11: Trauma and Human Bonds.* Hillsdale, NJ, Analytic Press, 2003, pp. 191–209.

76. Schore AN: "Effects of a Secure Attachment Relationship on Right Brain Development, Affect Regulation, and Infant Mental Health." *Infant Mental Health Journal* 22:7–66, 2001.

77. Teicher MH, Polcari A, Andersen SL, et al.: "Neurobiological Effects of Childhood Stress and Trauma," in *September 11: Trauma and Human Bonds.* Hillsdale, NJ, Analytic Press, 2003, pp. 211–237.

78. Fonagy P, Target M: "Attachment and Reflective Function: Their Role in Self-Organization." *Development and Psychopathology* 9:679–700, 1997.

79. Fonagy P, Gergely G, Jurist EL, et al.: *Affect Regulation, Mentalization, and the Development of the Self.* New York, Other Press, 2002.

80. Fonagy P, Target M: "Evolution of the Interpersonal Interpretive Function: Clues for Effective Preventive Intervention in Early Childhood," in *September 11: Trauma and Human Bonds.* Hillsdale, NJ, Analytic Press, 2003, pp. 99–113.

81. Fonagy P: "Thinking About Thinking: Some Clinical and Theoretical Considerations in the Treatment of a Borderline Patient." *International Journal of Psycho-Analysis* 72:639–656, 1991.

82. Allen JG: "Mentalizing." *Bulletin of the Menninger Clinic* 67:87–108, 2003.

83. Allen JG, Bleiberg E, Haslam-Hopwood GTG: *Mentalizing as a Compass for Treatment.* Houston, TX, The Menninger Clinic, 2003.

84. Gergely G, Watson JS: "The Social Biofeedback Theory of Parental Affect-Mirroring: The Development of Emotional Self-Awareness and Self-Control in Infancy." *International Journal of Psycho-Analysis* 77:1181–1212, 1996.

85. Gergely G, Watson JS: "Early Social-Emotional Development: Contingency Perception and the Social Biofeedback Model," in *Early Social Cognition: Understanding Others in the First Months of Life.* Edited by Rochat P. Hillsdale, NJ, Erlbaum, 1999, pp. 101–137.

86. Fonagy P, Redfern S, Charman A: "The Relationship Between Belief-Desire Reasoning and a Projective Measure of Attachment Security (SAT)." *British Journal of Developmental Psychology* 15:51–61, 1997.

87. Meins E: *Security of Attachment and the Social Development of Cognition.* East Sussex, UK, Psychology Press, 1997.

88. Dunn J: "The Emanuel Miller Memorial Lecture 1995: Children's Relationships: Bridging the Divide Between Cognitive and Social Development." *Journal of Child Psychology and Psychiatry* 37:507–518, 1996.

89. Fonagy P, Steele M, Steele H, et al.: "Attachment, the Reflective Self, and Borderline States: The Predictive Specificity of the Adult Attachment Interview and Pathological Emotional Development," in *Attachment Theory: Social, Developmental, and Clinical Perspectives.* Edited by Goldberg S, Muir R, Kerr J. Hillsdale, NJ, Analytic Press, 1995, pp. 233–278.

90. Ainsworth MDS, Blehar MC, Waters E, et al.: *Patterns of Attachment: A Psychological Study of the Strange Situation.* Hillsdale, NJ, Erlbaum, 1978.

91. Solomon J, George C: "The Measurement of Attachment Security in Infancy and Childhood," in *Handbook of Attachment: Theory, Research, and Clinical Applications.* New York, Guilford, 1999, pp. 287–316.

92. Vaughn BE, Bost KK: "Attachment and Temperament: Redundant, Independent, or Interacting Influences on Interpersonal Adaptation and Personality Development?" in *Handbook of Attachment: Theory, Research, and Clinical Applications.* New York, Guilford, 1999, pp. 198–225.

93. Belsky J: "Interactional and Contextual Determinants of Attachment Security," in *Handbook of Attachment: Theory, Research, and Clinical Applications.* New York, Guilford, 1999, pp. 249–264.

94. Winnicott DW: *Collected Papers: Through Paediatrics to Psycho-Analysis.* London, Tavistock, 1958.

95. Fox NA, Card JA: "Psychophysiological Measures in the Study of Attachment," in *Handbook of Attachment: Theory, Research, and Clinical Applications.* New York, Guilford, 1999, pp. 226–245.

96. Weinfield NS, Sroufe LA, Egeland B, et al.: "The Nature of Individual Differences in Infant-Caregiver Attachment," in *Handbook of Attachment: Theory, Research, and Clinical Applications.* New York, Guilford, 1999, pp. 68-88.

97. Main M: "Recent Studies in Attachment: Overview, With Selected Implications for Clinical Work," in *Attachment Theory: Social, Developmental, and Clinical Perspectives.* Edited by Goldberg S, Muir R, Kerr J. Hillsdale, NJ, Analytic Press, 1995, pp. 407–474 .

98. Main M, Solomon J: "Procedures for Identifying Infants as Disorganized/Disoriented During the Ainsworth Strange Situation," in *Attachment in the Preschool Years: Theory, Research, and Intervention.* Edited by Greenberg MT, Cicchetti D, Cummings EM. Chicago, IL, University of Chicago Press, 1990, pp. 121–160 .

99. van Ijzendoorn MH, Schuengel C, Bakermans-Kranenburg MJ: "Disorganized Attachment in Early Childhood: Meta-Analysis of Precursors, Concomitants, and Sequelae." *Development and Psychopathology* 11:225–249, 1999.

100. Main M, Hesse E: "Parents' Unresolved Traumatic Experiences Are Related to Infant Disorganized Attachment Status: Is Frightened and/or Frightening Parental Behavior the Linking Mechanism?" in *Attachment in the Preschool Years: Theory, Research, and Intervention.* Edited by Greenberg MT, Cicchetti D, Cummings EM. Chicago, IL, University of Chicago Press, 1990, pp. 161–182.

101. Allen JG, Huntoon J, Fultz J, et al.: "A Model for Brief Assessment of Attachment and Its Application to Women in Inpatient Treatment for Trauma-Related Psychiatric Disorders." *Journal of Personality Assessment* 76:420–446, 2001.

102. Main M: "Attachment Theory: Eighteen Points With Suggestions for Future Studies," in *Handbook of Attachment: Theory, Research, and Clinical Applications.* New York, Guilford, 1999, pp. 845–887.

103. Steele H, Steele M, Fonagy P: "Associations Among Attachment Classifications of Mothers, Fathers, and Their Infants." *Child Development* 67:541–555, 1996.

104. Ainsworth MDS: "Attachments Beyond Infancy." *American Psychologist* 44:709–716, 1989.

105. Lichtenberg JD: *Psychoanalysis and Motivation.* Hillsdale, NJ, Analytic Press, 1989.

106. Melson GF: "Studying Children's Attachment to Their Pets: A Conceptual and Methodological Review." *Anthrozoos* 4:91–99, 1988.

107. Brown S-E, Katcher AH: "The Contribution of Attachment to Pets and Attachment to Nature to Dissociation and Absorption." *Dissociation* 10:125–129, 1997.

108. Scott JP: "The Emotional Basis of Attachment and Separation," in *Attachment and the Therapeutic Processes: Essays in Honor of Otto Allen Will, Jr., M.D.* Edited by Sacksteder JL, Schwartz DP, Akabane Y. Madison, CT, International University Press, 1987, pp. 43–62.

109. Thompson RA: "Early Attachment and Later Development," in *Handbook of Attachment: Theory, Research, and Clinical Applications.* New York, Guilford, 1999, pp. 265–286.

110. Howes C: "Attachment Relationships in the Context of Multiple Caregivers," in *Handbook of Attachment: Theory, Research, and Clinical Applications.* New York, Guilford, 1999, pp. 671–687.

111. Stein H, Koontz AD, Fonagy P, et al.: "Adult Attachment: What Are the Underlying Dimensions?" *Psychology and Psychotherapy* 75:77–91, 2002.

112. Scarr S: "Developmental Theories for the 1990s: Development and Individual Differences." *Child Development* 63:1–19, 1992.

113. Long AA: *Epictetus: A Stoic and Socratic Guide to Life.* New York, Oxford University Press, 2002.

114. Lebell S: *Epictetus: The Art of Living.* New York, HarperCollins, 1995.

115. Feldman Barrett L, Gross J, Christensen TC, et al.: "Knowing What You're Feeling and Knowing What to Do About It: Mapping the Relation Between Emotion Differentiation and Emotion Regulation." *Cognition and Emotion* 15:713–724, 2001.

116. Darwin C: *The Expression of Emotion in Man and Animals* (1872). Chicago, IL, University of Chicago Press, 1965.

117. Nussbaum MC: *Upheavals of Thought: The Intelligence of the Emotions.* Cambridge, UK, Cambridge University Press, 2001.

118. Damasio A: *The Feeling of What Happens: Body and Emotion in the Making of Consciousness.* New York, Harcourt Brace, 1999.

119. Levenson RW: "The Intrapersonal Functions of Emotion." *Cognition and Emotion* 13:481–504, 1999.

120. Parrott WG: "The Functional Utility of Negative Emotions," in *The Wisdom in Feeling: Psychological Processes in Emotional Intelligence.* Edited by Feldman Barrett L, Salovey P. New York, Guilford, 2002, pp. 341–359.

121. Mayr E: *One Long Argument: Charles Darwin and the Genesis of Modern Evolutionary Thought.* Cambridge, MA, Harvard University Press, 1991.

122. Mayr E: *Toward a New Philosophy of Biology: Observations of an Evolutionist.* Cambridge, MA, Harvard University Press, 1988.

123. Keltner D, Ekman P, Gonzaga GC, et al.: "Facial Expression of Emotion," in *Handbook of Affective Sciences.* Edited by Davidson RJ, Scherer KR, Goldsmith HH. New York, Oxford University Press, 2003, pp. 415–432.

124. Janig W: "The Autonomic Nervous System and Its Coordination by the Brain," in *Handbook of Affective Sciences.* Edited by Davidson RJ, Scherer KR, Goldsmith HH. New York, Oxford University Press, 2003, pp. 135–186.

125. Damasio A: *Looking for Spinoza: Joy, Sorrow, and the Feeling Brain.* New York, Harcourt, 2003.

126. Ekman P: *Emotions Revealed.* New York, Holt, 2003.

127. Ketter TA, Wang PW, Lembke A, et al.: "Physiological and Pharmacological Induction of Affect," in *Handbook of Affective Sciences.* Edited by Davidson RJ, Scherer KR, Goldsmith HH. New York, Oxford University Press, 2003, pp. 930–962.

128. Buss AH: "Personality: Primate Heritage and Human Distinctiveness," in *Personality Structure in the Life Course: Essays on Personology in the Murray Tradition.* Edited by Zucker RA, Rabin AI, Aronoff J. New York, Springer, 1992, pp. 57–100.

129. Kagan J: "Behavioral Inhibition as a Temperamental Category," in *Handbook of Affective Sciences.* Edited by Davidson RJ, Scherer KR, Goldsmith HH. New York, Oxford University Press, 2003, pp. 320–331.

130. Ovsiew F, Yudofsky SC: "Aggression: A Neuroscientific Perspective," in *Rage, Power, and Aggression.* Edited by Glick RA, Roose SP. New Haven, CT, Yale University Press, 1993, pp. 213–230.

131. Akiskal HS: "Toward a Temperament-Based Approach to Depression: Implications for Neurobiological Research," in *Depression and Mania: From Neurobiology to Temperament.* Edited by Gessa GL, Fratta W, Pani L, et al. New York, Raven, 1995, pp. 99–112.

132. Watson D: *Mood and Temperament.* New York, Guilford, 2000.

133. Ellsworth PC, Scherer KR: "Appraisal Processes in Emotion," in *Handbook of Affective Sciences.* Edited by Davidson RJ, Scherer KR, Goldsmith HH. New York, Oxford University Press, 2003, pp. 572–595.

134. Davidson RJ: "Affective Style, Psychopathology, and Resilience: Brain Mechanisms and Plasticity." *American Psychologist* 55:1196–1214, 2000.

135. Levenson RW: "Autonomic Specificity and Emotion," in *Handbook of Affective Sciences.* Edited by Davidson RJ, Scherer KR, Goldsmith HH. New York, Oxford University Press, 2003, pp. 212–224.

136. Scherer KR, Johnstone T, Klasmeyer G: "Vocal Expression of Emotion," in *Handbook of Affective Sciences.* Edited by Davidson RJ, Scherer KR, Goldsmith HH. New York, Oxford University Press, 2003, pp. 433–456.

137. Panksepp J: *Affective Neuroscience: The Foundations of Human and Animal Emotions.* New York, Oxford University Press, 1998.

138. Baron-Cohen S: *Mindblindness: An Essay on Autism and Theory of Mind.* Cambridge, MA, MIT Press, 1995.

139. Dunn J: "Emotional Development in Early Childhood: A Social Relationship Perspective," in *Handbook of Affective Sciences.* Edited by Davidson RJ, Scherer KR, Goldsmith HH. New York, Oxford University Press, 2003, pp. 332–346.

140. Eisenberg N, Losoya S, Spinrad T: "Affect and Prosocial Responding," in *Handbook of Affective Sciences*. Edited by Davidson RJ, Scherer KR, Goldsmith HH. New York, Oxford University Press, 2003, pp. 787–803.

141. Haidt J: "The Moral Emotions," in *Handbook of Affective Sciences*. Edited by Davidson RJ, Scherer KR, Goldsmith HH. New York, Oxford University Press, 2003, pp. 852–870.

142. Epstein J: *Envy*. New York, Oxford University Press, 2003.

143. Solomon RC: *Spirituality for the Skeptic: The Thoughtful Love of Life*. New York, Oxford University Press, 2002.

144. Lazarus RS: *Psychological Stress and the Coping Process*. New York, McGraw-Hill, 1966.

145. Ohman A, Wiens S: "On the Automaticity of Autonomic Responses in Emotion: An Evolutionary Perspective," in *Handbook of Affective Sciences*. Edited by Davidson RJ, Scherer KR, Goldsmith HH. New York, Oxford University Press, 2003, pp. 256–275.

146. Pavlov IP: *Conditioned Reflexes and Psychiatry*. New York, International Publishers, 1941.

147. Davidson RJ, Pizzagalli D, Nitschke JB, et al.: "Parsing the Subcomponents of Emotion and Disorders of Emotion: Perspectives From Affective Neuroscience," in *Handbook of Affective Sciences*. Edited by Davidson RJ, Scherer KR, Goldsmith HH. New York, Oxford University Press, 2003, pp. 8–24.

148. Lewis L, Kelly KA, Allen JG: *Restoring Hope and Trust: An Illustrated Guide to Mastering Trauma*. Baltimore, MD, Sidran Press, 2004.

149. Mineka S, Rafaeli E, Yovel I: "Cognitive Biases in Emotional Disorders: Information Processing and Social-Cognitive Perspectives," in *Handbook of Affective Sciences*. Edited by Davidson RJ, Scherer KR, Goldsmith HH. New York, Oxford University Press, 2003, pp. 976–1009.

150. Gray JA: "The Neuropsychological Basis of Anxiety," in *Handbook of Anxiety Disorders*. Edited by Last CG, Hersen M. New York, Pergamon, 1988, pp. 10–37.

151. Barlow DH: "The Nature of Anxiety: Anxiety, Depression, and Emotional Disorders," in *Chronic Anxiety: Generalized Anxiety Disorder and Mixed Anxiety-Depression*. Edited by Rapee DM, Barlow DH. New York, Guilford, 1991, pp. 1–28.

152. Dawkins R: *The Selfish Gene*. New York, Oxford University Press, 1989.

153. Falsetti SA, Resnick HS, Dansky BS, et al.: "The Relationship of Stress to Panic Disorder: Cause or Effect?" in *Does Stress Cause Psychiatric Illness?* Edited by Mazure CM. Washington, DC, American Psychiatric Press, 1995, pp. 111–147.

154. Freed S, Craske MG, Greher MR: "Nocturnal Panic and Trauma." *Depression and Anxiety* 9:141–145, 1999.

155. Falsetti SA, Resick PA: "Cognitive Behavioral Treatment of PTSD With Comorbid Panic Attacks." *Journal of Contemporary Psychotherapy* 30:163–179, 2000.

156. Taylor S, Koch WJ, McNally RJ: "How Does Anxiety Sensitivity Vary Across the Anxiety Disorders?" *Journal of Anxiety Disorders* 6:249–259, 1992.

157. Grayling AC: *Meditations for the Humanist: Ethics for a Secular Age*. New York, Oxford University Press, 2002.

158. Berkowitz L: "Affect, Aggression, and Antisocial Behavior," in *Handbook of Affective Sciences*. Edited by Davidson RJ, Scherer KR, Goldsmith HH. New York, Oxford University Press, 2003, pp. 804–823.

159. Oliver JE: "Intergenerational Transmission of Child Abuse: Rates, Research, and Clinical Implications." *American Journal of Psychiatry* 150:1315–1324, 1993.

160. Lerner HG: *The Dance of Anger: A Woman's Guide to Changing the Patterns of Intimate Relationships.* New York, Harper & Row, 1985.

161. Lewis M: "The Development of Anger and Rage," in *Rage, Power, and Aggression.* Edited by Glick RA, Roose SP. New Haven, CT, Yale University Press, 1993, pp. 148–168.

162. Card C: *The Atrocity Paradigm: A Theory of Evil.* New York, Oxford University Press, 2002.

163. Parens H: "A View of the Development of Hostility in Early Life," in *Affect: Psychoanalytic Perspectives.* Edited by Shapiro T, Emde RN. Madison, CT, International Universities Press, 1992, pp. 75–108.

164. Horwitz L: "The Capacity to Forgive: Intrapsychic and Developmental Perspectives." *Journal of the American Psychoanalytic Association,* in press.

165. Murphy JG: *Getting Even: Forgiveness and Its Limits.* New York, Oxford University Press, 2003.

166. Connor KM, Davidson JRT, Lee LC: "Spirituality, Resilience, and Anger in Survivors of Violent Trauma: A Community Survey." *Journal of Traumatic Stress* 16:487–494, 2003.

167. Novaco RW: *Anger Control: The Development and Evaluation of an Experimental Treatment.* Lexington, MA, DC Heath, 1975.

168. Novaco RW, Chemtob CM: "Anger and Trauma: Conceptualization, Assessment, and Treatment," in *Cognitive-Behavioral Therapies for Trauma.* Edited by Follette VM, Ruzek JI, Abueg FR. New York, Guilford, 1998, pp. 162–190.

169. Novaco RW: "Anger and Coping With Stress: Cognitive Behavioral Interventions," in *Cognitive Behavior Therapy: Research and Application.* Edited by Forfeyt JP, Rathjen DP. New York, Plenum, 1978, pp. 135–173.

170. Aristotle: *Ethics.* London, Penguin, 1976.

171. Harter S: *The Construction of the Self: A Developmental Perspective.* New York, Guilford, 1999.

172. Nathanson DL: *Shame and Pride: Affect, Sex, and the Birth of the Self.* New York, WW Norton, 1992.

173. Lewis CS: *Mere Christianity.* New York, Simon & Schuster, 1980.

174. Clark MS, Brissette I: "Two Types of Close Relationships and Their Influence on People's Emotional Lives," in *Handbook of Affective Sciences.* Edited by Davidson RJ, Scherer KR, Goldsmith HH. New York, Oxford University Press, 2003, pp. 824–835.

175. Zerbe KJ: *The Body Betrayed: Women, Eating Disorders, and Treatment.* Washington, DC, American Psychiatric Press, 1993.

176. Bowlby J: *Attachment and Loss: Separation, Vol. 2.* New York, Basic Books, 1973.

177. van der Kolk BA: "The Body Keeps the Score: Memory and the Evolving Psychobiology of Posttraumatic Stress." *Harvard Review of Psychiatry* 1:253–265, 1994.

178. Eichenbaum H: *The Cognitive Neuroscience of Memory: An Introduction.* New York, Oxford University Press, 2002.

179. Schacter DL: *Searching for Memory: The Brain, the Mind, and the Past.* New York, Basic Books, 1996.

180. Pillemer DB: *Momentous Events, Vivid Memories.* Cambridge, MA, Harvard University Press, 1998.

181. Schacter DL: "The Seven Sins of Memory: Insights From Psychology and Cognitive Neuroscience." *American Psychologist* 54:182–203, 1999.

182. Frankel FH: "The Concept of Flashbacks in Historical Perspective." *International Journal of Clinical and Experimental Hypnosis* 42:321–336, 1994.

183. Pitman RK, Orr SP: "The Black Hole of Trauma." *Biological Psychiatry* 27:469–471, 1990.

184. Wegner DM: "When the Antidote Is the Poison: Ironic Mental Control Processes." *Psychological Science* 8:148–150, 1997.

185. Post RM, Weiss SRB, Li H, et al.: "Neural Plasticity and Emotional Memory." *Development and Psychopathology* 10:829–855, 1998.

186. Saakvitne KW, Gamble S, Pearlman LA, et al.: *Risking Connection: A Training Curriculum for Working With Survivors of Childhood Abuse.* Lutherville, MD, Sidran, 2000.

187. Beck AT, Rush AJ, Shaw BF, et al.: *Cognitive Therapy of Depression.* New York, Guilford, 1979.

188. Freud S: "The Aetiology of Hysteria" (1896), in *The Standard Edition of the Complete Psychological Works of Sigmund Freud,* Vol. 3. Translated and edited by Strachey J. London, Hogarth Press, 1962, pp. 187–221.

189. Freud S: *The Origins of Psycho-Analysis: Letters to Wilhelm Fliess, Drafts and Notes, 1887–1902.* New York, Basic Books, 1954.

190. Freud S: "New Introductory Lectures on Psycho-Analysis" (1933), in *The Standard Edition of the Complete Psychological Works of Sigmund Freud,* Vol. 22. Translated and edited by Strachey J. London, Hogarth Press, 1964, pp. 1–182.

191. Grinker RR, Spiegel JP: *Men Under Stress.* Philadelphia, PA, Blakiston, 1945.

192. Kardiner A: *The Traumatic Neuroses of War.* Washington, DC, National Research Council, 1941.

193. Ferenczi S: "Confusion of Tongues Between the Adult and the Child." *International Journal of Psycho-Analysis* 30:225–230, 1949.

194. Sinnett K: "Foreword." *Bulletin of the Menninger Clinic* 57:281–284, 1993.

195. Loftus EF: "The Reality of Repressed Memories." *American Psychologist* 48:518–537, 1993.

196. Alpert JL, Brown LS, Ceci SJ, et al.: *Working Group on Investigation of Memories of Childhood Abuse: Final Report.* Washington, DC, American Psychological Association, 1996.

197. Brown D, Scheflin AW, Hammond DC: *Memory, Trauma Treatment, and the Law.* New York, WW Norton, 1998.

198. Morton J, Andrews B, Bekerian D, et al.: "Recovered Memories: The Report of the Working Party of the British Psychological Society," in *The Recovered Memory/False Memory Debate.* Edited by Pezdek K, Banks WP. New York, Academic Press, 1996, pp. 373–392.

199. McGaugh JL, Cahill L: "Emotion and Memory: Central and Peripheral Contributions," in *Handbook of Affective Sciences.* Edited by Davidson RJ, Scherer KR, Goldsmith HH. New York, Oxford University Press, 2003, pp. 93–116.

200. Brewin CR, Andrews B: "Recovered Memories of Trauma: Phenomenology and Cognitive Mechanisms." *Clinical Psychology Review* 18:949–970, 1998.

201. Williams LM, Banyard VL: "Perspectives on Adult Memories of Childhood Sexual Abuse: A Research Review," in *American Psychiatric Press Review of Psychiatry,* Vol. 16. Edited by Dickstein LJ, Riba MB, Oldham JM. Washington, DC, American Psychiatric Press, 1997, pp. 123–151.

202. Chu JA, Frey LM, Ganzel BL, et al.: "Memories of Childhood Abuse: Dissociation, Amnesia, and Corroboration." *American Journal of Psychiatry* 156:749–755, 1999.

203. Brown R, Kulick J: "Flashbulb Memories." *Cognition* 5:73–99, 1977.

204. Loftus EF, Loftus GR: "On the Permanence of Stored Information in the Human Brain." *American Psychologist* 35:409–420, 1980.

205. Allen JG: "The Spectrum of Accuracy in Memories of Childhood Trauma." *Harvard Review of Psychiatry* 3:84–95, 1995.

206. Rubin DC: "On the Retention Function for Autobiographical Memory." *Journal of Verbal Learning and Verbal Behavior* 21:21–28, 1982.

207. Pillemer DB, White SH: "Childhood Events Recalled by Children and Adults," in *Advances in Child Development and Behavior,* Vol. 21. Edited by Reese HW. New York, Academic Press, 1989, pp. 297–340.

208. Usher JA, Neisser U: "Childhood Amnesia and the Beginnings of Memory for Four Early Life Events." *Journal of Experimental Psychology: General* 122:155–165, 1993.

209. Reiker PP, Carmen E: "The Victim-to-Patient Process: The Disconfirmation and Transformation of Abuse." *American Journal of Orthopsychiatry* 56:360–370, 1986.

210. Lynn SJ, Rhue JW: "Fantasy Proneness: Hypnosis, Developmental Antecedents, and Psychopathology." *American Psychologist* 43:35–44, 1988.

211. Allen JG, Console DA, Lewis L: "Dissociative Detachment and Memory Impairment: Reversible Amnesia or Encoding Failure?" *Comprehensive Psychiatry* 40:160–171, 1999.

212. Steinberg M: *Handbook for the Assessment of Dissociation: A Clinical Guide.* Washington, DC, American Psychiatric Press, 1995.

213. LeDoux J: *The Emotional Brain.* New York, Simon & Schuster, 1996.

214. Pope HG, Hudson JI: "Can Memories of Childhood Sexual Abuse Be Repressed?" *Psychological Medicine* 25:121–126, 1995.

215. Holmes DS: "The Evidence for Repression: An Examination of Sixty Years of Research," in *Repression and Dissociation: Implications for Personality Theory, Psychopathology, and Health.* Edited by Singer JL. Chicago, IL, University of Chicago Press, 1990, pp. 85–102.

216. Neisser U: "Time Present and Time Past," in *Practical Aspects of Memory: Current Research and Issues.* Edited by Gruneberg MM, Morris PE, Sykes RN. New York, Wiley, 1988, pp. 545–560.

217. Moscovitch M: "Confabulation," in *Memory Distortion: How Minds, Brains, and Societies Reconstruct the Past.* Edited by Schacter DL. Cambridge, MA, Harvard University Press, 1995, pp. 226–251.

218. Christianson S: "Remembering Emotional Events: Potential Mechanisms," in *The Handbook of Emotion and Memory: Research and Theory.* Edited by Christianson S. Hillsdale, NJ, Erlbaum, 1992, pp. 307–340.

219. Barclay CR, Wellman HM: "Accuracies and Inaccuracies in Autobiographical Memories." *Journal of Memory and Language* 25:93–103, 1986.

220. van der Hart O, Brown P: "Abreaction Re-evaluated." *Dissociation* 5:127–140, 1992.

221. Janoff-Bulman R: *Shattered Assumptions: Towards a New Psychology of Trauma.* New York, Free Press, 1992.

222. Spence DP: *Narrative Truth and Historical Truth: Meaning and Interpretation in Psychoanalysis*. New York, WW Norton, 1982.

223. Kluft RP: "Multiple Personality Disorder: A Contemporary Perspective." *Harvard Mental Health Letter* 10:5–7, 1993.

224. Brown DP, Fromm E: *Hypnotherapy and Hypnoanalysis*. Hillsdale, NJ, Erlbaum, 1986.

225. Gabbard GO, Wilkinson SM: *Management of Countertransference With Borderline Patients*. Washington, DC, American Psychiatric Press, 1994.

226. Mollon P: *Remembering Trauma: A Psychotherapist's Guide to Memory and Illusion*. Chichester, UK, Wiley, 1998.

227. Thomas L: *Late Night Thoughts on Listening to Mahler's Ninth Symphony*. New York, Viking, 1983.

228. Herman JL: "Complex PTSD: A Syndrome in Survivors of Prolonged and Repeated Trauma." *Journal of Traumatic Stress* 5:377–391, 1992.

229. Blatt SJ, Blass RB: "Relatedness and Self-Definition: Two Primary Dimensions in Personality Development, Psychopathology, and Psychotherapy," in *Interface of Psychoanalysis and Psychology*. Edited by Barron JW, Eagle MN, Wolitzky DL. Washington, DC, American Psychological Association, 1992, pp. 399–428.

230. James W: *The Principles of Psychology* (1890). New York, Dover, 1950.

231. Dennett DC: *Freedom Evolves*. London, Penguin, 2003.

232. Bruner J: *Acts of Meaning*. Cambridge, MA, Harvard University Press, 1990.

233. Dennett DC: *Consciousness Explained*. Boston, MA, Little, Brown, 1991.

234. Modell AH: "The Private Self and Private Space," in *The Annual of Psychoanalysis*, Vol. 20. Edited by Winer JA. Hillsdale, NJ, Analytic Press, 1992, pp. 1–14.

235. Taylor SE: *Positive Illusions: Creative Self-Deception and the Healthy Mind*. New York, Basic Books, 1989.

236. Kabat-Zinn J: *Full Catastrophe Living: Using the Wisdom of Your Body and Mind to Face Stress, Pain, and Illness*. New York, Delta, 1990.

237. Stern DN: *The Interpersonal World of the Infant: A View From Psychoanalysis and Developmental Psychology*. New York, Basic Books, 1985.

238. Seligman MEP: *Helplessness: On Depression, Development, and Death*. San Francisco, WH Freeman, 1975.

239. Freud S: "The Ego and the Id" (1923), in *Standard Edition of the Complete Psychological Works of Sigmund Freud*, Vol. 19. Translated and edited by Strachey J. London, Hogarth Press, 1961, pp. 12–66

240. Ehrenberg DB: *The Intimate Edge: Extending the Reach of Psychoanalytic Interaction*. New York, WW Norton, 1992.

241. Reis HT, Gable SL: "Toward a Positive Psychology of Relationships," in *Flourishing: Positive Psychology and the Life Well-Lived*. Edited by Keyes CL, Haidt J. Washington, DC, American Psychological Association, 2003, pp. 129–159.

242. Slade A, Aber JL: "Attachments, Drives, and Development: Conflicts and Convergences in Theory," in *Interface of Psychoanalysis and Psychology*. Edited by Barron JW, Eagle MN, Wolitzky DL. Washington, DC, American Psychological Association, 1992, pp.154–185.

243. Fonagy P, Target M: "Perspectives on the Recovered Memories Debate," in *Recovered Memories of Abuse: True or False?* Edited by Sandler J, Fonagy P. Madison, CT, International Universities Press, 1997, pp. 183–237.

244. MacIntyre A: *Dependent Rational Animals: Why Human Beings Need the Virtues*. Chicago, IL, Open Court, 1999.

245. Freud A: *The Ego and the Mechanisms of Defence* (1936). New York, International Universities Press, 1946.

246. Lewis DO: "From Abuse to Violence: Psychophysiological Consequences of Maltreatment." *Journal of the American Academy of Child and Adolescent Psychiatry* 31:383–391, 1992.

247. Davies JM, Frawley MG: *Treating the Adult Survivor of Childhood Sexual Abuse.* New York, Basic Books, 1994.

248. Freud S: "Beyond the Pleasure Principle" (1920), in *The Standard Edition of the Complete Psychological Works of Sigmund Freud,* Vol. 18. Translated and edited by Strachey J. London, Hogarth Press, 1964, pp. 7–64.

249. Freud S: "Remembering, Repeating, and Working-Through" (1914), in *The Standard Edition of the Complete Psychological Works of Sigmund Freud,* Vol. 12. Translated and edited by Strachey J. London, Hogarth Press, 1958, pp. 147–156.

250. Terr L: "What Happens to Early Memories of Trauma? A Study of Twenty Children Under Age Five at the Time of Documented Traumatic Events." *Journal of the American Academy of Child and Adolescent Psychiatry* 27:96–104, 1988.

251. Dutton DG, Painter S: "Emotional Attachments in Abusive Relationships: A Test of Traumatic Bonding Theory." *Violence and Victims* 8:105–120, 1993.

252. Strentz T: "The Stockholm Syndrome: Law Enforcement Policy and Hostage Behavior," in *Victims of Terrorism.* Edited by Ochberg FM, Soskis DA. Boulder, CO, Westview Press, 1982, pp. 149–163.

253. Dutton D, Painter SL: "Traumatic Bonding: The Development of Emotional Attachments in Battered Women and Other Relationships of Intermittent Abuse." *Victimology* 6:139–155, 1981.

254. Symonds M: "Victim Responses to Terror: Understanding and Treatment," in *Victims of Terrorism.* Edited by Ochberg FM, Soskis DA. Boulder, CO, Westview Press, 1982, pp. 95–103.

255. Henderson AJZ, Bartholomew K, Dutton DG: "He Loves Me; He Loves Me Not: Attachment and Separation Resolution of Abused Women." *Journal of Family Violence* 12:169–191, 1997.

256. Enns CZ, Campbell J, Courtois CA: "Recommendations for Working With Domestic Violence Survivors, With Special Attention to Memory Issues and Posttraumatic Processes." *Psychotherapy* 34:459–477, 1997.

257. Allen JG, Coyne L, Console DA: "Course of Illness Following Specialized Inpatient Treatment for Women With Trauma-Related Psychopathology." *Bulletin of the Menninger Clinic* 64:235–256, 2000.

258. Ryff CD, Singer B: "Flourishing Under Fire: Resilience as a Prototype of Challenged Thriving," in *Flourishing: Positive Psychology and the Life Well-Lived.* Edited by Keyes CL, Haidt J. Washington, DC, American Psychological Association, 2003, pp. 15–36.

259. Stein H, Allen JG, Hill J: "Roles and Relationships: A Psychoeducational Approach to Reviewing Strengths and Difficulties in Adulthood Functioning." *Bulletin of the Menninger Clinic* 67:281–313, 2003.

260. Hill J, Harrington R, Fudge H, et al.: "Adult Personality Functioning Assessment (APFA): An Investigator-Based Standardised Interview." *British Journal of Psychiatry* 155:24–35, 1989.

261. Bremner JD: *Does Stress Damage the Brain? Understanding Trauma-Related Disorders From a Mind-Body Perspective.* New York, WW Norton, 2002.

262. Dunman RS, Malberg J, Thome J: "Neural Plasticity to Stress and Antidepressant Treatment." *Biological Psychiatry* 46:1181–1191, 1999.

263. Shelton RC: "Cellular Mechanisms in the Vulnerability to Depression and Response to Antidepressants." *Psychiatric Clinics of North America* 23:713–729, 2000.

264. McEwen BS: *The End of Stress as We Know It.* Washington, DC, Joseph Henry Press, 2002.

265. Allen JG: "Coping With the Catch 22s of Depression: A Guide for Educating Patients." *Bulletin of the Menninger Clinic* 66:103–144, 2002.

266. Parsons T: "Illness and the Role of the Physician: A Sociological Perspective." *American Journal of Orthopsychiatry* 21:452–460, 1951.

267. Cannon WB: *Bodily Changes in Pain, Hunger, Fear and Rage: An Account of Recent Researches Into the Function of Emotional Excitement.* Boston, MA, Charles T. Branford, 1953.

268. Fanselow MS, Lester LS: "A Functional Behavioristic Approach to Aversively Motivated Behavior: Predatory Imminence as a Determinant of the Topography of Defensive Behavior," in *Evolution and Learning.* Edited by Bolles RC, Beecher MD. Hillsdale, NJ, Erlbaum, 1988, pp. 185–212.

269. Post RM, Weiss SRB, Smith M, et al.: "Kindling Versus Quenching: Implications for the Evolution and Treatment of Posttraumatic Stress Disorder," in *Psychobiology of Posttraumatic Stress Disorder (Annals of the New York Academy of Sciences,* Vol. 821). Edited by Yehuda R, McFarlane AC. New York, New York Academy of Sciences, 1997, pp. 285–295.

270. Krystal JH, Kosten RR, Southwick S, et al.: "Neurobiological Aspects of PTSD: Review of Clinical and Preclinical Studies." *Behavior Therapy* 20:177–198, 1989.

271. Aston-Jones G, Valentino RJ, Van Bockstaele EJ, et al.: "Locus Coeruleus, Stress, and PTSD: Neurobiological and Clinical Parallels," in *Catecholamine Function in Posttraumatic Stress Disorder: Emerging Concepts.* Edited by Murburg MM. Washington, DC, American Psychiatric Press, 1994, pp. 17–62.

272. LaBar KS, LeDoux JE: "Emotional Learning Circuits in Animals and Humans," in *Handbook of Affective Sciences.* Edited by Davidson RJ, Scherer KR, Goldsmith HH. New York, Oxford University Press, 2003, pp. 52–65.

273. Rauch SL: "Neuroimaging and the Neurobiology of Anxiety Disorders," in *Handbook of Affective Sciences.* Edited by Davidson RJ, Scherer KR, Goldsmith HH. New York, Oxford University Press, 2003, pp. 963–975.

274. Goldberg E: *The Executive Brain: Frontal Lobes and the Civilized Mind.* New York, Oxford University Press, 2001.

275. Arnsten AFT: "The Biology of Being Frazzled." *Science* 280:1711–1712, 1998.

276. Mayes LC: "A Developmental Perspective on the Regulation of Arousal States." *Seminars in Perinatology* 24:267–279, 2000.

277. van der Kolk BA, Burbridge JA, Suzuki J: "The Psychobiology of Traumatic Memory: Clinical Implications of Neuroimaging Studies," in *Psychobiology of Posttraumatic Stress Disorder (Annals of the New York Academy of Sciences,* Vol. 821). Edited by Yehuda R, McFarlane AC. New York, New York Academy of Sciences, 1997, pp. 99–113.

278. Yehuda R: "Neuroendocrinology of Trauma and Posttraumatic Stress Disorder," in *Psychological Trauma.* Edited by Yehuda R. Washington, DC, American Psychiatric Press, 1998, pp. 97–131.

279. Nemeroff CB: "The Neurobiology of Depression." *Scientific American* 278:42–49, 1998.
280. Bremner JD, Vythilingam M, Vermetten E, et al.: "MRI and PET Study of Deficits in Hippocampal Structure and Function in Women With Childhood Sexual Abuse and Posttraumatic Stress Disorder." *American Journal of Psychiatry* 160:924–932, 2003.
281. Sapolsky RM: "Stress, Glucocorticoids, and Damage to the Nervous System: The Current State of Confusion." *Stress* 1:1–19, 1996.
282. Southwick SM, Yehuda R, Morgan CAI: "Clinical Studies of Neurotransmitter Alterations in Post-Traumatic Stress Disorder," in *Neurobiological and Clinical Consequences of Stress: From Normal Adaptation to Post-Traumatic Stress Disorder.* Edited by Friedman MJ, Charney DS, Deutch AY. Philadelphia, PA, Lippincott-Raven, 1995, pp. 335–349.
283. Pitman RK, Orr SP, van der Kolk BA, et al.: "Analgesia: A New Dependent Variable for the Biological Study of Posttraumatic Stress Disorder," in *Posttraumatic Stress Disorder: Etiology, Phenomenology, and Treatment.* Edited by Wolf ME, Mosnaim AD. Washington, DC, American Psychiatric Press, 1990, pp. 140–147.
284. Morange M: *The Misunderstood Gene.* Cambridge, MA, Harvard University Press, 2001.
285. Davidson JRT, Tupler LA, Wilson WH, et al.: "A Family Study of Chronic Post-traumatic Stress Disorder Following Rape Trauma." *Journal of Psychiatric Research* 32:301–309, 1998.
286. Kendler KS, Neale M, Kessler R, et al.: "A Twin Study of Recent Life Events and Difficulties." *Archives of General Psychiatry* 50:789–796, 1993.
287. McEwen BS, Seeman T: "Stress and Affect: Applicability of the Concepts of Allostasis and Allostatic Load," in *Handbook of Affective Sciences.* Edited by Davidson RJ, Scherer KR, Goldsmith HH. New York, Oxford University Press, 2003, pp. 1117–1137.
288. Weiner H: *Perturbing the Organism: The Biology of Stressful Experience.* Chicago, IL, University of Chicago Press, 1992.
289. McCauley J, Kern DE, Kolodner K, et al.: "Clinical Characteristics of Women with a History of Childhood Abuse." *Journal of the American Medical Association* 277:1362–1368, 1997.
290. Andreski P, Chilcoat H, Breslau N: "Post-traumatic Stress Disorder and Somatization Symptoms: A Prospective Study." *Psychiatry Research* 79:131–138, 1998.
291. Zerbe KJ: *Women's Mental Health in Primary Care.* Philadelphia, PA, WB Saunders, 1999.
292. Friedman MJ, Schnurr PP: "The Relationship Between Trauma, Post-Traumatic Stress Disorder, and Physical Health," in *Neurobiological and Clinical Consequences of Stress: From Normal Adaptation to Post-Traumatic Stress Disorder.* Edited by Friedman MJ, Charney DS, Deutch AY. Philadelphia, PA, Lippincott-Raven, 1995, pp.507–524.
293. Burgess AW, Holmstrom LL: "Rape Trauma Syndrome." *American Journal of Psychiatry* 131:981–986, 1974.
294. Westerlund E: *Women's Sexuality After Childhood Incest.* New York, WW Norton, 1992.
295. Kaplan HS: *The New Sex Therapy: Active Treatment of Sexual Dysfunctions.* New York, Brunner/Mazel, 1974.

296. Bolen JD: "Sexuality-Focused Treatment With Survivors and Their Partners," in *Treatment of Adult Survivors of Incest*. Edited by Paddison PL. Washington, DC, American Psychiatric Press, 1993, pp. 55–75.

297. Thase ME, Jindal R, Howland RH: "Biological Aspects of Depression," in *Handbook of Depression*. Edited by Gotlib IH, Hammen C. New York, Guilford, 2002, pp. 192–218.

298. Post RM: "Transduction of Psychosocial Stress Into the Neurobiology of Recurrent Affective Disorder." *American Journal of Psychiatry* 149:999–1010, 1992.

299. Solomon A: *The Noonday Demon: An Atlas of Depression*. New York, Simon & Schuster, 2001.

300. Keller MB, Shapiro RW: "'Double Depression': Superimposition of Acute Depressive Episodes on Chronic Depressive Disorders." *American Journal of Psychiatry* 139:438–442, 1982.

301. Phillips KA, Gunderson JG, Triebwasser J, et al.: "Reliability and Validity of Depressive Personality Disorder." *American Journal of Psychiatry* 155:1044–1048, 1998.

302. Wallace J, Schneider T, McGuffin P: "Genetics of Depression," in *Handbook of Depression*. Edited by Gotlib IH, Hammen C. New York, Guilford, 2002, pp. 169–191.

303. Akiskal HS: "Temperamental Foundation of Affective Disorders," in *Interpersonal Factors in the Origin and Course of Affective Disorders*. Edited by Mundt C, Goldstein MJ, Hahlweg K, et al. London, Gaskell, 1996, pp. 3–30.

304. Hatfield E, Cacioppo JT, Rapson RL: *Emotional Contagion*. Cambridge, UK, Cambridge University Press, 1994.

305. Newport DJ, Stowe ZN, Nemeroff CB: "Parental Depression: Animal Models of an Adverse Life Event." *American Journal of Psychiatry* 159:1265–1283, 2002.

306. Field T: "Prenatal Effects of Maternal Depression," in *Children of Depressed Parents: Mechanisms of Risk and Implications for Treatment*. Edited by Goodman SH, Gotlib IH. Washington, DC, American Psychological Association, 2002, pp. 59–88.

307. Ashman SB, Dawson G: "Maternal Depression, Infant Psychobiological Development, and Risk for Depression," in *Children of Depressed Parents: Mechanisms of Risk and Implications for Treatment*. Edited by Goodman SH, Gotlib IH. Washington, DC, American Psychological Association, 2002, pp. 37–58.

308. Hossain Z, Field T, Gonzalez J, et al.: "Infants of 'Depressed' Mothers Interact Better With Their Nondepressed Fathers." *Infant Mental Health Journal* 15:348–357, 1994.

309. Pelaez-Nogueras M, Field T, Cigales M, et al.: "Infants of Depressed Mothers Show Less 'Depressed' Behavior With Their Nursery Teachers." *Infant Mental Health Journal* 15:358–367, 1994.

310. Nolen-Hoeksema S: "Gender Differences in Depression," in *Handbook of Depression*. Edited by Gotlib IH, Hammen C. New York, Guilford, 2002, pp. 492–509.

311. Plotsky PM, Owens MJ, Nemeroff CB: "Psychoneuroendocrinology of Depression: Hypothalamic-Pituitary-Adrenal Axis." *Psychiatric Clinics of North America* 21:293–307, 1998.

312. Bernet CZ, Stein MB: "Relationship of Childhood Maltreatment to the Onset and Course of Major Depression in Adulthood." *Depression and Anxiety* 9:169–174, 1999.

313. Bifulco A, Brown GW, Moran P, et al.: "Predicting Depression in Women: The Role of Past and Present Vulnerability." *Psychological Medicine* 28:39–50, 1998.

314. Hammen C: *Depression*. East Sussex, UK, Psychology Press, 1997.

315. Lewinsohn PM, Essau CA: "Depression in Adolescents," in *Handbook of Depression*. Edited by Gotlib IH, Hammen C. New York, Guilford, 2002, pp. 541–559.

316. Judd LL, Akiskal HS, Maser JD, et al.: "Major Depressive Disorder: A Prospective Study of Residual Subthreshold Depressive Symptoms as Predictor of Rapid Relapse." *Journal of Affective Disorders* 50:97–108, 1998.

317. Brown GW, Harris TO: *Social Origins of Depression: A Study of Psychiatric Disorder in Women*. New York, Free Press, 1978.

318. Kendler KS, Karkowski LM, Prescott CA: "Causal Relationships Between Stressful Life Events and the Onset of Major Depression." *American Journal of Psychiatry* 156:837–841, 1999.

319. Breslau N, Davis G, Adreski P, et al.: "Epidemiological Findings on Posttraumatic Stress Disorder and Co-Morbid Disorders in the General Population," in *Adversity, Stress, and Psychopathology*. Edited by Dohrenwend BP. New York, Oxford University Press, 1998, pp. 319–330.

320. Comijs HC, Pot AM, Smit JH, et al.: "Elder Abuse in the Community: Prevalence and Consequences." *Journal of the American Geriatrics Society* 46:885–888, 1998.

321. Lachs MS, Williams CS, O'Brien S, et al.: "The Mortality of Elder Mistreatment." *Journal of the American Medical Association* 280:428–342, 1998.

322. Aarts PGH, Op den Velde W: "Prior Traumatization and the Process of Aging: Theory and Clinical Implications," in *Traumatic Stress: The Effects of Overwhelming Experience on Mind, Body, and Society*. Edited by van der Kolk BA, McFarlane AC, Weisaeth L. New York, Guilford Press, 1996, pp. 359–377.

323. Leary MR: "The Self and Emotion: The Role of Self-Reflection in the Generation and Regulation of Affective Experience," in *Handbook of Affective Sciences*. Edited by Davidson RJ, Scherer KR, Goldsmith HH. New York, Oxford University Press, 2003, pp. 773–786.

324. Flett GL, Hewitt PL, Oliver JM, et al.: "Perfectionism in Children and Their Parents: A Developmental Analysis," in *Perfectionism: Theory, Research, and Treatment*. Edited by Flett GL, Hewitt PL. Washington, DC, American Psychological Association, 2002, pp. 89–132.

325. Neese RM: "Is Depression an Adaptation?" *Archives of General Psychiatry* 57:14–20, 2000.

326. Dubovsky SL: *Mind-Body Deceptions: The Psychosomatics of Everyday Life*. New York, WW Norton, 1997.

327. Gilbert P: *Depression: The Evolution of Powerlessness*. New York, Guilford, 1992.

328. Kudryavtseva NN, Avgustinovich DF: "Behavioral and Physiological Markers of Experimental Depression Induced by Social Conflicts (DISC)." *Aggressive Behavior* 24:271–286, 1998.

329. Zetzel ER: "Depression and the Incapacity to Bear It," in *Drives, Affects, Behavior*, Vol. 2. Edited by Schur M. New York, International Universities Press, 1965, pp. 243–274.

330. Keller MB, Lavori PW, Mueller TI, et al.: "Time to Recovery, Chronicity, and Levels of Psychopathology in Major Depression." *Archives of General Psychiatry* 49:809–816, 1992.

331. Solomon DA, Keller MB, Leon AC, et al.: "Recovery From Major Depression: A 10-Year Prospective Follow-Up Across Multiple Episodes." *Archives of General Psychiatry* 54:1001–1006, 1997.

332. Murray CJL, Lopez AD: "Executive Summary," in *The Global Burden of Disease: A Comprehensive Assessment of Mortality and Disability From Diseases, Injuries, and Risk Factors in 1990 and Projected to 2020.* Geneva and Boston, World Health Organization and Harvard School of Public Health, 1996, pp. 1–43.

333. Wells KB, Sturm R, Sherbourne CD, et al.: *Caring for Depression.* Cambridge, MA, Harvard University Press, 1996.

334. Carver CS, Scheier MF: *On the Self-Regulation of Behavior.* Cambridge, UK, Cambridge University Press, 1998.

335. Breslau N, Roth T, Rosenthal L, et al.: "Sleep Disturbance and Psychiatric Diagnosis: A Longitudinal Epidemiological Study of Young Adults." *Biological Psychiatry* 39:411–418, 1996.

336. Allen JG, Console DA, Brethour JR Jr, et al.: "Screening for Trauma-Related Sleep Disturbance in Women Admitted for Specialized Inpatient Treatment." *Journal of Trauma and Dissociation* 1:59–86, 2000.

337. Rolls ET: *The Brain and Emotion.* New York, Oxford University Press, 1999.

338. Thayer RE: *Calm Energy: How People Regulate Mood With Food and Exercise.* New York, Oxford University Press, 2001.

339. Babyak M, Blumenthal JA, Herman S, et al.: "Exercise Treatment for Major Depression: Maintenance of Therapeutic Benefit at 10 Months." *Psychosomatic Medicine* 62:633–638, 2000.

340. Meehl PE: "Hedonic Capacity: Some Conjectures." *Bulletin of the Menninger Clinic* 39:295–307, 1975.

341. Lewinsohn PM, Munoz RF, Youngren MA, et al.: *Control Your Depression.* New York, Simon & Schuster, 1986.

342. Hollon SD, Haman KL, Brown LL: "Cognitive-Behavioral Treatment of Depression," in *Handbook of Depression.* Edited by Gotlib IH, Hammen C. New York, Guilford, 2002, pp. 383–403.

343. Teasdale JD, Barnard PJ: *Affect, Cognition, and Change: Re-Modelling Depressive Thought.* Hillsdale, NJ, Erlbaum, 1993.

344. Ingram RE, Miranda J, Segal ZV: *Cognitive Vulnerability to Depression.* New York, Guilford, 1998.

345. Peterson C, Chang EC: "Optimism and Flourishing," in *Flourishing: Positive Psychology and the Life Well-Lived.* Edited by Keyes CL, Haidt J. Washington, DC, American Psychological Association, 2003, pp. 55–79.

346. Brown GW: "Loss and Depressive Disorders," in *Adversity, Stress, and Psychopathology.* Edited by Dohrenwend BP. New York, Oxford University Press, 1998, pp. 358–370.

347. Lyubomirsky S, Nolen-Hoeksema S: "Self-Perpetuating Properties of Dysphoric Rumination." *Journal of Personality and Social Psychology* 65:339–349, 1993.

348. Drevets WC, Videen TO, Price JL, et al.: "A Functional Anatomical Study of Unipolar Depression." *Journal of Neuroscience* 12:3628–3641, 1992.

349. Elliott R, Baker C, Rogers RD, et al.: "Prefrontal Dysfunction in Depressed Patients Performing a Complex Planning Task: A Study Using Positron Emission Tomography." *Psychological Medicine* 27:931–942, 1997.

350. Segal ZV, Williams JMG, Teasdale JD: *Mindfulness-Based Cognitive Therapy for Depression: A New Approach to Preventing Relapse.* New York, Guilford, 2002.

351. Joiner TE: "Depression in Its Interpersonal Context," in *Handbook of Depression*. Edited by Gotlib IH, Hammen C. New York, Guilford, 2002, pp. 295–313.

352. Potthoff JG, Holahan CJ, Joiner TE: "Reassurance Seeking, Stress Generation, and Depressive Symptoms: An Integrative Model." *Journal of Personality and Social Psychology* 68:664–670, 1995.

353. Coyne JC, Burchill SAL, Stiles WB: "An Interactional Perspective on Depression," in *Handbook of Social and Clinical Psychology*. Edited by Snyder CR, Forsyth DR. New York, Pergamon, 1991, pp. 327–349.

354. McNally RJ, Saigh PA: "On the Distinction Between Traumatic Simple Phobia and Posttraumatic Stress Disorder," in *Posttraumatic Stress Disorder: DSM-IV and Beyond*. Edited by Davidson JRT, Foa EB. Washington, DC, American Psychiatric Press, 1993, pp. 207–212.

355. Trimble MR: "Post-traumatic Stress Disorder: History of a Concept," in *Trauma and Its Wake: The Study and Treatment of Post-Traumatic Stress Disorder*. Edited by Figley CR. New York, Brunner/Mazel, 1985, pp. 5–14.

356. Kulka RA, Schlenger WE, Fairbank JA, et al.: *Trauma and the Vietnam War Generation: Report of Findings from the National Vietnam Veterans Readjustment Study*. New York, Brunner/Mazel, 1990.

357. Lindemann E: "Symptomatology and Management of Acute Grief." *American Journal of Psychiatry* 101:141–148, 1944.

358. Finkelhor D: *Child Sexual Abuse: New Theory and Research*. New York, Free Press, 1984.

359. Breslau N: "Epidemiology of Trauma and Posttraumatic Stress Disorder," in *Psychological Trauma*. Edited by Yehuda R. Washington, DC, American Psychiatric Press, 1998, pp. 1–29.

360. Drell MJ, Siegel CH, Gaensbauer TJ: "Post-Traumatic Stress Disorder," in *Handbook of Infant Mental Health*. Edited by Zeanah CH. New York, Guilford, 1993, pp. 291–304.

361. Brewin CR, Dalgleish T, Joseph S: "A Dual Representation Theory of Posttraumatic Stress Disorder." *Psychological Review* 103:670–686, 1996.

362. McCaffrey RJ, Fairbank JA: "Behavioral Assessment and Treatment of Accident-Related Posttraumatic Stress Disorder: Two Case Studies." *Behavior Therapy* 16:406–416, 1985.

363. Hartmann E: "Nightmare After Trauma as a Paradigm for All Dreams: A New Approach to the Nature and Functions of Dreaming." *Psychiatry* 61:223–238, 1998.

364. Burnstein A: "Posttraumatic Flashbacks, Dream Disturbances, and Mental Imagery." *Journal of Clinical Psychiatry* 46:374–378, 1985.

365. Ross RJ, Ball WA, Dinges DF, et al.: "Motor Dysfunction During Sleep in Posttraumatic Stress Disorder." *Sleep* 17:723–732, 1994.

366. Krakow B, Germain A, Warner TD, et al.: "The Relationship of Sleep Quality and Posttraumatic Stress to Potential Sleep Disorders in Sexual Assault Survivors With Nightmares, Insomnia, and PTSD." *Journal of Traumatic Stress* 14:647–665, 2001.

367. Craske MG, Rowe MK: "Nocturnal Panic." *Clinical Psychology: Science and Practice* 4:153–174, 1997.

368. Krakow B, Hollifield M, Schrader R, et al.: "A Controlled Study of Imagery Rehearsal for Chronic Nightmares in Sexual Assault Survivors With PTSD: A Preliminary Report." *Journal of Traumatic Stress* 13:589–609, 2000.

369. de Loos WS: "Psychosomatic Manifestations of Chronic Posttraumatic Stress Disorder," in *Posttraumatic Stress Disorder: Etiology, Phenomenology, and Treatment*. Edited by Wolf ME, Mosnaim AD. Washington, DC, American Psychiatric Press, 1990, pp. 94–104.

370. Friedman MJ: "Interrelationships Between Biological Mechanisms and Pharmacotherapy of Posttraumatic Stress Disorder," in *Posttraumatic Stress Disorder: Etiology, Phenomenology, and Treatment*. Edited by Wolf ME, Mosnaim AD. Washington, DC, American Psychiatric Press, 1990, pp. 204–225.

371. Horowitz MJ: *Stress Response Syndromes: PTSD, Grief, and Adjustment Disorders*. Northvale, NJ, Jason Aronson, 1997.

372. Foa EB, Riggs DS, Gershuny BS: "Arousal, Numbing, and Intrusion: Symptom Structure of PTSD Following Assault." *American Journal of Psychiatry* 152:116–120, 1995.

373. Litz BT, Gray MJ: "Emotional Numbing in Posttraumatic Stress Disorder: Current and Future Research Directions." *Australian and New Zealand Journal of Psychiatry* 36:198–204, 2002.

374. Nishith P, Mechanic MB, Resick PA: "Prior Interpersonal Trauma: The Contribution to Current PTSD Symptoms in Female Rape Victims." *Journal of Abnormal Psychology* 109:20–25, 2000.

375. Glodich A, Allen JG, Arnold L: "Protocol for a Trauma-Based Psychoeducational Group Intervention to Decrease Risk-Taking, Reenactment, and Further Violence Exposure: Application to the Public High School Setting." *Journal of Child and Adolescent Group Psychotherapy* 11:87–107, 2002.

376. Blank AS Jr: "The Longitudinal Course of Posttraumatic Stress Disorder," in *Posttraumatic Stress Disorder: DSM-IV and Beyond*. Edited by Davidson JRT, Foa EB. Washington, DC, American Psychiatric Press, 1993, pp. 3–22.

377. Marmar CR, Weiss DS, Schlenger WE, et al.: "Peritraumatic Dissociation and Posttraumatic Stress in Male Vietnam Theater Veterans." *American Journal of Psychiatry* 151:902–907, 1994.

378. Solomon Z, Laror N, McFarlane AC: "Acute Posttraumatic Reactions in Soldiers and Civilians," in *Traumatic Stress: The Effects of Overwhelming Experience on Mind, Body, and Society*. Edited by van der Kolk BA, McFarlane AC, Weisaeth L. New York, Guilford Press, 1996, pp. 102–114.

379. Brewin CR, Andrews B, Rose S, et al.: "Acute Stress Disorder and Posttraumatic Stress Disorder in Victims of Violent Crime." *American Journal of Psychiatry* 156:360–366, 1999.

380. Marshall RD, Spitzer R, Liebowitz MR: "Review and Critique of the New DSM-IV Diagnosis of Acute Stress Disorder." *American Journal of Psychiatry* 156:1677–1685, 1999.

381. Kessler RC, Sonnega A, Bromet E, et al.: "Posttraumatic Stress Disorder in the National Comorbidity Survey." *Archives of General Psychiatry* 52:1048–1060, 1995.

382. Goodwin JM: "Applying to Adult Incest Victims What We Have Learned From Victimized Children," in *Incest-Related Syndromes of Adult Psychopathology*. Edited by Kluft RP. Washington, DC, American Psychiatric Press, 1990, pp. 55–74.

383. True WR, Rice J, Eisen SA, et al.: "A Twin Study of Genetic and Environmental Contributions to Liability for Posttraumatic Stress Symptoms." *Archives of General Psychiatry* 50:257–264, 1991.

384. Breslau N, Davis GC, Andreski P, et al.: "Traumatic Events and Posttraumatic Stress Disorder in an Urban Population of Young Adults." *Archives of General Psychiatry* 48:216–222, 1991.

385. Davidson JRT: "Issues in the Diagnosis of Posttraumatic Stress Disorder," in *American Psychiatric Press Review of Psychiatry,* Vol. 12. Edited by Oldham JM, Riba MB, Tasman A. Washington, DC, American Psychiatric Press, 1993, pp. 141–155.

386. Bremner JD, Southwick SM, Johnson DR, et al.: "Childhood Physical Abuse and Combat-Related Posttraumatic Stress Disorder in Vietnam Veterans." *American Journal of Psychiatry* 150:235–239, 1993.

387. Foy DW, Resnick HS, Sipprelle RC, et al.: "Premilitary, Military, and Postmilitary Factors in the Development of Combat-Related Posttraumatic Stress Disorder." *Behavior Therapist* 10:3–9, 1987.

388. Boman B: "Are All Vietnam Veterans Like John Rambo?" in *Posttraumatic Stress Disorder: Etiology, Phenomenology, and Treatment.* Edited by Wolf ME, Mosnaim AD. Washington, DC, American Psychiatric Press, 1990, pp. 80–93.

389. Campbell R, Sefl T, Barnes HE, et al.: "Community Services for Rape Survivors: Enhancing Psychological Well-Being or Increasing Trauma?" *Journal of Consulting and Clinical Psychology* 67:847–858, 1999.

390. Flach F: "The Resilience Hypothesis and Posttraumatic Stress Disorder," in *Posttraumatic Stress Disorder: Etiology, Phenomenology, and Treatment.* Edited by Wolf ME, Mosnaim AD. Washington, DC, American Psychiatric Press, 1990, pp. 36–45.

391. Menninger K: *The Vital Balance.* New York, Viking, 1963.

392. Shalev AY: "Treating Survivors in the Immediate Aftermath of Traumatic Events, in *Treating Trauma Survivors With PTSD.* Edited by Yehuda R. Washington, DC, American Psychiatric Publishing, 2002, pp. 157–188.

393. Mitchell JT, Everly GS: *Critical Incident Stress Debriefing: An Operations Manual for the Prevention of Traumatic Stress Among Emergency Services and Disaster Workers.* Ellicott City, MD, Chevron, 1995.

394. Rose S, Bisson J: "Brief Early Psychological Interventions Following Trauma: A Systematic Review of the Literature. *Journal of Traumatic Stress* 11:697–710, 1998.

395. Raphael B, Wilson J, Meldrum L, et al.: "Acute Preventive Interventions," in *Traumatic Stress: The Effects of Overwhelming Experience on Mind, Body, and Society.* Edited by van der Kolk BA, McFarlane AC, Weisaeth L. New York, Guilford Press, 1996, pp. 463–479.

396. Kluft RP: "Discussion: A Specialist's Perspective on Multiple Personality Disorder." *Psychoanalytic Inquiry* 12:139–171, 1992.

397. Chu JA: "Dissociative Symptomatology in Adult Patients With Histories of Childhood Physical and Sexual Abuse," in *Trauma, Memory, and Dissociation.* Edited by Bremner JD, Marmar CR. Washington, DC, American Psychiatric Press, 1998, pp. 179–203.

398. Ellason JW, Ross CA, Fuchs DL: "Lifetime Axis I and II Comorbidity and Childhood Trauma History in Dissociative Identity Disorder." *Psychiatry* 59:255–266, 1996.

399. Coons PM: "Depersonalization and Derealization," in *Handbook of Dissociation: Theoretical, Empirical, and Clinical Perspectives.* Edited by Michelson LK, Ray WJ. New York, Plenum, 1996, pp. 291–305.

400. Steinberg M, Schnall M: *The Stranger in the Mirror: Dissociation—The Hidden Epidemic.* New York, HarperCollins, 2000.

401. Marmar CR, Weiss DS, Metzler TJ: "The Peritraumatic Dissociative Experiences Questionnaire," in *Assessing Psychological Trauma and PTSD.* Edited by Wilson JP, Keane TM. New York, Guilford, 1997, pp. 412–428.

402. Ursano RJ, Fullerton CS, Epstein RS, et al.: "Acute and Chronic Posttraumatic Stress Disorder in Motor Vehicle Accident Victims." *American Journal of Psychiatry* 156:589–595, 1999.

403. Cardena E, Spiegel D: "Dissociative Reactions to the San Francisco Bay Area Earthquake of 1989." *American Journal of Psychiatry* 150:474–478, 1993.

404. Marmar CR, Weiss DS, Metzler TJ, et al.: "Characteristics of Emergency Services Personnel Related to Peritraumatic Dissociation During Critical Incident Exposure." *American Journal of Psychiatry* 153:94–102, 1996.

405. Shalev AY, Peri T, Canetti L, et al.: "Predictors of PTSD in Injured Trauma Survivors: A Prospective Study." *American Journal of Psychiatry* 153:219–225, 1996.

406. Dancu CV, Riggs DS, Hearst-Ikeda D, et al.: "Dissociative Experiences and Posttraumatic Stress Disorder Among Female Victims of Criminal Assault and Rape." *Journal of Traumatic Stress* 9:253–267, 1996.

407. Marmar CR, Weiss DS, Metzler TJ, et al.: "Longitudinal Course and Predictors of Continuing Distress Following Critical Incident Exposure in Emergency Services Personnel." *Journal of Nervous and Mental Disease* 187:15–22, 1999.

408. Marshall GN, Schell TL: "Reappraising the Link Between Peritraumatic Dissociation and PTSD Symptom Severity: Evidence From a Longitudinal Study of Community Violence Survivors. *Journal of Abnormal Psychology* 111:626–636, 2002.

409. Halligan SL, Michael T, Clark DM, et al.: "Posttraumatic Stress Disorder Following Assault: The Role of Cognitive Processing, Trauma Memory, and Appraisals." *Journal of Consulting and Clinical Psychology* 71:419-431, 2003.

410. Main M, Morgan H: "Disorganization and Disorientation in Infant Strange Situation Behavior: Phenotypic Resemblance to Dissociative States," in *Handbook of Dissociation: Theoretical, Empirical, and Clinical Perspectives.* Edited by Michelson LK, Ray WJ. New York, Plenum, 1996, pp. 107–138.

411. Hesse E: "The Adult Attachment Interview: Historical and Current Perspectives," *Handbook of Attachment: Theory, Research, and Clinical Applications.* Edited by Cassidy J, Shaver PR. New York, Guilford, 1999, pp. 395–433.

412. Carlson EA: "A Prospective Longitudinal Study of Attachment Disorganization/Disorientation." *Child Development* 69:1107–1128, 1998.

413. Baars BJ: *A Cognitive Theory of Consciousness.* New York, Cambridge University Press, 1988.

414. Tellegen A, Atkinson G: "Openness to Absorbing and Self-Altering Experiences ('Absorption'), a Trait Related to Hypnotic Susceptibility." *Journal of Abnormal Psychology* 83:268–277, 1974.

415. Waller NG, Putnam FW, Carlson EB: "Types of Dissociation and Dissociative Types: A Taxometric Analysis of Dissociative Experiences." *Psychological Methods* 1:300–321, 1996.

416. Roche SM, McConkey KM: "Absorption: Nature, Assessment, and Correlates." *Journal of Personality and Social Psychology* 59:91–101, 1990.

417. Allen JG, Coyne L, Console DA: "Dissociative Detachment Relates to Psychotic Symptoms and Personality Decompensation." *Comprehensive Psychiatry* 38:327–334, 1997.

418. Simeon D, Gross S, Guralnik O, et al.: "Feeling Unreal: 30 Cases of DSM-III-R Depersonalization Disorder." *American Journal of Psychiatry* 154:1107–1113, 1997.

419. Armstrong D: "What Is Consciousness?" in *The Nature of Consciousness: Philosophical Debates*. Edited by Block N, Flanagan O, Guzeldere G. Cambridge, MA, MIT Press, 1997, pp. 721–728.

420. Janet P: *The Major Symptoms of Hysteria: Fifteen Lectures Given in the Medical School of Harvard University*. New York, Macmillan, 1907.

421. van der Hart O, Friedman B: "A Reader's Guide to Pierre Janet on Dissociation: A Neglected Intellectual Heritage." *Dissociation* 2:3–16, 1989.

422. Terr L: *Unchained Memories: True Stories of Traumatic Memories, Lost and Found*. New York, Basic Books, 1994.

423. Kihlstrom JF, Schacter DL: "Functional Disorders of Autobiographical Memory," in *Handbook of Memory Disorders*. Edited by Baddeley AD, Wilson BA, Watts FN. New York, Wiley, 1995, pp. 337–364.

424. Cardena E, Spiegel D: "Diagnostic Issues, Criteria, and Comorbidity of Dissociative Disorders," in *Handbook of Dissociation: Theoretical, Empirical, and Clinical Perspectives*. Edited by Michelson LK, Ray WJ. New York, Plenum, 1996, pp. 227–250.

425. Putnam FW: "The Switch Process in Multiple Personality Disorder and Other State-Change Disorders." *Dissociation* 1:24–32, 1988.

426. Davidson J, Allen JG, Smith WH: "Complexities in the Hospital Treatment of a Patient With Multiple Personality Disorder." *Bulletin of the Menninger Clinic* 51:561–568, 1987.

427. Ellenberger HF: *The Discovery of the Unconscious: The History and Evolution of Dynamic Psychiatry*. New York, Basic Books, 1970.

428. Rifkin A, Ghisalbert D, Dimatou S, et al.: "Dissociative Identity Disorder in Psychiatric Inpatients." *American Journal of Psychiatry* 155:844–855, 1998.

429. Ross CA, Anderson G, Fleisher WP, et al.: "The Frequency of Multiple Personality Disorder Among Psychiatric Inpatients." *American Journal of Psychiatry* 148:1717–1720, 1991.

430. Cormier JF, Thelen MH: "Professional Skepticism of Multiple Personality Disorder." *Professional Psychology: Research and Practice* 29:163–167, 1998.

431. Pope HG, Oliva PS, Hudson JI, et al.: "Attitudes Toward DSM-IV Dissociative Disorder Diagnoses Among Board-Certified American Psychiatrists." *American Journal of Psychiatry* 156:321–323, 1999.

432. Putnam FW: "Discussion: Are Alter Personalities Fragments or Figments? *Psychoanalytic Inquiry* 12:95–111, 1992.

433. Putnam FW, Helmers K, Horowitz LA, et al.: "Hypnotizability and Dissociativity in Sexually Abused Girls." *Child Abuse and Neglect* 19:645–655, 1995.

434. Goodwin JM, Sachs RG: "Child Abuse in the Etiology of Dissociative Disorders," in *Handbook of Dissociation: Theoretical, Empirical, and Clinical Perspectives*. Edited by Michelson LK, Ray WJ. New York, Plenum, 1996, pp. 91–105.

435. Irwin HJ: "Proneness to Dissociation and Traumatic Childhood Events." *Journal of Nervous and Mental Disease* 182:456–460, 1994.

436. Nijenhuis ERS, Spinhoven P, van Dyck R, et al.: "Degree of Somatoform and Psychological Dissociation in Dissociative Disorder Is Correlated With Reported Trauma." *Journal of Traumatic Stress* 11:711–730, 1999.

437. Anderson CL, Alexander PC: "The Relationship Between Attachment and Dissociation in Adult Survivors of Incest." *Psychiatry* 59:240–254, 1996.

438. Jang KL, Paris J, Zweig-Frank H, et al.: "Twin Study of Dissociative Experience." *Journal of Nervous and Mental Disease* 186:345–351, 1998.

439. Waller NG, Ross CA: "The Prevalence and Biometric Structure of Pathological Dissociation in the General Population: Taxometric and Behavior Genetic Findings." *Journal of Abnormal Psychology* 106:499–510, 1997.

440. Tellegen A, Lykken DT, Bouchard TJ, et al.: "Personality Similarity in Twins Reared Apart and Together." *Journal of Personality and Social Psychology* 54:1031–1039, 1988.

441. Krystal JH, Bennett A, Bremner JD, et al.: "Toward a Cognitive Neuroscience of Dissociation and Altered Memory Functions in Post-Traumatic Stress Disorder," in *Neurobiological and Clinical Consequences of Stress: From Normal Adaptation to Post-Traumatic Stress Disorder.* Edited by Friedman MJ, Charney DS, Deutch AY. Philadelphia, PA, Lippincott-Raven, 1995, pp. 239–269.

442. Good MI: "The Concept of an Organic Dissociative Syndrome: What Is the Evidence?" *Harvard Review of Psychiatry* 1:145–157, 1993.

443. Bowman ES, Markland ON: "The Contribution of Life Events to Pseudoseizure Occurrence in Adults." *Bulletin of the Menninger Clinic* 63:70–88, 1999.

444. Levey M: *The Life and Death of Mozart.* New York, Stein & Day, 1971.

445. Bliss EL: *Multiple Personality, Allied Disorders, and Hypnosis.* New York, Oxford University Press, 1986.

446. Maldonado JR, Spiegel D: "Trauma, Dissociation, and Hypnotizability," in *Trauma, Memory, and Dissociation.* Edited by Bremner JD, Marmar CR. Washington, DC, American Psychiatric Press, 1998, pp. 57–106.

447. Vermetten E, Bremner JD, Spiegel D: "Dissociation and Hypnotizability: A Conceptual and Methodological Perspective on Two Distinct Concepts," in *Trauma, Memory, and Dissociation.* Edited by Bremner JD, Marmar CR. Washington, DC, American Psychiatric Press, 1998, pp. 107–159.

448. Nijenhuis ERS, Vanderlinden J, Spinhoven P: "Animal Defensive Reactions as a Model for Trauma-Induced Dissociative Reactions." *Journal of Traumatic Stress* 11:243–260, 1998.

449. Gallup GGJ: "Animal Hypnosis: Factual Status of a Fictional Concept." *Psychological Bulletin* 81:836–853, 1974.

450. Munich RL: "Efforts to Preserve the Mind in Contemporary Hospital Treatment." *Bulletin of the Menninger Clinic* 76:167–186, 2003.

451. Steinberg M, Bancroft J, Buchanan J: "Multiple Personality Disorder in Criminal Law." *Bulletin of the American Academy of Psychiatry and the Law* 21:345–356, 1993.

452. Kluft RP: "Basic Principles in Conducting the Psychotherapy of Multiple Personality Disorder," in *Current Perspectives on Multiple Personality Disorder.* Edited by Kluft RP, Fine CG. Washington, DC, American Psychiatric Press, 1993, pp. 19–50.

453. Halleck SL: "Dissociative Phenomena and the Question of Responsibility." *International Journal of Clinical and Experimental Hypnosis* 38:298–314, 1990.

454. Beahrs JO: "Why Dissociative Disordered Patients Are Fundamentally Responsible: A Master Class Commentary." *International Journal of Clinical and Experimental Hypnosis* 42:93–96, 1994.

455. Michelson LK, Ray WJ (eds.): *Handbook of Dissociation: Theoretical, Empirical, and Clinical Perspectives.* New York, Plenum, 1996.

456. Bradley SJ: *Affect Regulation and the Development of Psychopathology.* New York, Guilford, 2000.

457. Goldstein A: *Addiction: From Biology to Drug Policy.* New York, Oxford University Press, 2001.

458. Mueller TI, Lavori PW, Keller MB, et al.: "Prognostic Effect of the Variable Course of Alcoholism on the 10-Year Course of Depression." *American Journal of Psychiatry* 151:701–706, 1994.

459. McFarlane AC: "Epidemiological Evidence About the Relationship Between PTSD and Alcohol Abuse: The Nature of the Association." *Addictive Behaviors* 23:813–825, 1998.

460. Bremner JD, Southwick SM, Darnell A, et al.: "Chronic PTSD in Vietnam Combat Veterans: Course of Illness and Substance Abuse." *American Journal of Psychiatry* 153:369–375, 1996.

461. Ruzek JI, Polusny MA, Abueg FR: "Assessment and Treatment of Concurrent Posttraumatic Stress Disorder and Substance Abuse," in *Cognitive-Behavioral Therapies for Trauma.* Edited by Follette VM, Ruzek JI, Abueg FR. New York, Guilford, 1998, pp. 226–255.

462. Sorg BA, Kalivas PW: "Stress and Neuronal Sensitization," in *Neurobiological and Clinical Consequences of Stress: From Normal Adaptation to Post-Traumatic Stress Disorder.* Edited by Friedman MJ, Charney DS, Deutch AY. Philadelphia, PA, Lippincott-Raven, 1995, pp. 83–102.

463. Brown PJ, Stout RL, Gannon-Rowley J: "Substance Use Disorder–PTSD Comorbidity: Patients' Perceptions of Symptom Interplay and Treatment Issues." *Journal of Substance Abuse Treatment* 15:445–448, 1998.

464. Norris F: "Epidemiology of Trauma: Frequency and Impact of Different Potentially Traumatic Events on Different Demographic Groups." *Journal of Consulting and Clinical Psychology* 60:409–418, 1992.

465. Brady KT, Dansky BS, Sonne SC, et al.: "Posttraumatic Stress Disorder and Cocaine Dependence: Order of Onset." *American Journal on Addictions* 7:128–135, 1998.

466. Resnick HS, Yehuda R, Acierno R: "Acute Post-Rape Plasma Cortisol, Alcohol Use, and PTSD Symptom Profile Among Recent Rape Victims," in *Psychobiology of Posttraumatic Stress Disorder (Annals of the New York Academy of Sciences, Vol. 821).* Edited by Yehuda R, McFarlane AC. New York, New York Academy of Sciences, 1997, pp. 433–436 .

467. Allen JG: "Substance Abuse Is a Catalyst for Depression." *Menninger Perspective* 33(1):17–20, 2003.

468. Stine SM, Kosten TR: "Complications of Chemical Abuse and Dependency," in *Neurobiological and Clinical Consequences of Stress: From Normal Adaptation to Post-Traumatic Stress Disorder.* Edited by Friedman MJ, Charney DS, Deutch AY. Philadelphia, PA, Lippincott-Raven, 1995, pp. 447–464.

469. Stewart SH, Pihl RO, Conrod PJ, et al.: "Functional Associations Among Trauma, PTSD, and Substance-Related Disorders." *Addictive Behaviors* 23:797–812, 1998.

470. Wechselblatt T, Gurnick G, Simon R: "Autonomy and Relatedness in the Development of Anorexia Nervosa: A Clinical Case Series Using Grounded Theory." *Bulletin of the Menninger Clinic* 64:91–123, 2000.

471. Fallon P, Wonderlich SA: "Sexual Abuse and Other Forms of Trauma," in *Handbook of Treatment for Eating Disorders*, 2nd Edition. Edited by Garner DM, Garfinkel PE. New York, Guilford, 1997, pp. 394–414 .

472. Dansky BS, Brewerton TD, Kilpatrick DG, et al.: "The National Women's Study: Relationship of Victimization and Posttraumatic Stress Disorder to Bulimia Nervosa." *International Journal of Eating Disorders* 21:231–228, 1997.

473. Mallinckrodt B, McCreary BA, Robertson AK: "Co-Occurrence of Eating Disorders and Incest: The Role of Attachment, Family Environment, and Social Competencies." *Journal of Counseling Psychology* 42:178–186, 1995.

474. Heatherton TF, Baumeister RF: "Binge Eating as Escape From Self-Awareness." *Psychological Bulletin* 110:86–108, 1991.

475. Rorty M, Yager J: "Histories of Childhood Trauma and Complex-Posttraumatic Sequelae in Women With Eating Disorders." *Psychiatric Clinics of North America* 19:773–791, 1996.

476. Swirsky D, Mitchell V: "The Binge-Purge Cycle as a Means of Dissociation: Somatic Trauma and Somatic Defense in Sexual Abuse and Bulimia." *Dissociation* 9:18–27, 1996.

477. Wonderlich SA, Brewerton TD, Jocic J, et al.: "Relationship of Childhood Sexual Abuse and Eating Disorders." *Journal of the American Academy of Child and Adolescent Psychiatry* 36:1107–1115, 1997.

478. Zerbe KJ: "Selves That Starve and Suffocate: The Continuum of Eating Disorders and Dissociative Phenomena." *Bulletin of the Menninger Clinic* 57:319–327, 1993.

479. Morgan HG, Burns-Cox CJ, Pocock H, et al.: "Deliberate Self-Harm: Clinical and Socio-Economic Characteristics of 368 Patients." *British Journal of Psychiatry* 127:564–574, 1975.

480. Zlotnick C, Mattia JI, Zimmerman M: "Clinical Correlates of Self-Mutilation in a Sample of General Psychiatric Patients." *Journal of Nervous and Mental Disease* 187:296–301, 1999.

481. Connors R: "Self-Injury in Trauma Survivors, 1: Functions and Meanings." *American Journal of Orthopsychiatry* 66:197–206, 1996.

482. Jones I, Daniels BA: "An Ethological Approach to Self-Injury." *British Journal of Psychiatry* 169:263–267, 1996.

483. Favazza AR, Conterio K: "Female Habitual Self-Mutilators." *Acta Psychiatrica Scandinavica* 79:283–289, 1989.

484. Romans SE, Martin JL, Anderson JC, et al.: "Sexual Abuse in Childhood and Deliberate Self-Harm." *American Journal of Psychiatry* 152:1336–1342, 1995.

485. Pitman R: Self-Mutilation in Combat-Related PTSD" (letter). *American Journal of Psychiatry* 147:123–124, 1990.

486. Greenspan GS, Samuel SE: "Self-Cutting After Rape." *American Journal of Psychiatry* 146:789–790, 1989.

487. Kraemer GW: "Psychobiology of Early Social Attachment in Rhesus Monkeys: Clinical Applications," in *The Integrative Neurobiology of Affiliation*. Edited by Carter CS, Lederhendler II, Kirkpatrick B. Cambridge, MA, MIT Press, 1999, pp. 373–390.

488. Kaplan LJ: *Female Perversions: The Temptations of Emma Bovary.* New York, Doubleday, 1991.

489. van der Kolk BA, Perry JC, Herman JL: "Childhood Origins of Self-Destructive Behavior." *American Journal of Psychiatry* 148:1666–1671, 1991.

490. Kemperman I, Russ MJ, Clark WC, et al.: "Pain Assessment in Self-Injurious Patients With Borderline Personality Disorder Using Signal Detection Theory." *Psychiatry Research* 70:175–183, 1997.

491. Glover H, Lader W, Walker-O'Keefe J, et al.: "Numbing Scale Scores in Female Psychiatric Inpatients Diagnosed With Self-Injurious Behavior, Dissociative Identity Disorder, and Major Depression." *Psychiatry Research* 70:115–123, 1997.

492. Osuch EA, Noll JG, Putnam FW: "The Motivations for Self-Injury in Psychiatric Inpatients." *Psychiatry* 62:334–346, 1999.

493. Walsh BW, Rosen PM: *Self-Mutilation: Theory, Research, and Treatment.* New York, Guilford, 1988.

494. Kemperman I, Russ MJ, Shearin E: "Self-Injurious Behavior and Mood Regulation in Borderline Patients." *Journal of Personality Disorders* 11:146–157, 1997.

495. Novotny P: "Self-Cutting." *Bulletin of the Menninger Clinic* 36:505–514, 1972.

496. Baumeister RF: "Suicide as Escape From Self." *Psychological Review* 97:90–113, 1990.

497. Blumenthal SJ: "An Overview and Synopsis of Risk Factors, Assessment, and Treatment of Suicidal Patients Over the Life Cycle," in *Suicide Over the Life Cycle: Risk Factors, Assessment, and Treatment of Suicidal Patients.* Edited by Blumenthal SJ, Kupfer DJ. Washington, DC, American Psychiatric Press, 1990, pp. 685–723 .

498. Harris EC, Barraclough B: "Suicide as an Outcome for Mental Disorders: A Meta-Analysis." *British Journal of Psychiatry* 170:205–228, 1997.

499. Soloff PH, Lynch KG, Kelly TM, et al.: "Characteristics of Suicide Attempts of Patients With Major Depressive Episode and Borderline Personality Disorder: A Comparative Study." *American Journal of Psychiatry* 157:601–608, 2000.

500. Mann JJ, Oquendo M, Underwood MD, et al.: "The Neurobiology of Suicide Risk: A Review for the Clinician." *Journal of Clinical Psychiatry* 60 (suppl 2):7–11, 1999.

501. Dubo ED, Zanarini MC, Lewis RE, et al.: "Childhood Antecedents of Self-Destructiveness in Borderline Personality Disorder." *Canadian Journal of Psychiatry* 42:63–69, 1997.

502. Williams M: *Cry of Pain: Understanding Suicide and Self-Harm.* London, Penguin, 1997.

503. Gabbard GO, Coyne L, Allen JG, et al.: "Intensive Inpatient Treatment of Severe Personality Disorders: A Treatment Evaluation Study." *Psychiatric Services* 51:893–898, 2000.

504. Parker G, Barrett E: "Personality and Personality Disorder: Current Issues and Directions." *Psychological Medicine* 30:1–9, 2000.

505. Johnson JG, Cohen P, Brown J, et al.: "Childhood Maltreatment Increases Risk for Personality Disorders During Early Adulthood." *Archives of General Psychiatry* 56:600–606, 1999.

506. Howell EF: "Masochism: A Bridge to the Other Side of Abuse." *Dissociation* 10:240–245, 1997.

507. Cooper AM: "The Narcissistic-Masochistic Character," in *Masochism: Current Psychoanalytic Perspectives.* Edited by Glick RA, Meyers DI. Hillsdale, NJ, Analytic Press, 1988, pp. 117–138.

508. Gabbard GO: "Challenges in the Analysis of Adult Patients With Histories of Childhood Sexual Abuse. *Canadian Journal of Psychoanalysis* 5:1–25, 1997.

509. Coyne JC, Ellard JH, Smith DAF: "Social Support, Interdependence, and the Dilemmas of Helping," in *Social Support: An Interactional View.* Edited by Sarason BA, Sarason IG, Pierce GR. New York, Wiley, 1990, pp. 129–149.

510. Paris J: *Borderline Personality Disorder: A Multidimensional Approach.* Washington, DC, American Psychiatric Press, 1994.

511. Gabbard GO: *Psychodynamic Psychiatry in Clinical Practice,* 3rd Edition. Washington, DC, American Psychiatric Press, 2000.

512. Gunderson JG: "The Borderline Patient's Intolerance of Aloneness: Insecure Attachments and Therapist Availability." *American Journal of Psychiatry* 153: 752–758, 1996.

513. Linehan MM: *Cognitive-Behavioral Treatment of Borderline Personality Disorder.* New York, Guilford, 1993.

514. Fonagy P, Target M, Gergely G, et al.: "The Developmental Roots of Borderline Personality Disorder in Early Attachment Relationships: A Theory and Some Evidence." *Psychoanalytic Inquiry* 23:412–459, 2003.

515. Patrick M, Hobson RP, Castle D, et al.: "Personality Disorder and the Mental Representation of Early Experience." *Development and Psychopathology* 6:375–388, 1994.

516. Bateman AW, Fonagy P: "The Development of an Attachment-Based Treatment Program for Borderline Personality Disorder." *Bulletin of the Menninger Clinic* 67:187–211, 2003.

517. Newman JP, Lorenz AR: "Response Modulation and Emotion Processing: Implications for Psychopathy and Other Dysregulatory Psychopathology," in *Handbook of Affective Sciences.* Edited by Davidson RJ, Scherer KR, Goldsmith HH. New York, Oxford University Press, 2003, pp. 904–929.

518. Feldman Barrett L, Salovey P (eds.): *The Wisdom in Feeling: Psychological Processes in Emotional Intelligence.* New York, Guilford, 2002.

519. Mayer JD, Salovey P: "What Is Emotional Intelligence?" in *Emotional Development and Emotional Intelligence.* Edited by Salovey P, Sluyter DJ. New York, Basic Books, 1997, pp. 3–31.

520. Salovey P, Bedell BT, Detweiler JB, et al.: "Coping Intelligently: Emotional Intelligence and the Coping Process," in *Coping: The Psychology of What Works.* Edited by Snyder CR. New York, Oxford University Press, 1999, pp. 141–164.

521. Robins CJ, Ivanoff AM, Linehan M: "Dialectical Behavior Therapy," in *Handbook of Personality Disorders.* Edited by Livesley WJ. New York, Guilford, 2001, pp. 437–459.

522. Scherer KR: "Introduction: Cognitive Components of Emotion," in *Handbook of Affective Sciences.* Edited by Davidson RJ, Scherer KR, Goldsmith HH. New York, Oxford University Press, 2003, pp. 563–571.

523. Stanton AL, Franz R: "Focusing on Emotion: An Adaptive Coping Strategy?" in *Coping: The Psychology of What Works.* Edited by Snyder CR. New York, Oxford University Press, 1999, pp. 90–118.

524. Kabat-Zinn J: *Wherever You Go, There You Are: Mindfulness Meditation in Everyday Life.* New York, Hyperion, 1994.

525. Gollwitzer PM: "Implementation Intentions: Strong Effects of Simple Plans." *American Psychologist* 54:493–503, 1999.

526. Hobson JA: *The Chemistry of Conscious States: How the Brain Changes Its Mind.* Boston, MA, Little, Brown, 1994.

527. Hauri P, Linde S: *No More Sleepless Nights.* New York, Wiley, 1996.

528. Dement WC: *The Promise of Sleep.* New York, Random House, 1999.

529. Cooper K: *Aerobics.* New York, Evans, 1968.

530. Bailey C: *Smart Exercise.* New York, Houghton Mifflin, 1994.

531. Benson H: *The Relaxation Response.* New York, William Morrow, 1975.

532. Fahrion SL, Norris PA: "Self-Regulation of Anxiety." *Bulletin of the Menninger Clinic* 54:217–231, 1990.

533. Fitzgerald SG, Gonzalez E: "Dissociative States Induced by Relaxation Training in a PTSD Combat Veteran: Failure to Identify Trigger Mechanisms." *Journal of Traumatic Stress* 7:111–115, 1994.

534. Kosslyn SM: *Image and Brain: The Resolution of the Imagery Debate.* Cambridge, MA, MIT Press, 1994.

535. Watts A: *The Way of Zen.* New York, Random House, 1957.

536. Murphy M, Donovan S: *The Physical and Psychological Effects of Meditation: A Review of Contemporary Meditation Research With a Comprehensive Bibliography, 1931–1988.* San Raphael, CA, Esalen Institute, 1988.

537. Kabat-Zinn J, Massion AO, Kristeller J, et al.: "Effectiveness of a Meditation-Based Stress Reduction Program in the Treatment of Anxiety Disorders." *American Journal of Psychiatry* 149:936–943, 1992.

538. Davidson RJ: "Toward a Biology of Positive Affect and Compassion," in *Visions of Compassion: Western Scientists and Tibetan Buddhists Examine Human Nature.* Edited by Davidson RJ, Harrington A. New York, Oxford University Press, 2002, pp. 107–130.

539. Shapiro DH Jr: "Overview: Clinical and Physiological Comparison of Meditation With Other Self-Control Strategies." *American Journal of Psychiatry* 139:267–274, 1982.

540. Goldstein J, Kornfield J: *Seeking the Heart of Wisdom: The Path of Insight Meditation.* Boston, MA, Shambhala, 1987.

541. Hahn TN: *The Miracle of Mindfulness: A Manual on Meditation.* Boston, MA, Beacon, 1975.

542. Lazarus AA: "Meditation: The Problems of Any Unimodal Technique," in *Meditation: Classic and Contemporary Perspectives.* Edited by Shapiro DH, Walsh RN. New York, Aldine, 1984, p. 691.

543. Hahn TN: *Peace Is Every Step: The Path of Mindfulness in Everyday Life.* New York, Bantam, 1991.

544. Kagan J: *Galen's Prophecy: Temperament in Human Nature.* New York, Basic Books, 1994.

545. Green EE, Green AM: "Biofeedback and States of Consciousness," in *Handbook of States of Consciousness.* Edited by Wolman BB, Ullman M. New York, Van Nostrand Reinhold, 1986, pp. 553–589.

546. Norris P: "Biofeedback, Voluntary Control, and Human Potential." *Biofeedback and Self-Regulation* 11:1–19, 1986.

547. Norris P: "Current Conceptual Trends in Biofeedback and Self-Regulation," in *Eastern and Western Approaches to Healing.* Edited by Sheikh A. New York, Wiley, 1989, pp. 264–295.

548. Peniston EG, Marrinan DA, Deming WA, et al.: "EEG Alpha-Theta Brainwave Synchronization in Vietnam Theater Veterans With Post-Traumatic Stress Disorder and Alcohol Abuse." *Advances in Medical Psychotherapy* 6:37–50, 1993.

549. Seligman MEP: "Foreword: The Past and Future of Positive Psychology," in *Flourishing: Positive Psychology and the Life Well-Lived*. Edited by Keyes CL, Haidt J. Washington, DC, American Psychological Association, 2003, pp. xi–xx.

550. Fredrickson B: "The Value of Positive Emotions." *American Scientist* 91:330–335, 2003.

551. Fredrickson B, Levenson RW: "Positive Emotions Speed Recovery From the Cardiovascular Sequelae of Negative Emotions." *Cognition and Emotion* 12:191–220, 1998.

552. Ekman P, Davidson RJ: "Voluntary Smiling Changes Regional Brain Activity." *Psychological Science* 4:342–345, 1993.

553. Folkman S, Moskowitz JT: "Positive Affect and the Other Side of Coping." *American Psychologist* 55:647–654, 2000.

554. Tedeschi RG: "Violence Transformed: Posttraumatic Growth in Survivors and Their Societies." *Aggression and Violent Behavior* 4:319–341, 1999.

555. Olds J, Milner P: "Positive Reinforcement Produced by Electrical Stimulation of Septal Area and Other Regions of the Rat Brain." *Journal of Comparative and Physiological Psychology* 47:419–427, 1954.

556. Olds J: "Self Stimulation of the Brain: Its Use to Study Local Effects of Hunger, Sex, and Drugs. *Science* 127:315–324, 1958.

557. Brazelton TB: "Touch as Touchstone: Summary of the Roundtable," in *Touch: The Foundation of Experience*. Edited by Barnard KE, Brazelton TB. Madison, CT, International Universities Press, 1990, pp. 561–566.

558. Depue RA, Collins PF: "Neurobiology of the Structure of Personality: Dopamine, Facilitation of Incentive Motivation, and Extraversion." *Behavioral and Brain Sciences* 22:491–569, 1999.

559. Emde RN: "Positive Emotions for Psychoanalytic Theory: Surprises From Infancy Research and New Directions," in *Affect: Psychoanalytic Perspectives*. Edited by Shapiro T, Emde RN. Madison, CT, International Universities Press, 1992, pp. 5–44.

560. Csikszentmihalyi M: *Flow: The Psychology of Optimal Experience*. New York, HarperCollins, 1990.

561. Nussbaum MC: "Compassion and Terror," in *Terrorism and International Justice*. Edited by Sterba JP. New York, Oxford University Press, 2003, pp. 229–252.

562. Comte-Sponville A: *A Small Treatise on the Great Virtues*. New York, Holt, 2001.

563. Swanton C: *Virtue Ethics: A Pluralistic View*. New York, Oxford, 2003.

564. Dawkins R: *Unweaving the Rainbow: Science, Delusion and the Appetite for Wonder*. New York, Houghton Mifflin, 1998.

565. Kopp CB, Neufeld SJ: "Emotional Development During Infancy," in *Handbook of Affective Sciences*. Edited by Davidson RJ, Scherer KR, Goldsmith HH. New York, Oxford University Press, 2003, pp. 347–374.

566. Meichenbaum D: *A Clinical Handbook/Practical Therapist Manual for Assessing and Treating Adults With Posttraumatic Stress Disorder (PTSD)*. Waterloo, ON, Canada, Institute Press, 1994.

567. van der Kolk BA: "Assessment and Treatment of Complex PTSD," in *Treating Trauma Survivors With PTSD*. Edited by Yehuda R. Washington, DC, American Psychiatric Publishing, 2002, pp. 127–156.

568. Peebles MJ: "Through a Glass Darkly: The Psychoanalytic Use of Hypnosis With Post-Traumatic Stress Disorder." *International Journal of Clinical and Experimental Hypnosis* 37:192–206, 1989.

569. van der Hart O, Spiegel D: "Hypnotic Assessment and Treatment of Trauma-Induced Psychoses: The Early Psychotherapy of H. Bruckink and Modern Views." *International Journal of Clinical and Experimental Hypnosis* 41:191–209, 1993.

570. Wagner AW, Linehan MM: "Dissociative Behavior," in *Cognitive-Behavioral Therapies for Trauma.* Edited by Follette VM, Ruzek JI, Abueg FR. New York, Guilford, 1998, pp. 191–225.

571. Linehan MM, Armstrong HE, Suarez A, et al.: "Cognitive-Behavioral Treatment of Chronically Parasuicidal Borderline Patients." *Archives of General Psychiatry* 48:1060–1064, 1991.

572. Linehan MM: *Skills Training Manual for Treating Borderline Personality Disorder.* New York, Guilford, 1993.

573. Luborsky L, Crits-Christoph P, Alexander L, et al.: "Two Helping Alliance Methods for Predicting Outcomes of Psychotherapy: A Counting Signs Versus a Global Rating Method." *Journal of Nervous and Mental Disease* 171:480–491, 1983.

574. Horwitz L, Gabbard GO, Allen JG, et al.: *Borderline Personality Disorder: Tailoring the Therapy to the Patient.* Washington, DC, American Psychiatric Press, 1996.

575. Frieswyk SH, Colson DB, Allen JG: "Conceptualizing the Therapeutic Alliance From a Psychoanalytic Perspective." *Psychotherapy* 21:460–464, 1984.

576. Chu JA: "The Therapeutic Roller Coaster: Dilemmas in the Treatment of Childhood Abuse Survivors." *Journal of Psychotherapy Practice and Research* 1:351–370, 1992.

577. Gutheil TG, Gabbard GO: "The Concept of Boundaries in Clinical Practice: Theoretical and Risk-Management Dimensions." *American Journal of Psychiatry* 150:188–196, 1993.

578. Gabbard GO (ed.): *Sexual Exploitation in Professional Relationships.* Washington, DC, American Psychiatric Press, 1989.

579. Kluft RP: "Incest and Subsequent Revictimization: The Case of Therapist-Patient Sexual Exploitation, With a Description of the Sitting Duck Syndrome," in *Incest-Related Syndromes of Adult Psychopathology.* Edited by Kluft RP. Washington, DC, American Psychiatric Press, 1990, pp. 263–287.

580. Foa EB, Keane TM, Friedman MJ: "Guidelines for the Treatment of PTSD." *Journal of Traumatic Stress* 13:539–588, 2000.

581. Roth A, Fonagy P: *What Works for Whom? A Critical Review of Psychotherapy Research,* 2nd Edition. New York, Guilford, 2004

582. Foa EB: "Psychological Processes Related to Recovery From a Trauma and Effective Treatment for PTSD," in *Psychobiology of Posttraumatic Stress Disorder* (*Annals of the New York Academy of Sciences,* Vol. 821). Edited by Yehuda R, McFarlane AC. New York, New York Academy of Sciences, 1997, pp. 410–424.

583. Freuh BC, De Arellano MA, Turner SM: "Systematic Desensitization as an Alternative Exposure Strategy for PTSD" (letter). *American Journal of Psychiatry* 154:287–288, 1997.

584. Blake DD, Sonnenberg RT: "Outcome Research on Behavioral and Cognitive-Behavioral Treatments for Trauma Survivors," in *Cognitive-Behavioral Therapies for Trauma*. Edited by Follette VM, Ruzek JI, Abueg FR. New York, Guilford, 1998, pp. 15–47.

585. Foa EB, Ehlers A, Clark DM, et al.: "The Post-Traumatic Cognitions Inventory (PTCI): Development and Validation." *Psychological Assessment* 11:303–314, 1999.

586. Resick PA, Schnicke MK: *Cognitive Processing Therapy for Rape Victims: A Treatment Manual*. London, Sage, 1993.

587. Shapiro F: *Eye Movement Desensitization and Reprocessing: Basic Principles, Protocols, and Procedures*. New York, Guilford, 1995.

588. Rothbaum BO: "A Controlled Study of Eye Movement Desensitization and Reprocessing in the Treatment of Posttraumatic Stress Disorder." *Bulletin of the Menninger Clinic* 61:317–334, 1997.

589. Wilson SA, Becker LA, Tinker RH: "Fifteen-Month Follow-Up of Eye Movement Desensitization and Reprocessing (EMDR) Treatment for Posttraumatic Stress Disorder and Psychological Trauma." *Journal of Consulting and Clinical Psychology* 65:1047–1056, 1997.

590. Lipke H: "Comment on Hembree and Foa (2003) and EMDR." *Journal of Traumatic Stress* 16:573–574, 2003.

591. Hembree EA, Cahill SP, Foa EB: "Response to 'Comment on Hembree and Foa (2003).'" *Journal of Traumatic Stress* 16:575–577, 2003.

592. Van Etten ML, Taylor S: "Comparative Efficacy of Treatments for Posttraumatic Stress Disorder: A Meta-Analysis." *Clinical Psychology and Psychotherapy* 5:126–144, 1998.

593. Pitman RK, Orr SP, Altman B, et al.: "Emotional Processing During Eye-Movement Desensitization and Reprocessing Therapy of Vietnam Veterans With Chronic Posttraumatic Stress Disorder." *Comprehensive Psychiatry* 37:419–429, 1996.

594. Marks I, Lovell K, Noshirvani H, et al.: "Treatment of Posttraumatic Stress Disorder by Exposure and/or Cognitive Restructuring." *Archives of General Psychiatry* 55:317–325, 1998.

595. Tarrier N, Pilgrim H, Sommerfield C, et al.: "A Randomized Trial of Cognitive Therapy and Imaginal Exposure in Treatment of Chronic Posttraumatic Stress Disorder." *Journal of Consulting and Clinical Psychology* 67:13–18, 1999.

596. Bryant RA, Moulds ML, Guthrie RM, et al.: "Imaginal Exposure Alone and Imaginal Exposure With Cognitive Restructuring in Treatment of Posttraumatic Stress Disorder." *Journal of Consulting and Clinical Psychology* 71:706–712, 2003.

597. Taylor S, Thordarson DS, Maxfield L, et al.: "Comparative Efficacy, Speed, and Adverse Effects of Three PTSD Treatments: Exposure Therapy, EMDR, and Relaxation Training." *Journal of Consulting and Clinical Psychology* 71:330–338, 2003.

598. Buchele BJ: "Group Psychotherapy for Persons With Multiple Personality and Dissociative Disorders." *Bulletin of the Menninger Clinic* 57:362–370, 1993.

599. Yalom ID: *The Theory and Practice of Group Psychotherapy*. New York, Basic Books, 1970.

600. Figley CR: *Helping Traumatized Families*. San Francisco, CA, Jossey-Bass, 1989.

601. Maltas CP: "Reenactment and Repair: Couples Therapy With Survivors of Childhood Sexual Abuse." *Harvard Review of Psychiatry* 3:351–355, 1996.

602. Tarrier N, Sommerfield C, Pilgrim H: "Relatives' Expressed Emotion (EE) and PTSD Treatment Outcome." *Psychological Medicine* 29:801–811, 1999.

603. Solomon P: "Moving From Psychoeducation to Family Education for Families of Adults With Serious Mental Illness." *Psychiatric Services* 47:1364–1370, 1996.

604. Porter S, Kelly KA, Grame CJ: "Family Treatment of Spouses and Children of Patients With Multiple Personality Disorder." *Bulletin of the Menninger Clinic* 57:371–379, 1993.

605. Roesler TA: "Reactions to Disclosure of Childhood Sexual Abuse: The Effect on Adult Symptoms." *Journal of Nervous and Mental Disease* 182:618–624, 1994.

606. Schatzow E, Herman JL: "Breaking Secrecy: Adult Survivors Disclose to Their Families." *Psychiatric Clinics of North America* 12:337–349, 1989.

607. Healy D: "The Antidepressant Drama," in *Treatment of Depression: Bridging the 21st Century.* Edited by Weissman MM. Washington, DC, American Psychiatric Press, 2001, pp. 7–34.

608. Mellman TA: "Rationale and Role for Medication in the Comprehensive Treatment of PTSD," in *Treating Trauma Survivors With PTSD.* Edited by Yehuda R. Washington, DC, American Psychiatric Publishing, 2002, pp. 63–74.

609. Hembree EA, Foa EB: "Interventions for Trauma-Related Emotional Disturbances in Adult Victims of Crime." *Journal of Traumatic Stress* 16:187–199, 2003.

610. Aghajanian GK: "Serotonin," in *Encyclopedia of Neuroscience.* Edited by Adelman G. Boston, MA, Birkhauser, 1987, pp. 1082–1083.

611. Yehuda R, Marshall R, Giller EL: "Psychopharmacological Treatment of Post-traumatic Stress Disorder," in *A Guide to Treatments That Work.* Edited by Nathan PE, Gorman JM. New York, Oxford University Press, 1998, pp. 377–397.

612. Friedman MJ, Southwick SM: "Towards Pharmacotherapy for Post-Traumatic Stress Disorder," in *Neurobiological and Clinical Consequences of Stress: From Normal Adaptation to Post-Traumatic Stress Disorder.* Edited by Friedman MJ, Charney DS, Deutch AY. Philadelphia, PA, Lippincott-Raven, 1995, pp. 465–481.

613. Friedman M: "Drug Treatment for PTSD: Answers and Questions," in *Psychobiology of Posttraumatic Stress Disorder* (*Annals of the New York Academy of Sciences,* Vol. 821). Edited by Yehuda R, McFarlane AC. New York, New York Academy of Sciences, 1997, pp. 359–371.

614. Hamner MB, Frueh C, Ulmer HG, et al.: "Psychotic Features and Illness Severity in Combat Veterans With Chronic Posttraumatic Stress Disorder." *Biological Psychiatry* 45:846–852, 1999.

615. Saporta JA, Case J: "The Role of Medications in Treating Adult Survivors of Childhood Trauma," in *Treatment of Adult Survivors of Incest.* Edited by Paddison PL. Washington, DC, American Psychiatric Press, 1993, pp. 101–134.

616. Davidson JRT: "Drug Therapy of Post-Traumatic Stress Disorder." *British Journal of Psychiatry* 160:309–314, 1992.

617. Kluft RP: "Hospital Treatment of Multiple Personality Disorder: An Overview." *Psychiatric Clinics of North America* 14:695–719, 1991.

618. Barach PM: "Draft of 'Recommendations for Treating Dissociative Identity Disorder.'" *International Society for the Study of Multiple Personality and Dissociation News* 11(5):14–19, 1993.

619. Allen JG, Coyne L, Logue AM: "Do Clinicians Agree About Who Needs Extended Psychiatric Hospitalization?" *Comprehensive Psychiatry* 31:355–362, 1990.

620. Johnson DR, Rosenheck R, Fontana A, et al.: "Outcome of Intensive Inpatient Treatment for Combat-Related Posttraumatic Stress Disorder." *American Journal of Psychiatry* 153:771–777, 1996.

621. Ellason JW, Ross CA: "Two-Year Follow-Up of Inpatients With Dissociative Identity Disorder." *American Journal of Psychiatry* 154:832–839, 1997.

622. Coates SW: "Introduction: Trauma and Human Bonds," in *September 11: Trauma and Human Bonds*. Edited by Coates SW, Rosenthal JL, Schachter DS. Hillsdale, NJ, Analytic Press, 2003, pp. 1–14.

623. Peterson C: "The Future of Optimism." *American Psychologist* 55:44–55, 2000.

624. Menninger KA: "Hope." *Bulletin of the Menninger Clinic* 51:447–462, 1987.

625. Snyder CR, Cheavens J, Michael ST: "Hoping," in *Coping: The Psychology of What Works*. Edited by Snyder CR. New York, Oxford University Press, 1999, pp. 205–231.

626. Snyder CR: *The Psychology of Hope*. New York, Free Press, 1994.

627. Groopman J: *The Anatomy of Hope: How People Prevail in the Face of Illness*. New York, Random House, 2004.

628. Pruyser PW: "Maintaining Hope in Adversity." *Bulletin of the Menninger Clinic* 51:463–474, 1987.

629. Nakamura J, Csikszentmihalyi M: "The Construction of Meaning Through Vital Engagement," in *Flourishing: Positive Psychology and the Life Well-Lived*. Edited by Keyes CL, Haidt J. Washington, DC, American Psychological Association, 2003, pp. 83–104.

630. Emmons RA: "Personal Goals, Life Meaning, and Virtue: Wellsprings of a Positive Life," in *Flourishing: Positive Psychology and the Life Well-Lived*. Edited by Keyes CL, Haidt J. Washington, DC, American Psychological Association, 2003, pp. 105–128.

631. Keyes CL: "Complete Mental Health: An Agenda for the 21st Century," in *Flourishing: Positive Psychology and the Life Well-Lived*. Edited by Keyes CL, Haidt J. Washington, DC, American Psychological Association, 2003, pp. 293–312.

632. Hadas M: *The Stoic Philosophy of Seneca: Essays and Letters*. New York, WW Norton, 1958.

633. Aurelius M: *Meditations*. New York, Modern Library, 2002.

634. Neiman S: *Evil in Modern Thought: An Alternative History of Philosophy*. Princeton, NJ, Princeton University Press, 2002.

635. Taliaferro C: *Contemporary Philosophy of Religion*. Malden, MA, Blackwell, 1998.

636. Falsetti SA, Resick PA, Davis JL: "Changes in Religious Beliefs Following Trauma." *Journal of Traumatic Stress* 16:391–398, 2003.

637. Means JJ: *Trauma and Evil: Healing the Wounded Soul*. Minneapolis, MN, Fortress Press, 2000.

638. Baumeister RF: *Evil: Inside Human Violence and Cruelty*. New York, WH Freeman, 1997.

639. de Waal F: *Good Natured: The Origins of Right and Wrong in Humans and Other Animals.* Cambridge, MA, Harvard University Press, 1996.

640. Sober E, Wilson DS: *Unto Others: The Evolution and Psychology of Unselfish Behavior.* Cambridge, MA, Harvard University Press, 1998.

641. Haidt J: "Elevation and the Positive Psychology of Morality," in *Flourishing: Positive Psychology and the Life Well-Lived.* Edited by Keyes CL, Haidt J. Washington, DC, American Psychological Association, 2003, pp. 275–289.

642. Piliavin JA: "Doing Well by Doing Good: Benefits for the Benefactor," in *Flourishing: Positive Psychology and the Life Well-Lived.* Edited by Keyes CL, Haidt J. Washington, DC, American Psychological Association, 2003, pp. 227–248.

SUGGESTED READINGS

Trauma, Memory, and Healing

Bifulco A, Moran P: *Wednesday's Child: Research Into Women's Experience of Neglect and Abuse in Childhood, and Adult Depression.* London, Routledge, 1998

Bowlby J: *A Secure Base: Parent-Child Attachment and Healthy Human Development.* New York, Basic Books, 1988

Herman JL: *Trauma and Recovery.* New York, Basic Books, 1992

Lewis L, Kelly KA, Allen JG: *Restoring Hope and Trust: An Illustrated Guide to Mastering Trauma.* Baltimore, MD, Sidran Press, 2004

Macnab F: *Traumas of Life: Their Treatment,* Vols. 1 and 2. Melbourne, Australia, Spectrum, 2000

Pillemer DB: *Momentous Events, Vivid Memories.* Cambridge, MA, Harvard University Press, 1998

Schacter DL: *Searching for Memory: The Brain, the Mind, and the Past.* New York, Basic Books, 1996

Steinberg M, Schnall M: *The Stranger in the Mirror: Dissociation—The Hidden Epidemic.* New York, HarperCollins, 2000

Vermilyea EG: *Growing Beyond Survival: A Self-Help Toolkit for Managing Traumatic Stress.* Baltimore, MD, Sidran Press, 2000

Walker LE: *The Battered Woman.* New York, Harper & Row, 1979

Williams M: *Cry of Pain: Understanding Suicide and Self-Harm.* London, Penguin, 1997

Zerbe KJ: *The Body Betrayed: Women, Eating Disorders, and Treatment.* Washington, DC, American Psychiatric Press, 1993

Emotion and Stress Regulation

Allen JG, Bleiberg E, Haslam-Hopwood T: *Mentalizing as a Compass for Treatment.* Houston, TX, The Menninger Clinic, 2003

Csikszentmihalyi M: *Flow: The Psychology of Optimal Experience.* New York, HarperCollins, 1990

Damasio A: *Looking for Spinoza: Joy, Sorrow, and the Feeling Brain.* New York, Harcourt, 2003

Dement WC: *The Promise of Sleep.* New York, Random House, 1999

Ekman P: *Emotions Revealed.* New York, Holt, 2003

Groopman J: *The Anatomy of Hope: How People Prevail in the Face of Illness.* New York, Random House, 2004

Hahn TN: *Peace is Every Step: The Path of Mindfulness in Everyday Life.* New York, Bantam Books, 1991

Hauri P, Linde S: *No More Sleepless Nights.* New York, Wiley, 1996

Kabat-Zinn J: *Full Catastrophe Living: Using the Wisdom of Your Body and Mind to Face Stress, Pain, and Illness.* New York, Delta, 1990

LeDoux J: *The Emotional Brain.* New York, Simon & Schuster, 1996

Lerner HG: *The Dance of Anger: A Woman's Guide to Changing the Patterns of Intimate Relationships.* New York, Harper & Row, 1985

McEwen BS: *The End of Stress as We Know It.* Washington, DC, Joseph Henry Press, 2002

Snyder CR: *The Psychology of Hope.* New York, Free Press, 1994

Thayer RE: *Calm Energy: How People Regulate Mood With Food and Exercise.* New York, Oxford University Press, 2001

Philosophy

Card C: *The Atrocity Paradigm: A Theory of Evil.* New York, Oxford University Press, 2002

Comte-Sponville A: *A Small Treatise on the Great Virtues.* Translated by Temerson C. New York, Holt, 2001

Grayling AC: *Meditations for the Humanist: Ethics for a Secular Age.* New York, Oxford University Press, 2002

Lebell S: *Epictetus: The Art of Living.* New York, HarperCollins, 1995

MacIntyre A: *Dependent Rational Animals: Why Human Beings Need the Virtues.* Chicago, Open Court, 1999

Murphy JG: *Getting Even: Forgiveness and Its Limits.* New York, Oxford University Press, 2003

Neiman S: *Evil in Modern Thought: An Alternative History of Philosophy.* Princeton, NJ, Princeton University Press, 2002

Nussbaum MC: *Upheavals of Thought: The Intelligence of the Emotions.* Cambridge, UK, Cambridge University Press, 2001

Solomon RC: *Spirituality for the Skeptic: The Thoughtful Love of Life.* New York, Oxford University Press, 2002

Woodruff P: *Reverence: Renewing a Forgotten Virtue.* New York, Oxford University Press, 2001

Professional Literature

Allen JG: *Traumatic Relationships and Serious Mental Disorders.* Chichester, UK, Wiley, 2001

Brown D, Scheflin AW, Hammond DC: *Memory, Trauma Treatment, and the Law.* New York, WW Norton, 1998

Cassidy J, Shaver PR (eds.): *Handbook of Attachment: Theory, Research, and Clinical Applications.* New York, Guilford, 1999

Coates SW, Rosenthal JL, Schechter DS (eds.): *September 11: Trauma and Human Bonds.* Hillsdale, NJ, Analytic Press, 2003

Davidson RJ, Scherer KR, Goldsmith HH (eds.): *Handbook of Affective Sciences.* New York, Oxford University Press, 2003

Eichenbaum H: *The Cognitive Neuroscience of Memory: An Introduction.* New York, Oxford University Press, 2002

Feldman Barrett L, Salovey P (eds.): *The Wisdom in Feeling: Psychological Processes in Emotional Intelligence.* New York, Guilford, 2002

Foa EB, Rothbaum BO: *Treating the Trauma of Rape: Cognitive-Behavioral Therapy for PTSD.* New York, Guilford, 1998

Fonagy P: *Attachment Theory and Psychoanalysis.* New York, Other Press, 2001

Fonagy P, Gergely G, Jurist EL, et al: *Affect Regulation, Mentalization, and the Development of the Self.* New York, Other Press, 2002

Horowitz MJ: *Stress Response Syndromes: PTSD, Grief, and Adjustment Disorders,* 3rd Edition. Northvale, NJ, Jason Aronson, 1997

Sandler J, Fonagy P (eds.): *Recovered Memories of Abuse: True or False?* Madison, CT, International Universities Press, 1997

van der Kolk BA, McFarlane AC, Weisaeth L (eds.): *Traumatic Stress: The Effects of Overwhelming Experience on Mind, Body, and Society.* New York, Guilford, 1996

Yehuda R (ed.): *Psychological Trauma.* Washington, DC, American Psychiatric Press, 1998

Yehuda R (ed.): *Treating Trauma Survivors With PTSD.* Washington, DC, American Psychiatric Publishing, 2002

INDEX

90/10 reaction, 59, 68, 122, 138,
    177, 179
    emotional regulation and, 223
    caregiver strain and, 267
    self-destructiveness and, 213, 217

A

Abandonment
    hostility and, 119
    preoccupied attachment and, 37
    self-destructive behavior and,
        210–211, 215–217
Abreaction. *See* Catharsis
Abuse.
    See Emotional abuse;
    Physical abuse; Psychological
    abuse; Sexual abuse
Acute stress disorder, 180–181
Addiction. *See also* Substance abuse
    aggression as, 66
    benzodiazepines and, 273
    eating as, 166
    self-injury as, 210
Agency
    hope and, 281–282, 287
    responsibility and, 201

self-as-agent and, 100–101
self-efficacy and, 105–107
Aggression.
    See Anger and aggression
Alcohol, 48, 123, 188, 209, 273.
    See also Substance abuse
    avoidance of shame with, 71
    in case examples, 18–19, 58, 211
    as conditioned stimulus for fear,
        58–59, 140–141
    depression and, 155
    dissociative symptoms and, 198
    emotion regulation and,
        76, 230, 278
    ill health and, 147, 150
    PTSD and, 179
    stress analogy and, 16
    substance abuse and, 206–207, 225
    suicide risk and, 212
Alienation, 128, 170, 210
Amnesia, 193–104.
    See also Dissociative disorders
    infantile, 91
Amphetamines, 207.
    See also Substance abuse
Amygdala, 140–143